Insulin Therapy

Guest Editors

JACK L. LEAHY, MD
WILLIAM T. CEFALU, MD

ENDOCRINOLOGY AND METABOLISM CLINICS OF NORTH AMERICA

www.endo.theclinics.com

Consulting Editor
DEREK LEROITH, MD, PhD

March 2012 • Volume 41 • Number 1

SAUNDERS an imprint of ELSEVIER, Inc.

W.B. SAUNDERS COMPANY
A Division of Elsevier Inc.

1600 John F. Kennedy Boulevard • Suite 1800 • Philadelphia, Pennsylvania 19103-2899

http://www.theclinics.com

ENDOCRINOLOGY AND METABOLISM CLINICS OF NORTH AMERICA Volume 41, Number 1
March 2012 ISSN 0889-8529, ISBN-13: 978-1-4557-3857-1

Editor: Pamela Hetherington
Developmental Editor: Teia Stone

Endocrinology and Metabolism Clinics of North America (ISSN 0889-8529) is published quarterly by Elsevier Inc., 360 Park Avenue South, New York, NY 10010-1710. Months of issue are March, June, September, and December. Periodicals postage paid at New York, NY and additional mailing offices. Subscription prices are USD 313.00 per year for US individuals, USD 536.00 per year for US institutions, USD 158.00 per year for US students and residents, USD 393.00 per year for Canadian individuals, USD 656.00 per year for Canadian institutions, USD 456.00 per year for international individuals, USD 656.00 per year for international institutions, and USD 233.00 per year for international and Canadian and foreign students/residents. To receive student/resident rate, orders must be accompanied by name of affiliated institution, date of term, and the signature of program/residency coordinator on institution letterhead. Orders will be billed at individual rate until proof of status is received. Foreign air speed delivery is included in all *Clinics* subscription prices. All prices are subject to change without notice. **POSTMASTER:** Send address changes to *Endocrinology and Metabolism Clinics of North America*, Elsevier Health Sciences Division, Subscription Customer Service, 3251 Riverport Lane, Maryland Heights, MO 63043. **Customer Service: Telephone: 1-800-654-2452** (U.S. and Canada); **1-314-447-8871** (outside U.S. and Canada). **Fax: 1-314-447-8029. E-mail: journalscustomerservice-usa@elsevier.com** (for print support); **journalsonlinesupport-usa@elsevier.com** (for online support).

Reprints. For copies of 100 or more, of articles in this publication, please contact the Commercial Rights Department, Elsevier Inc., 360 Park Avenue South, New York, NY 10010-1710; phone: (+1) 212-633-3813; fax: (+1) 212-462-1935; e-mail: reprints@elsevier.com.

Endocrinology and Metabolism Clinics of North America is covered in *MEDLINE/PubMed (Index Medicus), EMBASE/Excerpta Medica, Current Contents/Clinical Medicine, Current Contents/Life Sciences, Science Citation Index, ISI/BIOMED, BIOSIS,* and *Chemical Abstracts.*

Printed in the United States of America.

Contributors

CONSULTING EDITOR

DEREK LEROITH, MD, PhD
Chief, Division of Endocrinology, Metabolism, and Bone Diseases, Department of Medicine, Mount Sinai School of Medicine, New York, New York

GUEST EDITORS

JACK L. LEAHY, MD
Professor of Medicine; Chief of Endocrinology, Diabetes and Metabolism, University of Vermont, Colchester, Vermont

WILLIAM T. CEFALU, MD
Associate Executive Director of Clinical Research, Douglas L. Manship, Sr. Professor of Diabetes, Pennington Biomedical Research Center, Baton Rouge; Chief, Joint Program on Diabetes, Endocrinology and Metabolism, Pennington Biomedical Research Center, Baton Rouge; Louisiana State University Health Science Center School of Medicine, New Orleans, Louisiana

AUTHORS

CARLA A. BORGOÑO, MD, PhD
Resident Physician, Internal Medicine Residency Training Program, Division of General Internal Medicine, Department of Medicine, University of Toronto, Toronto, Canada

ELE FERRANNINI, MD
Professor of Medicine, Department of Internal Medicine, University of Pisa School of Medicine, Pisa, Italy

SATISH K. GARG, MD
Professor of Medicine and Pediatrics, Barbara Davis Center for Childhood Diabetes; School of Medicine, University of Colorado Denver; Editor in Chief, *Diabetes Technology & Therapeutics*, Aurora, Colorado

ROMAN HOVORKA, PhD
Institute of Metabolic Science, Addenbrookes Hospital, University of Cambridge, Cambridge, United Kingdom

JACK L. LEAHY, MD
Professor of Medicine; Chief of Endocrinology, Diabetes and Metabolism, University of Vermont, Colchester, Vermont

ANTHONY L. MCCALL, MD, PhD, FACP
James M. Moss Professor of Diabetes in Internal Medicine, Division of Endocrinology, University of Virginia School of Medicine, Charlottesville, Virginia

MARIE E. MCDONNELL, MD
Assistant Professor of Medicine, Department of Medicine, Boston University School of Medicine, Boston, Massachusetts

AIDAN MCELDUFF, FRACP
Clinical Associate Professor, Discipline of Medicine, Sydney University, Sydney; Northern Sydney Endocrine Centre, St Leonards, New South Wales, Australia

EMILY G. MOSER, BA
Barbara Davis Center for Childhood Diabetes; School of Medicine, University of Colorado Denver, Aurora, Colorado

ROBERT G. MOSES, MD
Illawarra Diabetes Service, Wollongong West, New South Wales, Australia

MATTHEW C. RIDDLE, MD
Professor of Medicine, Division of Endocrinology, Diabetes and Clinical Nutrition, Department of Medicine, Oregon Health and Science University, Portland, Oregon

BRIANA E. ROCKLER, BA
Barbara Davis Center for Childhood Diabetes; School of Medicine, University of Colorado Denver, Aurora, Colorado

KRISTIN A. SIKES, MSN, APRN, CDE
Yale Children's Diabetes Program, New Haven, Connecticut

SEAN M. SWITZER, BA
Barbara Davis Center for Childhood Diabetes; School of Medicine, University of Colorado Denver, Aurora, Colorado

WILLIAM V. TAMBORLANE, MD
Department of Pediatrics, Yale University School of Medicine, New Haven, Connecticut

HOOD THABIT, MD
Institute of Metabolic Science, Addenbrookes Hospital, University of Cambridge, Cambridge, United Kingdom; Faculty of Medicine, University of Malaya, Kuala Lumpur, Malaysia

GUILLERMO E. UMPIERREZ, MD
Professor of Medicine, Department of Medicine, Emory University School of Medicine, Atlanta, Georgia

KEVIN C.J. YUEN, MD
Assistant Professor of Medicine, Division of Endocrinology, Diabetes and Clinical Nutrition, Department of Medicine, Oregon Health and Science University, Portland, Oregon

BERNARD ZINMAN, MD
Senior Scientist, Samuel Lunenfeld Research Institute; Director, Leadership Sinai Centre for Diabetes, Mount Sinai Hospital; Professor of Medicine, University of Toronto, Toronto, Ontario, Canada

Contents

> This article highlights selected milestones in insulin discovery and its continued development as a pivotal therapy for diabetes. The last 90 years have witnessed tremendous progress in insulin therapy, from the initial crude, yet life-saving, animal insulin extracts to novel human insulin analogues. Although the complete physiologic replacement of insulin is inherently difficult to achieve with open-loop subcutaneously administered insulin, the continued development of improved injectable insulin formulations with superior pharmacokinetics and pharmacodynamics will enhance glucose control, and represents important clinical advances in the treatment of both type 1 and type 2 diabetes.

> An input-output schematization of plasma glucose homeostasis provides quantitative information on glucose fluxes and their control by insulin. Insulin action is dependent on the target tissue, the route of delivery, and the kinetics of insulin activation and deactivation, which are different for glucose production and disposal and are a function of insulin resistance. Under normal conditions, the closed-loop control of minute-by-minute insulin release by arterial glucose levels protects against both hyperglycemia and hypoglycemia. Open-loop insulin therapy faces the complexities of insulin pharmacokinetics and pharmacodynamics. Insulin therapy thus remains defiantly empiric.

> Recent large clinical trials have shown that intensive glycemic control can reduce microvascular complications, but appropriate and safe glycemic goals to improve macrovascular outcomes in patients with type 2 diabetes remain poorly defined. This article surveys recent epidemiologic studies and interventional trials, examines the current understanding of the natural history of type 2 diabetes, and proposes new goals and tactics for optimizing insulin therapy.

> Hypoglycemia is the most important and common side effect of insulin therapy. It is also the rate limiting factor in safely achieving excellent glycemic control. A three-fold increased risk of severe hypoglycemia occurs in both type 1 and type 2 diabetes with tight glucose control. This dictates a need to individualize therapy and glycemia goals to minimize this risk. Several ways to reduce hypoglycemia risk are recognized and discussed. They include frequent monitoring of blood sugars with home blood glucose tests and sometimes continuous glucose monitoring (CGM) in order to identify hypoglycemia particularly in hypoglycemia unawareness. Considerations include prompt measured hypoglycemia treatment, attempts to reduce glycemic variability, balancing basal and meal insulin therapy, a pattern therapy approach and use of a physiological mimicry with insulin analogues in a flexible manner. Methods to achieve adequate control while focusing on minimizing the risk of hypoglycemia are delineated in this article.

> There has been a significant increase in the prevalence of type 1 diabetes mellitus and type 2 diabetes mellitus in the past decade. The International Diabetes Foundation reported that there will be more than a half-billion people with diabetes by 2030, largely in emerging economies. Improved glucose control reduces microvascular and macrovascular complications and can be accomplished with intensive diabetes management. Continuous glucose monitors allow further improvement. The best way to emulate normal physiology is the development of an artificial pancreas. Early versions of closed-loop technology may be available in the United States in the next 3 to 5 years.

> Advances in diabetes technology have led to significant improvements in the quality of life and care received by individuals with diabetes. Despite this, achieving tight glycemic control through intensive insulin therapy and modern insulin regimens is challenging because of the barrier of hypoglycemia, the most feared complication of insulin therapy as reported by patients, caregivers, and physicians. This article outlines the individual components of the closed-loop system together with the existing clinical evidence. The artificial pancreas prototypes currently used in clinical studies are reviewed as well as obstacles and limitations facing the technology.

> Health care providers and patients have lots of choice to treat type 2 diabetes, but the blood glucose improvement is limited. The one therapy with unlimited potential (at least theoretically) is insulin. Many studies show that

glucose control is achievable with insulin safely in most patients with type 2 diabetes. Effective diabetes management at the primary care or specialty level requires a belief in the importance of insulin therapy in uncontrolled patients with type 2 diabetes. This review details the theories, observed outcomes, and how-tos regarding insulin use in type 2 diabetes.

Insulin therapy is the mainstay of treatment in children and adolescents with type 1 diabetes (T1D) and is a key component in the treatment of type 2 diabetes (T2D) in this population as well. A major aim of current insulin replacement therapy is to simulate the normal pattern of insulin secretion as closely as possible. This aim can best be achieved with basal-bolus therapy using multiple daily injections (MDI) or continuous insulin infusion (CSII) pump therapy. Only a few years ago, options for insulin formulations were limited. There are now more than 10 varieties of biosynthetic human and analogue insulin.

Insulin therapy is essential for optimal glycemic control during pregnancy in women with type 1 diabetes and is frequently required to optimize control in women with type 2 diabetes. Less commonly, women with gestational diabetes mellitus (GDM) require insulin for glycemic control. However, because of its greater prevalence, GDM is the most common reason for insulin use in pregnancy. The most frequently used insulin regimen in pregnancy is a basal/bolus combination of long- and short-acting insulin preparations. There is no evidence base to support one treatment regimen over another. Therapy should be individualized and based on local expertise.

It has long been established that hyperglycemia with or without a prior diagnosis of diabetes increases both mortality and disease-specific morbidity in hospitalized patients and that goal-directed insulin therapy can improve outcomes. This article reviews the pathophysiology of hyperglycemia during illness, the mechanisms for increased complications and mortality due to hyperglycemia and hypoglycemia, and beneficial mechanistic effects of insulin therapy and provides updated recommendations for the inpatient management of diabetes in the critical care setting and in the general medicine and surgical settings.

ENDOCRINOLOGY AND METABOLISM CLINICS OF NORTH AMERICA

Foreword

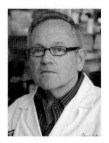

Derek LeRoith, MD, PhD
Consulting Editor

This issue, edited by Drs Leahy and Cefalu, covers a very important aspect of diabetes care, namely, insulin therapy. As the reader will perceive, the topics chosen and authors contributing bring the latest developments in our understanding of the newer developments and use of insulin in both types of diabetes.

Drs Borgoño and Zinman take us through the discovery of insulin, the early preparations, and the more recent advances in the molecular preparations of analogue insulins. They describe how the new analogue insulins, both short-acting and long-acting, when used appropriately better simulate to some degree the normal physiology; at least that's the intention. Also, they discuss the controversy surrounding the long-acting insulin glargine and whether it carries a potential to worsen cancer risk and conclude from the data presented in the literature that it remains unclear. Finally, they present all of the more recent preclinical and early clinical studies with the newest analogue or modified insulins that are being developed—superfast insulins, and basal insulins that may act longer than what is presently available.

In an article that is critical for our understanding of physiological control of glucose, Dr Ferrannini describes how fasting blood glucose is controlled primarily by hepatic glucose production, whereas postprandial blood glucose levels are normally maintained through a reduction in hepatic glucose production and simultaneously enhanced glucose clearance either dependent or independent of insulin action on peripheral tissues. He goes on to discuss the high precision of the normal feedback system between endogenous insulin secretion and its effect on target tissues, in particular the liver, that is extremely sensitive to insulin's effect of inhibiting hepatic glucose output and is usually bathed in higher concentrations of insulin than are the peripheral tissues. Thus it is not surprising that developing the perfect closed loop system to emulate the natural system remains a major challenge.

The article by Drs Riddle and Yuen critically assesses what has been learned from large clinical trials regarding the balance between safety and effectiveness of insulin therapy. They describe the effects of intensive insulin therapy in type 1 diabetes and the positive outcomes regarding microangiopathic complications. This is followed by a description of the mixed results from the outcomes of intensified control of type 2 diabetes, where microangiopathy was reduced but macrovascular complications were

Endocrinol Metab Clin N Am 41 (2012) ix–xi
doi:10.1016/j.ecl.2012.03.005
0889-8529/12/$ – see front matter © 2012 Elsevier Inc. All rights reserved.

not. On the other hand, 10-year follow-up studies of both type 1 (Diabetes Control and Complications Trial) and type 2 diabetics (UKPDS), after the trials had ceased, showed improved macrovascular outcomes, highlighting the very important understanding that early intensive therapy can result in later positive results, the so-called "metabolic memory or legacy" effect. Finally they discuss the variable results with therapy intensification in later stage type 2 diabetes (ACCORD, ADVANCE, VADT trials), and the authors posit, as do many others, that intensive insulin therapy should be individualized, but that early tight metabolic control can have positive results. On the other hand, in established disease with undoubtedly the presence of cardiovascular disease, metabolic control should be approached more cautiously.

An up-to-date analysis of the progress that is occurring with closed loop insulin delivery systems is discussed in an article by Drs Thabit and Hovorka. They suggest that the closed loop system that couples minute-by-minute glucose monitoring with insulin delivery could be the bridge to the cure, until stem cell therapy or islet cell transplantation become a reality. Multiple technical advances have occurred and devices been developed for real-time glucose monitoring as well as for insulin delivery and these are discussed in detail in the article. Also discussed are that overnight and low-glucose suspend systems are rapidly becoming a clinical reality with the potential to eliminate the nighttime hypoglycemia that is devastating for some patients.

One of the major issues with intensified insulin therapy is hypoglycemia, which often leads to noncompliance in patients with both type 1 diabetes and those patients with type 2 diabetes using insulin. As discussed by Dr McCall in his article, hypoglycemia also has significant consequences, namely, injury to both brain and heart as well as the possibility of precipitating sudden death. Particularly important in this context is the phenomenon of hypoglycemic unawareness with defective counterregulatory hormone responses that often occurs with longstanding type 1 diabetes and occasionally in type 2 patients. Also, he discusses current strategies to reduce the risks of hypoglycemia, and how SBGM and more advanced monitoring devices hold promise for preventing this devastating complication of correct insulin use in our patients.

The importance of intensive insulin therapy for tight metabolic control in type 1 diabetes has been demonstrated most definitively by the Diabetes Control and Complications Trial. In this trial the tight control prevented microvascular disease during the period of the trial and macrovascular protection was seen years later. In their article Drs Switzer, Moser, Rockler, and Garg discuss the various paradigms used in type 1 diabetes to achieve such tight metabolic control. These include multiple daily injections of insulin, particularly with the new analogue insulins, or alternatively using continuous subcutaneous insulin infusions. They also highlight the importance of blood glucose monitoring that is traditionally performed by finger stick methodology (SBGM). On the other hand, their in-depth discussion of continuous blood glucose monitoring as well as the possibility of closed-loop pump systems shows the power of new technology.

Type 2 diabetes is known to be a progressive disorder that after years of treatment with oral hypoglycemic agents eventuates in the need for insulin to correct the metabolic derangements. Dr Leahy describes the initiation of basal insulin, which is often the first step in introducing insulin therapy. Also, for intensifying therapy he compares the basal bolus regimen to the premixed insulin regimen, concluding that one-by-one additions of mealtime insulin injections to basal insulin may be the best approach. While insulin pumps may avoid the multiple injections, they are seldom used in patients with type 2 diabetes. On the other hand, the addition of incretin therapies to insulin therapy has begun to make its mark in uncontrolled type 2 diabetes.

Drs McElduff and Moses discuss the use of insulin therapy in gestational diabetes and during pregnancy in women with type 1 and type 2 diabetes. Despite the focus over the last two decades on successful pregnancies in type 1 diabetes, nevertheless the large majority of diabetic pregnancies include gestational diabetes in the prediabetic population and in women with type 2 diabetics; these two conditions are becoming more common due to the obesity epidemic that leads to earlier onset of type 2 diabetes. In their article, the authors discuss in a very practical manner the management of diabetes-related pregnancy, and in particular, the commonly used analogue insulins, the importance of glucose control, the avoidance of hypoglycemia and ketacidosis, and the use of insulin pumps primarily by type 1 diabetics.

In their article on insulin therapy in children and adolescents Drs Tamborlane and Sikes describe in more depth the indications for insulin administration using pumps and monitoring devices in a pediatric population. They describe the value and use of basal-bolus regimens and analogue insulins. Most important are the practical aspects of initiating insulin therapy in children using the continuous insulin infusion devices (CSII), which also includes calorie counting and dosing with insulin. There are issues with CSII devices such as "stacking," where too many boluses are given and too often; glucose monitoring can avoid this issue. Also, pump failure could lead to ketoacidosis since only rapid-acting insulins are used; here again, BG monitoring is critical to avoid this complication.

Drs McDonnell and Umpierrez discuss the use of insulin in hospitalized patients. Initially there was interest in maintaining very tight blood glucose control in hospitalized patients, whether diabetic or nondiabetic, due to convincing evidence that hyperglycemia was associated with increased morbidity and mortality. More recently the focus has shifted to concern over hypoglycemic events being linked to excess morbidity and mortality, and the authors carefully discuss the current recommendations that take more of a middle-of-the-road approach.

The consulting editor and staff wish to thank Drs Leahy and Cefalu for compiling a very topical issue, with outstanding contributions from experts in the field, who have provided practical information as well as basic understanding of the role of insulin in research and practice.

Derek LeRoith, MD, PhD
Division of Endocrinology, Metabolism, and Bone Diseases
Department of Medicine
Mount Sinai School of Medicine
One Gustave L. Levy Place
Box 1055, Altran 4-36
New York, NY 10029, USA

E-mail address:
derek.leroith@mssm.edu

Preface

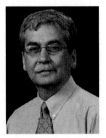 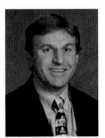

Jack L. Leahy, MD   William T. Cefalu, MD
Guest Editors

In 2002, the editors of this volume, Jack Leahy and Will Cefalu, edited a book entitled *Insulin Therapy*. It was made up of chapters from experts in the field regarding insulin physiology and therapy, and, in particular, the *how to's* and *why's* regarding insulin usage in various patient populations. We did that project because of the lack of a centralized source of up-to-date information on this key subject. Now, 10 years later, the need for a comprehensive sourcebook for insulin therapy is even greater. Much has happened in those 10 years. Insulin analogues are firmly established, and new increasingly innovative insulins and delivery devices are coming. Technology has become an everyday part of type 1 diabetes—pumps, sensors, meters with computer programs to crunch the data, and soon (hopefully) automatic suspend closed loop systems. In type 2 diabetes, insulin therapy has stood the test of time despite new classes of pharmaceuticals having tried to make it obsolete. Just the opposite! Starting insulin in patients failing other therapies is common practice for primary care providers, and numerous studies from around the world have shown insulin in type 2 diabetes is generally safe and effective, and, most importantly, well-accepted by patients. The major discussion point today is not whether to use insulin in type 2 diabetes, but how early, and what to do if the starting program—basal or premixed insulin—fails? Particularly exciting are the recent studies combining a GLP-1 receptor agonist with a basal insulin, or adding a single injection of mealtime insulin to basal insulin rather than a full basal-bolus program. Also, important studies have tested how to optimize insulin therapy in children, in pregnancy, and in hospitalized patients. And there has been enormous discussion about goals of treatment, and prevention of hypoglycemia.

All of these topics are covered in the various articles of this volume. We have assembled an outstanding group of authors, all recognized as leaders in their field, and we, the editors, want to thank them for their excellent contributions.

Endocrinol Metab Clin N Am 41 (2012) xiii–xiv
doi:10.1016/j.ecl.2012.03.006

Jack L. Leahy, MD
Division of Endocrinology, Diabetes and Metabolism
Department of Medicine
University of Vermont
Colchester Research Facility, Room 110
208 South Park Drive
Colchester, VT 05446, USA

William T. Cefalu, MD
Pennington Biomedical Research Center
6400 Perkins Road
Baton Rouge, LA 70810, USA

Louisiana State University Health Science Center
School of Medicine
433 Bolivar Street
New Orleans, LA 70112, USA

E-mail addresses:
jleahy@uvm.edu (J.L. Leahy)
William.cefalu@pbrc.edu (W.T. Cefalu)

Insulins: Past, Present, and Future

Carla A. Borgoño, MD, PhD[a], Bernard Zinman, MD[b],*

KEYWORDS

• Injectable insulin • Insulin analogues • Pharmacokinetics

DISCOVERY AND EVOLUTION OF INSULIN

Since its discovery and first clinical use in the 1920s, insulin therapy has revolutionized the treatment and natural history of both type 1 and type 2 diabetes mellitus. This article highlights selected milestones in insulin discovery and its continued development as a pivotal therapy for diabetes (**Fig. 1**).

The history of insulin begins at the turn of the twentieth century, with the culmination of early landmark research on endocrine pancreas (patho)physiology, which provided the intellectual and methodological framework for insulin discovery. In 1890, von Mering and Minkowski[1] identified the crucial link between the pancreas and diabetes as evidenced by the diabetic phenotype they induced in dogs after pancreatectomy. Subsequent histologic observations during 1900-1901 of hyaline changes in the islets of Langerhans from patients with diabetes by Opie,[2] coupled with the pioneering animal pancreatic duct ligation experiments of Ssobolew[3] from 1900 to 1902, resulting in atrophied acinar cells accompanied by normal, intact islets and a nondiabetic phenotype, collectively implicated the pancreatic islets in the etiology of diabetes. Physiologist Sharpey-Schäfer[4] hypothesized that pancreatic islets might produce an "internal secretion" or hormone involved in glucose homeostasis. Consequently, the first 2 decades of the twentieth century witnessed numerous attempts to isolate this internal secretion. Although several investigators prepared and administered pancreatic extracts with transient hypoglycemic effects in animals and even humans, adverse side effects ultimately precluded their clinical utility.[5–9]

In 1920, the pathologist Barron[10] recognized that pancreatic duct obstruction, whether secondary to pancreatolithiasis in a rare post-mortem case or pancreatic duct ligation in prior animal experiments, led to atrophy of the exocrine but not

C.B. has nothing to disclose. B.Z. has received honoraria and/or research support from Eli Lilly, Novo Nordisk, Sanofi, and Halozyme.
a Division of General Internal Medicine, Department of Medicine, University of Toronto, 200 Elizabeth Street, Toronto, Ontario, Canada M5G 2C4
b Leadership Sinai Centre for Diabetes, Mount Sinai Hospital, 60 Murray Street, Suite L5-024, Mail Box 17, Toronto, Ontario, Canada M5T 3L9
* Corresponding author.
E-mail address: zinman@lunenfeld.ca

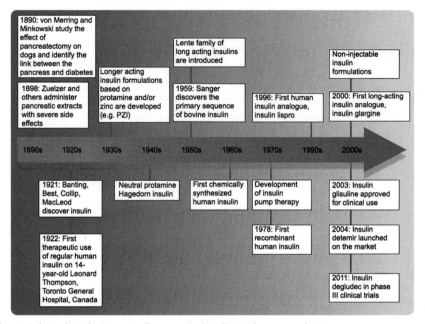

Fig. 1. Selected evolutionary milestones in insulin replacement therapy.

endocrine pancreas. Primarily inspired by Barron's paper, Frederick G. Banting conceived of a novel method of isolating the internal secretion by deliberately inducing atrophy of the acinar cells of the exocrine pancreas via duct ligation in dogs, to diminish the potentially destructive effect of digestive enzymes on the islet hormone.[11] In the summer of 1921, assisted by Charles H. Best in the laboratory of John J.R. MacLeod at the University of Toronto, Banting became the first to demonstrate that pancreatic islet extracts consistently reduced hyperglycemia and glycosuria in depancreatized, diabetic dogs.[12] Later that year, with the expertise of biochemist James B. Collip, a novel protocol was developed to purify what they later named "insulin" (Latin: *insula*, island), from pancreatic islets of whole bovine pancreata without the need for pancreatic duct ligation experiments.[13] The first successful therapeutic use of pancreas extracts of bovine insulin occurred at the Toronto General Hospital on January 11, 1922 on a 14-year-old patient, Leonard Thompson, who was admitted with type 1 diabetes.[13] Even this very unphysiologic rather crude form of insulin therapy rapidly transformed type 1 diabetes from an inevitably fatal condition to a chronic metabolic disease characterized by significant risk of hypoglycemia, diabetic ketoacidosis, and ultimately the long-term complications associated with diabetes. In 1923, the Nobel Prize in Medicine and Physiology was jointly awarded to Banting and MacLeod for what is considered one of the greatest advancements in modern medicine.

Insulin therapy has significantly evolved since 1922, with major improvements in insulin purification, production, formulation, regimens, and delivery systems. Until the 1980s animal insulins, extracted from either bovine or porcine pancreata, comprised all commercially available insulin formulations. Such soluble, "regular," animal insulin products were initially very impure, leading to immunologic reactions (eg, insulin allergy, immune-mediated lipoatrophy at the injection site, and antibody-mediated insulin resistance) and significant variability in pharmacokinetics and pharmacodynamics. Early advances in purification techniques led to better-quality products with more consistent biological action. To prolong the glucose-lowering effects of insulin and reduce the number of daily injections required with soluble regular insulin, longer-acting preparations were designed by combining insulin with zinc and/or basic proteins (protamines) to delay subcutaneous absorption. These formulations included prot-amine insulin and protamine zinc insulin (PZI) developed in the 1930s,[14–16] isophane neutral protamine Hagedorn (NPH) launched in the 1940s[17] and the trilogy of "lente" insulins introduced during the 1950s.[18] Among the latter, NPH insulin has retained its clinical utility to this day, as a twice-daily insulin, used alone or in conjunction with soluble insulin as a premixed product.[19] During the 1950s, Sanger[20] elucidated the primary structure of bovine insulin. Through advances in protein chromatography tech-niques, the 1970s witnessed the production of highly purified animal insulin, denoted monocomponent or single-peak insulin.[21] Although chemically synthesized human insulin was first produced in the 1960s[22–26] and studied in preliminary clinical trials,[27] this breakthrough was overshadowed by the advent of recombinant DNA technology in the late 1970s, which gave rise to recombinant human insulin in 1978, a much more commercially viable product.[28] This milestone marked a new era in the evolution of insulin therapy and peptide drug development in general. Since the 1980s, insulin replacement strategies have been incrementally optimized, with the development of structurally modified, so-called designer insulin analogues,[29,30] the evaluation of alter-native delivery routes (eg, nasal, pulmonary inhaled, oral, peritoneal insulin formula-tions),[31] continuous subcutaneous insulin infusion therapy (ie, insulin pumps),[32,33] and most recently the potential to use continuous glucose monitoring with glucose sensor technology (ie, closed-loop insulin delivery, also referred to as the artificial pancreas).[34,35] The remainder of this article focuses on current and future injectable insulin preparations.

INSULIN PHYSIOLOGY

Endogenous insulin, a 51-amino-acid anabolic hormone comprising 2 peptide chains (A and B; **Fig. 2**A), is a key regulator of glucose, protein, and fat homeostasis. Insulin is synthesized as proinsulin, then processed and secreted by pancreatic β cells of the islets of Langerhans into the portal circulation via the hepatic vein, whereby the liver extracts a substantial fraction before entering the systemic circulation.[36] To maintain euglycemia (ie, plasma glucose between 3.5 and 7.0 mmol/L), insulin release occurs both (1) at a constitutive, basal rate and (2) in short-lived large bursts, secondary to physiologic stimuli related to nutrient intake and mediated in great part by the gastro-intestinal system incretin hormones GLP1 and GIP. Basal insulin secretion occurs during fasting/resting states, to inhibit hepatic glycogenolysis, ketogenesis, and gluconeogenesis, and accounts for approximately 40% of total insulin output in a 24-hour period. Stimulated insulin secretion occurs when plasma glucose levels rise to above 4.4 to 5.6 mmol/L (80–100 mg/dL), particularly after meals (postprandial) to restore euglycemia via promotion of peripheral glucose uptake and fuel storage. In addition, insulin secretion in response to a meal occurs in 2 phases: an initial transient surge (first phase) followed by a prolonged steady increase (second phase). Although glucose is the most potent insulin secretagogue, additional dietary nutrients (eg, amino acids), enteric hormones (eg, incretins), and neural signals are also implicated in insulin regulation. In healthy individuals, plasma glucose and insulin excursions occur in parallel and are tightly linked throughout the day, thereby ensuring adequate glucoregulation (**Fig. 3**).

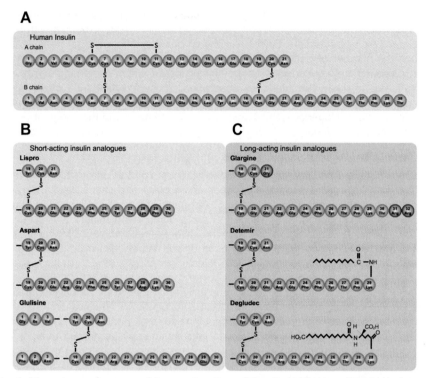

Fig. 2. The primary structure of human insulin and insulin analogues. (*A*) Native human insulin; (*B*) rapid-acting insulin analogues (lispro, aspart, glulisine); (*C*) long-acting insulin analogues (glargine, detemir, degludec). Modifications of each insulin analogue are shown.

GOALS OF INSULIN THERAPY

In using insulin it would of course be ideal if it could be supplied so as to imitate the natural process.

—*J.J.R. Macleod and W.R. Campbell, 1925*

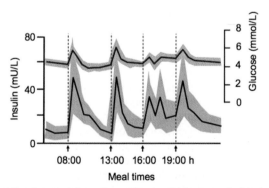

Fig. 3. Glucose and insulin excursions throughout a 24-hour period in healthy individuals. Mean levels with 95% confidence intervals are shown. (*Adapted from* Owens DR, Zinman B, Bolli GB. Insulins today and beyond. Lancet 2001;358:739–46.)

Insulin administration is the sole pharmacologic treatment currently available for patients with type 1 diabetes, and represents an important therapy for many patients with type 2 diabetes. Unfortunately, despite many important advances in the 90 years since its discovery, physiologic insulin replacement remains an elusive goal.[37] Indeed, despite the advent of novel insulin formulations, treatment regimens, delivery systems, continuous glucose monitoring, and multidisciplinary educational programs, diabetes remains a major cause of morbidity and mortality worldwide.[38,39] The latter is attributed to the significant microvascular and macrovascular complications associated with this disease.[38,39] However, as demonstrated by several epidemiologic studies and clinical trials, including the landmark Diabetes Control and Complications Trial (DCCT)[40] and the UK Prospective Diabetes Study (UKPDS),[41] the risk of diabetic complications can be prevented and substantially reduced with intensive glycemic control (**Table 1**).[40–49]

Given this unequivocal evidence, the fundamental treatment goals in diabetes care are to strive for optimal glycemic control and minimize the risk of hypoglycemia. To achieve these goals, the aim of insulin therapy is to approximate the physiologic insulin profile (see **Fig. 3**) via insulin replacement. However, this is often hindered by patient-related (eg, noncompliance) and treatment-related factors.[37,41,50] In fact, it is inherently impossible to replace insulin physiologically.[37] Compared with its endogenous portal secretion from the pancreas, exogenous insulin is administered peripherally via subcutaneous injection, leading to peripheral hyperinsulinemia and portal hypoinsulinemia. Moreover, the variability of subcutaneous insulin absorption and the risk of hypoglycemia further complicate insulin therapy and the attainment of optimal glycemic targets.

INSULIN PREPARATIONS IN CLINICAL USE

Insulin replacement and supplementation strategies aim to replicate endogenous stimulated and basal insulin release by the healthy pancreas (see **Fig. 3**), such that excursions in postmeal blood glucose are minimal and hepatic glucose production between meals is appropriately suppressed, respectively. Thus, insulin replacement regimens comprise 2 components: a basal (fasting) and bolus (meal/prandial) insulin preparation. Commercially available insulin formulations are classified as rapid-, short-, intermediate-, or long-acting products based on their pharmacokinetic properties, including onset, peak, and duration of action, summarized in **Table 2**. Accordingly,

Table 1
Various guidelines on optimal glycemic targets for patients with diabetes

Organization	HbA$_{1c}$ (%)	FPG		Postprandial PG		References
		mmol/L	mg/dL	mmol/L	mg/dL	
CDA	≤7.0	4.0–7.0	72–126	5.0–10.0[a]	90–180	177
ADA	≤7.0	3.9–7.2	70–130	<10.0	<180	178
AACE	≤6.5	<6.1	<110	<7.8	<140	179
ESC-EASD	≤6.5	—	—	—	—	180
IDF	<6.5	5.5	<100	7.8	<140	181

Abbreviations: ADA, American Diabetes Association; AACE, American Association of Clinical Endocrinologists; CDA, Canadian Diabetes Association; ESC, European Society of Cardiology; EASD, European Association for the Study of Diabetes; FPG, fasting plasma glucose; HbA$_{1c}$, hemoglobin A$_{1c}$; IDF, International Diabetes Federation; PG, plasma glucose.
[a] Target of 5.0 to 8.0 mmol/L if HbA$_{1c}$ targets are not being met.

Table 2
Pharmacokinetic parameters of currently available insulin preparations

Insulin	Trade Name	Manufacturer	Action Profile (h)		
			Onset	Peak	Duration
Rapid-acting					
Lispro	Humalog	Eli Lilly	0.2–0.5	0.5–2	3–4
Aspart	Novorapid	Novo Nordisk	0.2–0.5	0.5–2	3–4
Glulisine	Apidra	Sanofi-Aventis	0.2–0.5	0.5–2	3–4
Short-acting					
Regular	Humulin R	Eli Lilly	0.5–1	2–4	6–8
	Novolin ge Toronto	Novo Nordisk			
Intermediate-acting					
Isophane insulin (NPH)	Humulin N	Eli Lilly	1.5–4	4–10	Up to 20
	Novolin N	Novo Nordisk			
Long-acting					
Glargine	Lantus	Sanofi-Aventis	1–3	No peak	Up to 24
Detemir	Levemir	Novo Nordisk	1–3	No peak	Up to 24
Premixed human insulins					
NPH/regular[a]					
70%/30%	Humulin 70/30	Eli Lilly	0.5–1	3–12	Up to 24
	Novolin 70/30	Novo Nordisk			
50%/50%	Humulin 50/50	Eli Lilly	0.5–1	2–12	Up to 24
	Novolin 50/50	Novo Nordisk			
Premixed insulin analogues					
NPL/Lispro					
75%/25%	Humalog Mix 75/25	Eli Lilly	0.2–0.5	1–4	24
50%/50%	Humalog Mix 50/50	Eli Lilly	0.2–0.5	1–4	24
IAP/Aspart					
70%/30%	Novolog Mix 30	Novo Nordisk	0.2–0.5	1–4	24

Abbreviations: IAP, insulin aspart protamine; NPH, neutral protamine Hagedorn; NPL, neutral protamine lispro.

[a] Mixtures with different proportions of NPH and regular insulin are available in Europe.

Modified from Mooradian AD, Bernbaum M, Albert SG. Narrative review: a rational approach to starting insulin therapy. Ann Intern Med 2006;145:125–34.

the rapid and short-acting insulin formulations are used as the bolus component of insulin therapy, whereas intermediate-acting and long-acting preparations act to replace endogenous basal insulin secretion. The unique pharmacokinetic parameters of individual insulin products depend primarily on rate and extent of absorption into the systemic circulation following subcutaneous injection.

Human Insulins

Short-acting human insulin

Regular human insulin, the first insulin product generated using recombinant DNA technology,[28] has traditionally been used as a bolus insulin to mimic the response of endogenous insulin to a meal and also to correct for premeal and intermeal hyperglycemia. Human insulin exists as a monomer at low concentrations and is best absorbed into the bloodstream following subcutaneous injection in this form. Although the peptide sequence and tertiary structure of regular recombinant human insulin is identical to that of its endogenous counterpart, the former tends to self-aggregate into quaternary structures of dimers and hexamers in solutions of higher concentration containing zinc ions.[51,52] This propensity to self-associate delays the absorption of regular human insulin, which must first dissociate into dimers and monomers in the subcutaneous space to effectively diffuse into the general circulation and exert its glucodynamic action. Consequently, the latter is reflected in its pharmacokinetic profile, which consists of a delayed onset of action (30–60 minutes after administration), relatively late peak effect (2–4 hours postinjection) and a longer duration of action (6–8 hours) compared with the sharper peak secretion of endogenous insulin that occurs following meal ingestion.[53] Thus, regular human insulin does not adequately replicate the documented physiologic postprandial insulin secretion, which may lead to early postprandial hyperglycemia and late hypoglycemia.[54] Given its delayed onset of action, regular insulin should be administered 30 minutes before meals. This recommendation is difficult to comply with in real life, as meal timing can vary substantially and thus premeal doses are often administered immediately before meals. As a result, the conventional use of regular human insulin as a bolus or mealtime insulin has decreased in favor of the novel, more rapid-acting insulin analogues.

Intermediate-acting human insulin

At present, the only conventional intermediate-acting human insulin in clinical use is isophane NPH insulin. Originally developed in the 1940s in an attempt to prolong the biological action of regular insulin preparations to better approximate basal insulin profiles and minimize insulin dosing frequency, NPH was initially composed of an animal-derived insulin suspended in a neutral pH solution of protamine and zinc.[17] This unique suspension allows for a significant delay in the absorption of insulin from the subcutaneous tissue, resulting in an onset of action 1.5 to 4 hours after injection, a pronounced peak 4 to 10 hours after administration, and a duration of up to 24 hours (see **Table 2**).[55,56] Of note, NPH insulin was subsequently reformulated using recombinant human insulin during the 1980s. However, NPH does not constitute an appropriate surrogate for endogenous basal insulin production, for several reasons. From a pharmacokinetic perspective, an ideal exogenous basal insulin product should be "peakless," whereas NPH displays a pronounced peak action profile.[55,57,58] Moreover, the fact that NPH must be evenly suspended before administration has led to wide interindividual and intraindividual variability in its absorption from the subcutaneous tissue depot.[51,59] Taken together, this often results in a failure to obtain consistent adequate glycemic control, with a range in blood glucose excursions from hypoglycemia (eg, particularly nocturnal hypoglycemia when injected in the evening) to hyperglycemia (eg, given its short duration of action). Despite these findings, NPH has retained clinical utility as a basal insulin when administered twice daily and in a premixed insulin preparation combined with regular human insulin.[60] Its main attribute at this time is its low cost compared with the newer basal analogues.

Human Insulin Analogues

Insulin analogues were designed to improve on the subcutaneously administered pharmacokinetic and pharmacodynamic inadequacies of conventional human insulin products that limit their clinical efficacy. Through targeted structural manipulation of the human insulin molecule (eg, amino acid substitutions, inversions, or additions) using recombinant technology protein bioengineering techniques, several insulin analogues with modified biochemical properties resulting in altered rates of self-aggregation and subsequent subcutaneous absorption into the bloodstream have been recently developed, without adversely affecting biological function (ie, affinity for the insulin receptor and subsequent signaling events).[29,30] In general, rapid-acting and long-acting insulin analogues have been modified to possess a weaker or stronger ability to self-associate and hence, a faster or slower diffusion rate following subcutaneous tissue injection, respectively. Thus, the pharmacodynamic properties of analogues of native insulin better approximate endogenous insulin secretion and ultimately would be expected to result in to superior clinical end points, including improved glycemic control with reduced hypoglycemic episodes alongside greater treatment satisfaction and overall enhanced quality of life from the patient perspective.

Rapid-acting insulin analogues

At present, there are 3 commercially available rapid-acting insulin analogues approved for clinical use as bolus or mealtime insulins, namely lispro, aspart, and glulisine. The β insulin chain of each rapid-acting insulin analogue has been structurally altered to impede self-aggregation of insulin molecules into multimeric complexes (**Fig. 2**B). With respect to insulin lispro, the first rapid-acting analogue developed in 1996, transposition of amino acids proline and lysine at positions B28 and B29 leads to a conformational change that augments steric hindrance between interfaces implicated in dimerization.[61,62] Substitution of proline at B28 by a negatively charged aspartic acid residue in the case of insulin aspart results in repulsion of monomers.[63,64] Regarding insulin glulisine, replacement of lysine at B29 for glutamine and aspartic acid at B3 for lysine simultaneously provides stability and a reduced ability to self-associate.[65–67] The ensuing pharmacokinetic profile, that is, a faster onset of action (10–30 minutes postadministration), peak of action (0.5–2 hours), and a shorter duration of action (3–5 hours) in comparison with regular human insulin, are comparable among the rapid-acting insulin analogues and more compatible with physiologic time-activity profiles of meal-stimulated insulin release.[68,69] Moreover, less variability between injection sites has been described for insulin analogues in comparison with regular insulin.[64,68,70]

In addition to superior pharmacokinetic parameters, rapid-acting insulin analogues also demonstrate enhanced clinical efficacy, including improved normalization of postprandial glucose excursions, a decrease in hypoglycemic events, with either modest or no significant reductions in hemoglobin A_{1c} (HbA_{1c}) levels in patients with type 1 and 2 diabetes, respectively, when compared with traditional human insulin.[71–81] However, the lack of a significant reduction in HbA_{1c} in patients using these analogues may be dependent, to some extent, on the accompanying basal insulin product used and on the initial level of glycemic control before treatment. In addition, most of the studies were not double blinded but rather the regular insulin was given as per protocol, 30 minutes before the meal, with the rapid-acting analogue being administered immediately before the meal. In fact, in real life most patients take their meal insulin just before the meal regardless of whether it is regular or a rapid-acting analogue, so the differences in pharmacokinetics and pharmacodynamics would be even greater. It is also likely that the reduction in very low values of glucose, that is, hypoglycemia with rapid-acting analogues, would tend to raise HbA_{1c}, masking its beneficial effect on overall glucose control.

Patients who use rapid-acting insulin analogues as opposed to regular insulin also report an enhancement in their quality of life.[82–85] For instance, from a practical standpoint, the rapid onset of action of insulins lispro, aspart, and glulisine allows for greater flexibility and convenience in the timing of administration, that is, either at mealtime or even immediately postprandially. The latter option also allows for better matching of insulin dose to carbohydrate load consumed, therefore improved control of postmeal glycemic fluctuations may be attained.

Potential clinical disadvantages related to the kinetic profile of rapid-acting insulin analogues include the risk of early postprandial hypoglycemia and preprandial hyperglycemia, compared with regular insulin.[86]

Long-acting insulin analogues

The long-acting insulin analogues currently licensed for basal insulin replacement and supplementation include insulins glargine and detemir. As shown in **Fig. 2**, the structure of each analogue has been uniquely altered to achieve prolonged absorption following subcutaneous injection and a relatively peakless 24-hour time-action profile, which is much more analogous to physiologic basal insulin release when compared with NPH insulin. In the case of insulin glargine, the first long-acting analogue of insulin introduced in 2000, modifications to both the α and β insulin chains, specifically the replacement of asparagine with glycine at position A21 and the addition of 2 arginine residues at position B30, respectively, results in a molecule that is less soluble at neutral, physiologic pH yet stable in the acidic pH of its storage solution (**Fig. 2C**).[87–89] Thus, when injected into the neutral milieu of the subcutaneous tissue, glargine forms an amorphous precipitate from which insulin molecules are slowly released into the circulation.[87–89] Insulin detemir, on the other hand, features 2 alterations within the β insulin chain: deletion of amino acid threonine at position B30 and acylation of a 14-carbon aliphatic fatty acid (myristolytic acid) to the ε-amino group of lysine at position B29, which enhances its affinity for albumin.[90,91] This process results in an insulin product with protracted action, due to sustained release from multimeric complexes within the subcutaneous tissues postinjection as well as from albumin to which it is reversibly bound.[91–93]

The ensuing pharmacokinetic profiles of insulins glargine and detemir are comparable.[94] Both long-acting analogues have an onset of action within 1 to 3 hours of administration and a relatively peakless, dose-dependent, mean duration of action of approximately 24 hours.[58,94–98] Accordingly, these analogues represent better surrogates for basal insulin replacement and supplementation. Despite the controversy, clinical experience tends to suggest that there are some patients who require twice-daily dosing with glargine and detemir to provide full basal coverage. This situation appears to be more evident with insulin detemir.

Furthermore, both glargine and detemir demonstrate less intersubject variability in rates of absorption at different injection sites along with a reduced incidence of hypoglycemia when compared with NPH insulin (**Fig. 4**).[78,99–110] Not surprisingly, in a treat-to-target study design, similar HbA$_{1c}$ levels were achieved with long-acting insulin analogues in comparison with NPH.[86,109–111] However, this effect can only be achieved at the expense of increased nocturnal hypoglycemia with the NPH insulin. Similarly, several recent clinical trials comparing basal-bolus insulin regimens comprising only insulin analogues (eg, detemir/aspart) versus traditional insulin preparations (eg, NPH/regular) have failed to show consistent reductions in HbA$_{1c}$ with the use of regimens comprising insulin analogue only.[76,112,113] Regarding insulin detemir, this analogue displays reduced within-subject variability in glycemia versus glargine[97,99,104] and is associated with less weight gain than NPH[105,114,115] and glargine[116,117] in patients with type 2 diabetes. However, these differences are small and are generally not regarded as being of great clinical significance.

Premixed Insulin Preparations

Two main classes of premixed insulin preparations are currently on the market: premixes of conventional insulin products and fixed-ratio mixes of insulin analogues.

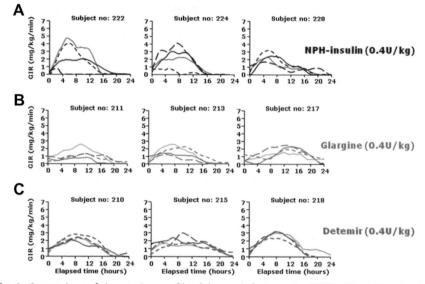

Fig. 4. Comparison of time-action profiles (glucose infusion rates [GIR]) of basal insulins (*A*) NPH, (*B*) glargine, and (*C*) detemir. The results of 4 euglycemic clamp studies per subject are shown in one plot. Intrasubject variability from highest to lowest: NPH > glargine > detemir. (*Adapted from* Heise T, Nosek L, Rønn BB, et al. Lower within-subject variability of insulin detemir in comparison to NPH insulin and insulin glargine in people with type 1 diabetes. Diabetes 2004;53:1614–20.)

With respect to the former, traditional short-acting and intermediate-acting human insulins have been combined in different ratios to form 2 preparations: Humulin 50/50 (comprising 50% NPH and 50% regular insulin) and Humulin or Novolin 70/30 (consisting of 70% NPH and 30% regular insulin). Regarding the latter, 3 formulations combining different ratios of rapid-acting insulin analogues are available: Humalog Mix 50/50 (a 50% neutral protamine lispro suspension with 50% insulin lispro), Humalog Mix 75/25 (75% neutral protamine lispro and 25% insulin lispro), and Novolog Mix 30 (70% protamine crystalline aspart and 30% insulin aspart). Of note, the protaminated forms of lispro (neutral protamine lispro [NPL, insulin lispro protamine]) and aspart (protamine crystalline aspart or insulin aspart protamine) are functionally identical to NPH.[118] The pharmacokinetic profiles of premixed insulin products are shown in **Table 2**.

Studies comparing the clinical efficacy of premixed human insulins and premixed insulin analogue preparations suggest that premixes of insulin analogues are superior in terms of controlling postprandial glucose excursions with less intrasubject variation, yet do not show consistent improvements in HbA_{1c} levels.[60,119–125] Premixed insulin products represent a convenient alternative to basal-bolus insulin therapy, with a decreased number of daily injections, and should be used only in patients with type 2 diabetes.[60,126]

CURRENT CONTROVERSIES IN THE USE OF INSULIN
Insulin Analogues and Cancer Risk

Despite the superiority in the clinical efficacy of insulin analogues over traditional insulin formulations, safety concerns have been raised regarding the putative carcinogenic potential of certain analogues. The rationale underlying the potential mitogenicity of analogues of insulin is that structural modifications to the native insulin molecule may result in perturbations of receptor binding sites (particularly the B10 and B26–B30 regions of the β chain),[127] and thus inadvertently lead to: (1) enhanced affinity toward the insulin-like growth factor (IGF-1) receptor, which shares greater than 50% amino-acid sequence similarity to the insulin receptor; and/or (2) altered binding kinetics (ie, prolonged occupancy time) of the insulin receptor, causing aberrant downstream signaling and promoting tumor development.[128–130] However, with respect to the rapid-acting insulin analogues, there is currently no compelling evidence that insulins lispro, aspart, and glulisine have increased mitogenic potential compared with regular human insulin.[86,131–133]

The main area of controversy revolves around the potential tumorigenic properties of long-acting insulin analogues, particularly insulin glargine. In vitro studies indicate that glargine has a higher affinity for the IGF-1 receptor and increased downstream proliferative and antiapoptotic effects in benign and malignant cell lines compared with human insulin and other analogues.[132–134] Similarly, the serum of patients treated with insulin glargine displayed greater mitogenic potency on human breast cancer cells compared with the serum of those treated with regular insulin or insulin detemir.[135] However, no difference in the mitogenic capacity of insulin glargine versus human insulin was reported in another study using normal and malignant breast epithelial cell lines,[136] nor did long-term glargine administration increase tumor development in murine models in vivo.[137] Recent data from observational studies and randomized control trials examining the risk of malignancy with insulin glargine are also equivocal. Several studies have identified an association between the use of glargine monotherapy and an increased incidence of malignancy, particularly breast cancer,[138,139] compared with the use of insulin products with and without glargine,[138–141] but were heavily criticized on methodological grounds.[142,143] Other studies have failed to show this association.[144–146] Furthermore, a recent cohort study by Suissa and colleagues[147] demonstrated that the incidence of breast cancer does not increase with short-term use (ie, <5 years) of insulin glargine in women with type 2 diabetes, but that a trend toward increased risk may be apparent with extended use (>5 years), in the context of long-standing insulin therapy before initiating treatment with glargine.

Of note, the other commercially available long-acting insulin analogue, detemir, displays a decreased affinity for IGF-1 compared with native human insulin, and hence does not possess increased mitogenicity in vitro.[132,134] However, a recent meta-analysis of data from randomized controlled trials on insulin detemir suggests that this analogue is associated with a lower or comparable cancer risk compared with NPH or glargine, respectively.[148]

Taken together, the evidence that long-acting insulin analogues promote cancer is limited. Indeed, this potential association may be confounded by the fact that diabetes and cancer share similar risk factors (eg, age, obesity) and comparable pathophysiologic mechanisms (eg, hyperinsulinemia, hyperglycemia, inflammation).[130,149] A consensus report by members of the American Diabetes Society and the American Cancer Society has recently been published on this subject.[149] In essence, further studies are warranted to establish the mitogenic potential and long-term safety of insulin analogues, so at present cancer risk should generally not be a major determinant when choosing appropriate therapeutic options for patients with diabetes.[149]

Insulin Analogues in Pregnancy

Owing to concerns of adverse side effects, including potential teratogenicity, embryo toxicity, immunogenicity with transplancental transfer, and mitogenicity, the use of insulin analogues for the management of hyperglycemia in pregnancy was initially limited.[150] Subsequent studies have shown that in addition to conventional human insulin preparations, the therapeutic use of rapid-acting insulin analogues lispro and aspart in pregnancy is safe and clinically efficacious, with no adverse maternal or fetal consequences reported.[151–155] To date, there are no published reports on insulin glulisine in pregnancy. Moreover, the safety of long-acting insulins glargine and detemir have not yet been extensively studied in this patient population and thus are not currently approved for use in pregnancy.[150,156–161]

FUTURE PERSPECTIVES

To optimize glycemic control in patients with type 1 or 2 diabetes and thus prevent the development and progression of long-term complications, insulin replacement and supplementation strategies must aim to replicate physiologic insulin excursions. To this end, 2 main approaches have evolved over the past 85 years to modify the kinetics of injectable exogenous insulin products: manipulation of the pharmaceutical formulation (eg, addition of zinc, protamine) and/or alteration of the insulin molecule itself (ie, the insulin analogues). However, as current exogenous insulin preparations are not ideal, several novel rapid-acting and long-acting insulin formulations are presently under development, which may broaden the therapeutic options for the management of patients with diabetes in the near future (**Table 3**).

Novel Insulin Formulations

In an effort to attain optimal postprandial glycemic targets, 2 novel ultra–rapid-acting insulin preparations, insulin-PH20 and Linjeta (formally VIAject), are currently under development in phase II and III trials, respectively. The insulin-PH20 (Halozyme Therapeutics, San Diego, CA) formulation contains one of the commercially available mealtime insulin products mixed with recombinant human hyaluronidase (rHuPH20). A recent phase I study revealed that coadministration of insulin (either regular human insulin or insulin lispro) with rHuPH20 results in faster absorption of insulin into the circulation, accelerated pharmacokinetic and glucodynamic effects, and decreased intersubject and intrasubject variability of metabolic activity compared with each insulin formulation alone.[162,163] Linjeta (Biodel Inc, Danbury, CT; www.biodel.com) is another unique insulin formulation comprising regular human insulin with ethylenediaminetetra-acetic acid and citric acid. The latter additives act to chelate zinc ions and prevent self-aggregation of insulin molecules into hexamers on injection into the subcutaneous tissue, thus maintaining insulin in a monomeric state. As anticipated, Linjeta displays a faster onset of action and peak effect, with reduced intraindividual variability of metabolic action compared with regular human insulin and/or insulin lispro in healthy subjects and patients with type 1 diabetes.[164–166]

With respect to basal insulin supplementation, 2 novel and potentially improved formulations of insulin glargine are currently in the pharmaceutical pipeline: LY2963016 (Eli Lilly, Indianapolis, IN) and BIOD-Adjustable Basal (Biodel). The latter is an altered preparation of glargine with a prolonged duration of action that can be premixed with other insulin products.[167,168] A new basal insulin formulation by Sanofi-Aventis (Bridgewater, NJ; www.sanofi.com) is also under development. Moreover, insulin lispro protamine, the basal component of several premixed insulin analogue preparations, is being investigated as a stand-alone basal insulin analogue in patients with type 1 and 2 diabetes.[169,170]

Another novel approach to delay insulin absorption involves chemically coupling the insulin molecule to poly(ethylene glycol) (PEG).[171] A PEGylated form of insulin lispro,

Table 3
Novel insulin preparations in development

Insulin	Manufacturer	Description	Phase
I. Rapid-acting			
Novel formulations			
Insulin-PH20	Halozyme Therapeutics	Prandial insulin products mixed with recombinant human hyaluronidase	Phase II
Linjeta	Biodel	Regular human insulin mixed with EDTA and citric acid	Phase III
II. Long-acting			
Novel formulations			
LY2963016	Eli Lilly	Novel preparation of insulin glargine	Phase III
BIOD-Adjustable Basal	Biodel	Novel preparation of insulin glargine	Phase I
Insulin lispro protamine	Eli Lilly	Protaminated form of insulin lispro	—
PEGylated insulin lispro	Eli Lilly	Insulin lispro linked to poly(ethylene glycol)	Phase III
FT-105	Flamel Technologies Inc	Insulin attached to polymer (polyglutamate peptide backbone linked to vitamin E molecules)	Phase I
"Smart" insulins SmartInsulin BIOD-Smart Basal	SmartCells Inc Biodel	Glucose-responsive insulin preparations	Preclinical
Novel analogues			
Degludec (IDeg)	Novo Nordisk	Two modifications of native insulin β chain: deletion of B30-threonine and addition of a 16-carbon fatty diacid B29-lysine	Phase III complete
LY2605541	Eli Lilly	No description given	Phase II

Abbreviation: EDTA, ethylenediaminetetra-acetic acid.

with a flatter, extended duration of action, has been developed by Eli Lilly and is currently entering phase III trials.

A unique ultra–long-acting basal insulin product, FT-105, is under development by Flamel Technologies Inc (Washington, DC; www.flamel.com). In this formulation, insulin is noncovalently bound to a polymer consisting of a polyglutamate peptide backbone linked to vitamin E molecule within a hydrogel,[172] which forms a depot of dense microparticles following subcutaneous injection, leading to the slow release of insulin molecules into the bloodstream. Preliminary results from a phase I clinical study indicate that FT-105 exhibits a prolonged duration of action, up to 48 hours, decreased intrasubject variability, and reduced hypoglycemic episodes when compared with insulin glargine (www.flamel.com).

Lastly, 2 unique glucose-responsive injectable "smart" insulin preparations that release insulin in proportion to ambient subcutaneous glucose levels are currently undergoing preclinical evaluation. SmartInsulin, a polymer developed by SmartCells Inc (Beverly, MA; www.smartinsulin.com), is composed of insulin reversibly bound to a glucose-binding molecule. Insulin is released from the SmartInsulin polymer in the presence of glucose, which competes with insulin for the binding sites on the glucose-binding molecule.[167] Another promising insulin preparation is BIOD-Smart-Basal, a formulation developed by Biodel that contains insulin glargine, glucose oxidase, and peroxidase. In the presence of glucose, glucose oxidase and peroxidase react to form gluconic acid, which lowers the pH and increases the solubility of insulin glargine, thereby promoting its release into the circulation.[168] Owing to their novel glucose-responsive mechanism, the smart insulin products may theoretically result in tighter glycemic control and a lower risk of both hypoglycemia and hyperglycemia compared with current insulin formulations.

Novel Insulin Analogues

The molecular structure of human insulin has been gradually refined over the past 2 decades, yielding several unique rapid-acting and long-acting insulin analogues with pharmacokinetic properties that closely imitate endogenous insulin profiles. The most promising novel analogue currently in clinical development is insulin degludec (IDeg; Novo Nordisk, Bagsvaerd, Denmark), an ultra–long-acting, basal insulin preparation. This analogue was generated through modification of the native insulin β chain at 2 locations: deletion of threonine at position B30 and addition of a 16-carbon fatty diacid to the lysine residue at position B29 via a glutamic acid spacer (see **Fig. 2**C). As a consequence, insulin degludec is able to self-aggregate and form large multihexamer complexes upon injection in subcutaneous tissues, which subsequently slowly dissociate into monomers that enter the circulation.[173] The result is a protracted action profile longer than 24 hours in duration.

Phase II clinical trials comparing once-daily insulin degludec to glargine indicate that both basal insulins provide comparable degrees of glycemic control; however, degludec is associated with lower rates of hypoglycemia in patients with type 1 diabetes[174] and superior postprandial glucose control compared with glargine in those with type 2 diabetes.[175] Another phase II proof-of-concept trial by Zinman and colleagues[176] reveals that insulin degludec, administered 3 times a week, results in similar glycemic control but no benefit with respect to hypoglycemia risk compared with insulin glargine, when injected once daily in insulin-naïve patients with type 2 diabetes. Degludec has also been studied in a premixed formulation with insulin aspart, denoted IDegAsp or Degludec Plus.[175] At present, phase III clinical trials evaluating the safety and efficacy of insulin degludec in type 1 and 2 diabetes have been completed, with publication of the final data pending.[168]

An additional novel candidate basal insulin analogue, LY2605541, developed by Eli Lilly, is presently undergoing phase II trials.

SUMMARY

The last 90 years have witnessed tremendous progress in insulin therapy, from the initial crude, yet life-saving, animal insulin extracts to novel human insulin analogues. Although the complete physiologic replacement of insulin is inherently difficult to achieve with open-loop subcutaneously administered insulin, the continued development of improved injectable insulin formulations with superior pharmacokinetics and pharmacodynamics will enhance glucose control, and represents important clinical advances in the treatment of both type 1 and type 2 diabetes.

REFERENCES

1. Von Mering J, Minkowski O. Diabetes mellitus nach pankreasexstirpation. Archiv für experimentelle Pathologie und Pharmakologie 1890;26:371–87 [in German].
2. Opie EL. The relation of diabetes mellitus to lesions of the pancreas. Hyaline degeneration of the islands of Langerhans. J Exp Med 1901;5:527–40.
3. Ssobolew LW. Zur normalen und pathologischen Morphologie der inneren Secretion der Bauchspeicheldrüse. Archiv für pathologische und anatomie und physiologie und für klinische medizine 1902;168:91–128 [in German].
4. Sharpey-Schäfer EA. An introduction to the Study of the endocrine glands and internal secretions: lane medical lectures, 1913. Palo Alto (CA): Stanford University; 1914.
5. Zuelzer G. Ueber versuche einer specifischen fermenttherapie des diabetes. Zeitschrift für experimentelle pathologie und therapie 1908;5:307–18 [in German].
6. Scott EL. On the influence of intravenous injections of an extract of the pancreas on experimental pancreatic diabetes. Am J Physiol 1912;29:306–10.
7. Kleiner IS. The action of intravenous injections of pancreas emulsions in experimental diabetes. J Biol Chem 1919;40:153–70.
8. Murlin JR, Kramer B. The influence of pancreatic and duodenal extracts on the glycosuria and the respiratory metabolism of depancreatized dogs. J Biol Chem 1913;15:365–83.
9. Paulesco NC. Action de l'extrait pancréatique injecté dans le sang, chez un animal diabétique. Comptes rendus des séances de la Société de biologie 1921;85:555–9 [in French].
10. Barron M. The relation of the islets of Langerhans to diabetes with special reference to cases of pancreatic lithiasis. Surg Gynecol Obstet 1920;31:437–48.
11. Banting FG. The history of insulin. Edinb Med J 1929;36:1–18.
12. Banting FG, Best CH. The internal secretion of the pancreas. J Lab Clin Med 1922;7:251–66.
13. Banting FG, Best CH, Collip JB, et al. Pancreatic extracts in the treatment of diabetes mellitus. Can Med Assoc J 1922;12:141–6.
14. Hagedorn HC, Jensen BN, Krarup NB, et al. Protamine insulinate. JAMA 1936;106:177–80.
15. Scott DA, Fisher AM. Studies on insulin with protamine. J Pharmacol Exp Therapeut 1936;58:78–92.
16. Himsworth HP. Protamine insulin and zinc protamine insulin. Br Med J 1937;1:541–6.
17. Krayenbuhl C, Rosenberg T. Crystalline protamine insulin. Rep Steno Mem Hosp Nord Insulinlab 1946;1:60–73.
18. Hallas-Moller K. The lente insulins. Diabetes 1956;5:7–14.
19. Oakley W, Hill D, Oakley N. Combined use of regular and crystalline protamine (NPH) insulins in the treatment of severe diabetes. Diabetes 1966;15:219–22.
20. Sanger F. Chemistry of insulin; determination of the structure of insulin opens the way to greater understanding of life processes. Science 1959;129:1340–4.
21. Markussen J, Damgaard U, Jorgensen KH, et al. Human monocomponent insulin. Chemistry and characteristics. Acta Med Scand Suppl 1983;671:99–105.

22. Meienhofer J, Schnabel E, Bremer H, et al. Synthesis of insulin chains and their combination to insulin-active preparations. Z Naturforsch B 1963;18:1120–1 [in German].
23. Kung YT, Du YC, Huang WT, et al. Total synthesis of crystalline insulin. Sci Sin 1966;15:544–61.
24. Katsoyannis PG, Tometsko A, Zalut C. Insulin peptides. XII. Human insulin generation by combination of synthetic A and B chains. J Am Chem Soc 1966;88:166–7.
25. Morihara K, Oka T, Tsuzuki H. Semi-synthesis of human insulin by trypsin-catalysed replacement of Ala-B30 by Thr in porcine insulin. Nature 1979;280:412–3.
26. Markussen J, Damgaard U, Pingel M, et al. Human insulin (Novo): chemistry and characteristics. Diabetes Care 1983;6(Suppl 1):4–8.
27. Teuscher A. The biological effect of purely synthetic human insulin in patients with diabetes mellitus. Schweiz Med Wochenschr 1979;109:743–7 [in German].
28. Keen H, Glynne A, Pickup JC, et al. Human insulin produced by recombinant DNA technology: safety and hypoglycaemic potency in healthy men. Lancet 1980;2:398–401.
29. Owens DR, Zinman B, Bolli GB. Insulins today and beyond. Lancet 2001;358: 739–46.
30. Hirsch IB. Insulin analogues. N Engl J Med 2005;352:174–83.
31. Owens DR, Zinman B, Bolli G. Alternative routes of insulin delivery. Diabet Med 2003;20:886–98.
32. Pickup JC, Keen H, Parsons JA, et al. Continuous subcutaneous insulin infusion: an approach to achieving normoglycaemia. Br Med J 1978;1:204–7.
33. Pickup J, Keen H. Continuous subcutaneous insulin infusion at 25 years: evidence base for the expanding use of insulin pump therapy in type 1 diabetes. Diabetes Care 2002;25:593–8.
34. Waldron-Lynch F, Herold KC. Continuous glucose monitoring: long live the revolution! Nat Clin Pract Endocrinol Metab 2009;5:82–3.
35. Hovorka R. Closed-loop insulin delivery: from bench to clinical practice. Nat Rev Endocrinol 2011;7:385–95.
36. Rojdmark S, Bloom G, Chou MC, et al. Hepatic extraction of exogenous insulin and glucagon in the dog. Endocrinology 1978;102:806–13.
37. Zinman B. The physiologic replacement of insulin. An elusive goal. N Engl J Med 1989;321:363–70.
38. Wild S, Roglic G, Green A, et al. Global prevalence of diabetes: estimates for the year 2000 and projections for 2030. Diabetes Care 2004;27:1047–53.
39. Zimmet P, Alberti KG, Shaw J. Global and societal implications of the diabetes epidemic. Nature 2001;414:782–7.
40. The effect of intensive treatment of diabetes on the development and progression of long-term complications in insulin-dependent diabetes mellitus. The Diabetes Control and Complications Trial Research Group. N Engl J Med 1993;329: 977–86.
41. Intensive blood-glucose control with sulphonylureas or insulin compared with conventional treatment and risk of complications in patients with type 2 diabetes (UKPDS 33). UK Prospective Diabetes Study (UKPDS) Group. Lancet 1998;352: 837–53.
42. Ohkubo Y, Kishikawa H, Araki E, et al. Intensive insulin therapy prevents the progression of diabetic microvascular complications in Japanese patients with non-insulin-dependent diabetes mellitus: a randomized prospective 6-year study. Diabetes Res Clin Pract 1995;28:103–17.

43. Retinopathy and nephropathy in patients with type 1 diabetes four years after a trial of intensive therapy. The Diabetes Control and Complications Trial/Epidemiology of Diabetes Interventions and Complications Research Group. N Engl J Med 2000;342:381–9.

44. Sustained effect of intensive treatment of type 1 diabetes mellitus on development and progression of diabetic nephropathy: the Epidemiology of Diabetes Interventions and Complications (EDIC) study. JAMA 2003;290:2159–67.

45. Nathan DM, Lachin J, Cleary P, et al. Intensive diabetes therapy and carotid intima-media thickness in type 1 diabetes mellitus. N Engl J Med 2003;348: 2294–303.

46. Patel A, MacMahon S, Chalmers J, et al. Intensive blood glucose control and vascular outcomes in patients with type 2 diabetes. N Engl J Med 2008;358: 2560–72.

47. Nathan DM, Cleary PA, Backlund JY, et al. Intensive diabetes treatment and cardiovascular disease in patients with type 1 diabetes. N Engl J Med 2005; 353:2643–53.

48. Stratton IM, Adler AI, Neil HA, et al. Association of glycaemia with macrovascular and microvascular complications of type 2 diabetes (UKPDS 35): prospective observational study. BMJ 2000;321:405–12.

49. Standl E, Balletshofer B, Dahl B, et al. Predictors of 10-year macrovascular and overall mortality in patients with NIDDM: the Munich General Practitioner Project. Diabetologia 1996;39:1540–5.

50. Hypoglycemia in the Diabetes Control and Complications Trial. The Diabetes Control and Complications Trial Research Group. Diabetes 1997;46:271–86.

51. Binder C, Lauritzen T, Faber O, et al. Insulin pharmacokinetics. Diabetes Care 1984;7:188–99.

52. Kang S, Brange J, Burch A, et al. Subcutaneous insulin absorption explained by insulin's physicochemical properties. Evidence from absorption studies of soluble human insulin and insulin analogues in humans. Diabetes Care 1991; 14:942–8.

53. Heinemann L, Richter B. Clinical pharmacology of human insulin. Diabetes Care 1993;16(Suppl 3):90–100.

54. Cryer PE. Banting lecture. Hypoglycemia: the limiting factor in the management of IDDM. Diabetes 1994;43:1378–89.

55. Starke AA, Heinemann L, Hohmann A, et al. The action profiles of human NPH insulin preparations. Diabet Med 1989;6:239–44.

56. Peterson GE. Intermediate and long-acting insulins: a review of NPH insulin, insulin glargine and insulin detemir. Curr Med Res Opin 2006;22:2613–9.

57. Bolli GB. The pharmacokinetic basis of insulin therapy in diabetes mellitus. Diabetes Res Clin Pract 1989;6:S3–15 [discussion: S15–6].

58. Lepore M, Pampanelli S, Fanelli C, et al. Pharmacokinetics and pharmacodynamics of subcutaneous injection of long-acting human insulin analog glargine, NPH insulin, and ultralente human insulin and continuous subcutaneous infusion of insulin lispro. Diabetes 2000;49:2142–8.

59. Jehle PM, Micheler C, Jehle DR, et al. Inadequate suspension of neutral protamine Hagendorn (NPH) insulin in pens. Lancet 1999;354:1604–7.

60. Mooradian AD, Bernbaum M, Albert SG. Narrative review: a rational approach to starting insulin therapy. Ann Intern Med 2006;145:125–34.

61. Holleman F, Hoekstra JB. Insulin lispro. N Engl J Med 1997;337:176–83.

62. Brems DN, Alter LA, Beckage MJ, et al. Altering the association properties of insulin by amino acid replacement. Protein Eng 1992;5:527–33.

63. Brange J, Owens DR, Kang S, et al. Monomeric insulins and their experimental and clinical implications. Diabetes Care 1990;13:923–54.

64. Mudaliar SR, Lindberg FA, Joyce M, et al. Insulin aspart (B28 asp-insulin): a fast-acting analog of human insulin: absorption kinetics and action profile compared with regular human insulin in healthy nondiabetic subjects. Diabetes Care 1999;22:1501–6.

65. Barlocco D. Insulin glulisine. Aventis pharma. Curr Opin Investig Drugs 2003;4: 1240–4.

66. Becker RH, Frick AD. Clinical pharmacokinetics and pharmacodynamics of insulin glulisine. Clin Pharmacokinet 2008;47:7–20.

67. Danne T, Becker RH, Heise T, et al. Pharmacokinetics, prandial glucose control, and safety of insulin glulisine in children and adolescents with type 1 diabetes. Diabetes Care 2005;28:2100–5.

68. Homko C, Deluzio A, Jimenez C, et al. Comparison of insulin aspart and lispro: pharmacokinetic and metabolic effects. Diabetes Care 2003;26:2027–31.

69. Becker RH, Frick AD, Burger F, et al. Insulin glulisine, a new rapid-acting insulin analogue, displays a rapid time-action profile in obese non-diabetic subjects. Exp Clin Endocrinol Diabetes 2005;113:435–43.

70. ter Braak EW, Woodworth JR, Bianchi R, et al. Injection site effects on the pharmacokinetics and glucodynamics of insulin lispro and regular insulin. Diabetes Care 1996;19:1437–40.

71. Anderson JH Jr, Brunelle RL, Koivisto VA, et al. Reduction of postprandial hyperglycemia and frequency of hypoglycemia in IDDM patients on insulin-analog treatment. Multicenter Insulin Lispro Study Group. Diabetes 1997;46:265–70.

72. Del Sindaco P, Ciofetta M, Lalli C, et al. Use of the short-acting insulin analogue lispro in intensive treatment of type 1 diabetes mellitus: importance of appropriate replacement of basal insulin and time-interval injection-meal. Diabet Med 1998;15:592–600.

73. Brange J, Volund A. Insulin analogs with improved pharmacokinetic profiles. Adv Drug Deliv Rev 1999;35:307–35.

74. Brunelle BL, Llewelyn J, Anderson JH Jr, et al. Meta-analysis of the effect of insulin lispro on severe hypoglycemia in patients with type 1 diabetes. Diabetes Care 1998;21:1726–31.

75. Home PD, Lindholm A, Hylleberg B, et al. Improved glycemic control with insulin aspart: a multicenter randomized double-blind crossover trial in type 1 diabetic patients. UK Insulin Aspart Study Group. Diabetes Care 1998;21:1904–9.

76. Hermansen K, Fontaine P, Kukolja KK, et al. Insulin analogues (insulin detemir and insulin aspart) versus traditional human insulins (NPH insulin and regular human insulin) in basal-bolus therapy for patients with type 1 diabetes. Diabetologia 2004;47:622–9.

77. Raskin P, Guthrie RA, Leiter L, et al. Use of insulin aspart, a fast-acting insulin analog, as the mealtime insulin in the management of patients with type 1 diabetes. Diabetes Care 2000;23:583–8.

78. Gough SC. A review of human and analogue insulin trials. Diabetes Res Clin Pract 2007;77:1–15.

79. Plank J, Siebenhofer A, Berghold A, et al. Systematic review and meta-analysis of short-acting insulin analogues in patients with diabetes mellitus. Arch Intern Med 2005;165:1337–44.

80. Rave K, Klein O, Frick AD, et al. Advantage of premeal-injected insulin glulisine compared with regular human insulin in subjects with type 1 diabetes. Diabetes Care 2006;29:1812–7.

81. Siebenhofer A, Plank J, Berghold A, et al. Short acting insulin analogues versus regular human insulin in patients with diabetes mellitus. Cochrane Database Syst Rev 2006;2:CD003287.
82. Kotsanos JG, Vignati L, Huster W, et al. Health-related quality-of-life results from multinational clinical trials of insulin lispro. Assessing benefits of a new diabetes therapy. Diabetes Care 1997;20:948–58.
83. Kamoi K, Miyakoshi M, Maruyama R. A quality-of-life assessment of intensive insulin therapy using insulin lispro switched from short-acting insulin and measured by an ITR-QOL questionnaire: a prospective comparison of multiple daily insulin injections and continuous subcutaneous insulin infusion. Diabetes Res Clin Pract 2004;64:19–25.
84. Grey M, Boland EA, Tamborlane WV. Use of lispro insulin and quality of life in adolescents on intensive therapy. Diabetes Educ 1999;25:934–41.
85. Bott U, Ebrahim S, Hirschberger S, et al. Effect of the rapid-acting insulin analogue insulin aspart on quality of life and treatment satisfaction in patients with Type 1 diabetes. Diabet Med 2003;20:626–34.
86. Miles HL, Acerini CL. Insulin analog preparations and their use in children and adolescents with type 1 diabetes mellitus. Paediatr Drugs 2008;10:163–76.
87. Bolli GB, Di Marchi RD, Park GD, et al. Insulin analogues and their potential in the management of diabetes mellitus. Diabetologia 1999;42:1151–67.
88. Bolli GB, Owens DR. Insulin glargine. Lancet 2000;356:443–5.
89. Buse J. Insulin glargine (HOE901): first responsibilities: understanding the data and ensuring safety. Diabetes Care 2000;23:576–8.
90. Barlocco D. Insulin detemir. Novo Nordisk. Curr Opin Investig Drugs 2003;4: 449–54.
91. Havelund S, Plum A, Ribel U, et al. The mechanism of protraction of insulin detemir, a long-acting, acylated analog of human insulin. Pharm Res 2004;21: 1498–504.
92. Kurtzhals P, Havelund S, Jonassen I, et al. Albumin binding of insulins acylated with fatty acids: characterization of the ligand-protein interaction and correlation between binding affinity and timing of the insulin effect in vivo. Biochem J 1995;312(Pt 3):725–31.
93. Markussen J, Havelund S, Kurtzhals P, et al. Soluble, fatty acid acylated insulins bind to albumin and show protracted action in pigs. Diabetologia 1996;39: 281–8.
94. Heise T, Pieber TR. Towards peakless, reproducible and long-acting insulins. An assessment of the basal analogues based on isoglycaemic clamp studies. Diabetes Obes Metab 2007;9:648–59.
95. Plank J, Bodenlenz M, Sinner F, et al. A double-blind, randomized, dose-response study investigating the pharmacodynamic and pharmacokinetic properties of the long-acting insulin analog detemir. Diabetes Care 2005;28: 1107–12.
96. Heinemann L, Linkeschova R, Rave K, et al. Time-action profile of the long-acting insulin analog insulin glargine (HOE901) in comparison with those of NPH insulin and placebo. Diabetes Care 2000;23:644–9.
97. Klein O, Lynge J, Endahl L, et al. Albumin-bound basal insulin analogues (insulin detemir and NN344): comparable time-action profiles but less variability than insulin glargine in type 2 diabetes. Diabetes Obes Metab 2007;9:290–9.
98. Heinemann L, Sinha K, Weyer C, et al. Time-action profile of the soluble, fatty acid acylated, long-acting insulin analogue NN304. Diabet Med 1999;16: 332–8.

99. Heise T, Nosek L, Rønn BB, et al. Lower within-subject variability of insulin detemir in comparison to NPH insulin and insulin glargine in people with type 1 diabetes. Diabetes 2004;53:1614–20.
100. Owens DR, Coates PA, Luzio SD, et al. Pharmacokinetics of 125I-labeled insulin glargine (HOE 901) in healthy men: comparison with NPH insulin and the influence of different subcutaneous injection sites. Diabetes Care 2000;23:813–9.
101. Ratner RE, Hirsch IB, Neifing JL, et al. Less hypoglycemia with insulin glargine in intensive insulin therapy for type 1 diabetes. U.S. Study Group of Insulin Glargine in Type 1 Diabetes. Diabetes Care 2000;23:639–43.
102. Riddle MC, Rosenstock J, Gerich J. The treat-to-target trial: randomized addition of glargine or human NPH insulin to oral therapy of type 2 diabetic patients. Diabetes Care 2003;26:3080–6.
103. Home P, Kurtzhals P. Insulin detemir: from concept to clinical experience. Expert Opin Pharmacother 2006;7:325–43.
104. Kølendorf K, Ross GP, Pavlic-Renar I, et al. Insulin detemir lowers the risk of hypoglycaemia and provides more consistent plasma glucose levels compared with NPH insulin in Type 1 diabetes. Diabet Med 2006;23:729–35.
105. Philis-Tsimikas A, Charpentier G, Clauson P, et al. Comparison of once-daily insulin detemir with NPH insulin added to a regimen of oral antidiabetic drugs in poorly controlled type 2 diabetes. Clin Ther 2006;28:1569–81.
106. Robertson KJ, Schoenle E, Gucev Z, et al. Insulin detemir compared with NPH insulin in children and adolescents with Type 1 diabetes. Diabet Med 2007;24: 27–34.
107. Bartley PC, Bogoev M, Larsen J, et al. Long-term efficacy and safety of insulin detemir compared to neutral protamine Hagedorn insulin in patients with type 1 diabetes using a treat-to-target basal-bolus regimen with insulin aspart at meals: a 2-year, randomized, controlled trial. Diabet Med 2008; 25:442–9.
108. Blonde L, Merilainen M, Karwe V, et al. Patient-directed titration for achieving glycaemic goals using a once-daily basal insulin analogue: an assessment of two different fasting plasma glucose targets - the TITRATE study. Diabetes Obes Metab 2009;11:623–31.
109. Garg S, Moser E, Dain MP, et al. Clinical experience with insulin glargine in type 1 diabetes. Diabetes Technol Ther 2010;12:835–46.
110. Horvath K, Jeitler K, Berghold A, et al. Long-acting insulin analogues versus NPH insulin (human isophane insulin) for type 2 diabetes mellitus. Cochrane Database Syst Rev 2007;2:CD005613.
111. Abrahamson MJ. Basal insulins: pharmacological properties and patient perspectives. Prim Care Diabetes 2010;4(Suppl 1):S19–23.
112. Murphy NP, Keane SM, Ong KK, et al. Randomized cross-over trial of insulin glargine plus lispro or NPH insulin plus regular human insulin in adolescents with type 1 diabetes on intensive insulin regimens. Diabetes Care 2003;26: 799–804.
113. Ashwell SG, Amiel SA, Bilous RW, et al. Improved glycaemic control with insulin glargine plus insulin lispro: a multicentre, randomized, cross-over trial in people with type 1 diabetes. Diabet Med 2006;23:285–92.
114. Raslová K, Bogoev M, Raz I, et al. Insulin detemir and insulin aspart: a promising basal-bolus regimen for type 2 diabetes. Diabetes Res Clin Pract 2004;66: 193–201.
115. Hermansen K, Davies M, Derezinski T, et al. A 26-week, randomized, parallel, treat-to-target trial comparing insulin detemir with NPH insulin as add-on

therapy to oral glucose-lowering drugs in insulin-naive people with type 2 diabetes. Diabetes Care 2006;29:1269-74.

116. Rosenstock J, Davies M, Home PD, et al. A randomised, 52-week, treat-to-target trial comparing insulin detemir with insulin glargine when administered as add-on to glucose-lowering drugs in insulin-naive people with type 2 diabetes. Diabetologia 2008;51:408-16.

117. Swinnen SG, Dain MP, Aronson R, et al. A 24-week, randomized, treat-to-target trial comparing initiation of insulin glargine once-daily with insulin detemir twice-daily in patients with type 2 diabetes inadequately controlled on oral glucose-lowering drugs. Diabetes Care 2010;33:1176-8.

118. DeWitt DE, Hirsch IB. Outpatient insulin therapy in type 1 and type 2 diabetes mellitus: scientific review. JAMA 2003;289:2254-64.

119. Yamada S, Watanabe M, Kitaoka A, et al. Switching from premixed human insulin to premixed insulin lispro: a prospective study comparing the effects on glucose control and quality of life. Intern Med 2007;46:1513-7.

120. Roach P, Yue L, Arora V. Improved postprandial glycemic control during treatment with Humalog Mix25, a novel protamine-based insulin lispro formulation. Humalog Mix25 Study Group. Diabetes Care 1999;22:1258-61.

121. Koivisto VA, Tuominen JA, Ebeling P. Lispro Mix25 insulin as premeal therapy in type 2 diabetic patients. Diabetes Care 1999;22:459-62.

122. Malone JK, Woodworth JR, Arora V, et al. Improved postprandial glycemic control with Humalog Mix75/25 after a standard test meal in patients with type 2 diabetes mellitus. Clin Ther 2000;22:222-30.

123. Kilo C, Mezitis N, Jain R, et al. Starting patients with type 2 diabetes on insulin therapy using once-daily injections of biphasic insulin aspart 70/30, biphasic human insulin 70/30, or NPH insulin in combination with metformin. J Diabet Complications 2003;17:307-13.

124. Mortensen H, Kocova M, Teng LY, et al. Biphasic insulin aspart vs. human insulin in adolescents with type 1 diabetes on multiple daily insulin injections. Pediatr Diabetes 2006;7:4-10.

125. Boehm BO, Home PD, Behrend C, et al. Premixed insulin aspart 30 vs. premixed human insulin 30/70 twice daily: a randomized trial in Type 1 and Type 2 diabetic patients. Diabet Med 2002;19:393-9.

126. Coscelli C, Calabrese G, Fedele D, et al. Use of premixed insulin among the elderly. Reduction of errors in patient preparation of mixtures. Diabetes Care 1992;15:1628-30.

127. Slieker LJ, Brooke GS, DiMarchi RD, et al. Modifications in the B10 and B26-30 regions of the B chain of human insulin alter affinity for the human IGF-I receptor more than for the insulin receptor. Diabetologia 1997;40(Suppl 2): S54-61.

128. Werner H, Weinstein D, Bentov I. Similarities and differences between insulin and IGF-I: structures, receptors, and signalling pathways. Arch Physiol Biochem 2008;114:17-22.

129. Yehezkel E, Weinstein D, Simon M, et al. Long-acting insulin analogues elicit atypical signalling events mediated by the insulin receptor and insulin-like growth factor-I receptor. Diabetologia 2010;53:2667-75.

130. Gerstein HC. Does insulin therapy promote, reduce, or have a neutral effect on cancers? JAMA 2010;303:446-7.

131. Hansen BF, Danielsen GM, Drejer K, et al. Sustained signalling from the insulin receptor after stimulation with insulin analogues exhibiting increased mitogenic potency. Biochem J 1996;315(Pt 1):271-9.

132. Kurtzhals P, Schäffer L, Sørensen A, et al. Correlations of receptor binding and metabolic and mitogenic potencies of insulin analogs designed for clinical use. Diabetes 2000;49:999–1005.

133. Sciacca L, Cassarino MF, Genua M, et al. Insulin analogues differently activate insulin receptor isoforms and post-receptor signalling. Diabetologia 2010;53: 1743–53.

134. Shukla A, Grisouard J, Ehemann V, et al. Analysis of signaling pathways related to cell proliferation stimulated by insulin analogs in human mammary epithelial cell lines. Endocr Relat Cancer 2009;16:429–41.

135. Mayer D, Chantelau E. Treatment with insulin glargine (Lantus) increases the proliferative potency of the serum of patients with type-1 diabetes: a pilot study on MCF-7 breast cancer cells. Arch Physiol Biochem 2010;116:73–8.

136. Staiger K, Hennige AM, Staiger H, et al. Comparison of the mitogenic potency of regular human insulin and its analogue glargine in normal and transformed human breast epithelial cells. Horm Metab Res 2007;39:65–7.

137. Stammberger I, Bube A, Durchfeld-Meyer B, et al. Evaluation of the carcinogenic potential of insulin glargine (LANTUS) in rats and mice. Int J Toxicol 2002;21:171–9.

138. Jonasson JM, Ljung R, Talbäck M, et al. Insulin glargine use and short-term incidence of malignancies—a population-based follow-up study in Sweden. Diabetologia 2009;52:1745–54.

139. Colhoun HM. Use of insulin glargine and cancer incidence in Scotland: a study from the Scottish Diabetes Research Network Epidemiology Group. Diabetologia 2009;52:1755–65.

140. Hemkens LG, Grouven U, Bender R, et al. Risk of malignancies in patients with diabetes treated with human insulin or insulin analogues: a cohort study. Diabetologia 2009;52:1732–44.

141. Mannucci E, Monami M, Balzi D, et al. Doses of insulin and its analogues and cancer occurrence in insulin-treated type 2 diabetic patients. Diabetes Care 2010;33:1997–2003.

142. Pocock SJ, Smeeth L. Insulin glargine and malignancy: an unwarranted alarm. Lancet 2009;374:511–3.

143. Hernandez-Diaz S, Adami HO. Diabetes therapy and cancer risk: causal effects and other plausible explanations. Diabetologia 2010;53:802–8.

144. Rosenstock J, Fonseca V, McGill JB, et al. Similar risk of malignancy with insulin glargine and neutral protamine Hagedorn (NPH) insulin in patients with type 2 diabetes: findings from a 5 year randomised, open-label study. Diabetologia 2009;52:1971–3.

145. Home PD, Lagarenne P. Combined randomised controlled trial experience of malignancies in studies using insulin glargine. Diabetologia 2009;52:2499–506.

146. Currie CJ, Poole CD, Gale EA. The influence of glucose-lowering therapies on cancer risk in type 2 diabetes. Diabetologia 2009;52:1766–77.

147. Suissa S, Azoulay L, Dell'Aniello S, et al. Long-term effects of insulin glargine on the risk of breast cancer. Diabetologia 2011;54:2254–62.

148. Dejgaard A, Lynggaard H, Rastam J, et al. No evidence of increased risk of malignancies in patients with diabetes treated with insulin detemir: a meta-analysis. Diabetologia 2009;52:2507–12.

149. Giovannucci E, Harlan DM, Archer MC, et al. Diabetes and cancer: a consensus report. Diabetes Care 2010;33:1674–85.

150. Lapolla A, Di Cianni G, Bruttomesso D, et al. Use of insulin detemir in pregnancy: a report on 10 type 1 diabetic women. Diabet Med 2009;26:1181–2.

151. Mecacci F, Carignani L, Cioni R, et al. Maternal metabolic control and perinatal outcome in women with gestational diabetes treated with regular or lispro insulin: comparison with non-diabetic pregnant women. Eur J Obstet Gynecol Reprod Biol 2003;111:19–24.
152. Jovanovic L, Ilic S, Pettitt DJ, et al. Metabolic and immunologic effects of insulin lispro in gestational diabetes. Diabetes Care 1999;22:1422–7.
153. Persson B, Swahn ML, Hjertberg R, et al. Insulin lispro therapy in pregnancies complicated by type 1 diabetes mellitus. Diabetes Res Clin Pract 2002;58:115–21.
154. Mathiesen ER, Kinsley B, Amiel SA, et al. Maternal glycemic control and hypoglycemia in type 1 diabetic pregnancy: a randomized trial of insulin aspart versus human insulin in 322 pregnant women. Diabetes Care 2007;30:771–6.
155. Singh SR, Ahmad F, Lal A, et al. Efficacy and safety of insulin analogues for the management of diabetes mellitus: a meta-analysis. CMAJ 2009;180:385–97.
156. Graves DE, White JC, Kirk JK. The use of insulin glargine with gestational diabetes mellitus. Diabetes Care 2006;29:471–2.
157. Price N, Bartlett C, Gillmer M. Use of insulin glargine during pregnancy: a case-control pilot study. BJOG 2007;114:453–7.
158. Gallen IW, Jaap A, Roland JM, et al. Survey of glargine use in 115 pregnant women with type 1 diabetes. Diabet Med 2008;25:165–9.
159. Di Cianni G, Torlone E, Lencioni C, et al. Perinatal outcomes associated with the use of glargine during pregnancy. Diabet Med 2008;25:993–6.
160. Fang YM, MacKeen D, Egan JF, et al. Insulin glargine compared with neutral protamine Hagedorn insulin in the treatment of pregnant diabetics. J Matern Fetal Neonatal Med 2009;22:249–53.
161. Torlone E, Di Cianni G, Mannino D, et al. Insulin analogs and pregnancy: an update. Acta Diabetol 2009;46:163–72.
162. Vaughn DE, Yocum RC, Muchmore DB, et al. Accelerated pharmacokinetics and glucodynamics of prandial insulins injected with recombinant human hyaluronidase. Diabetes Technol Ther 2009;11:345–52.
163. Muchmore DB, Vaughn DE. Review of the mechanism of action and clinical efficacy of recombinant human hyaluronidase coadministration with current prandial insulin formulations. J Diabetes Sci Technol 2010;4:419–28.
164. Steiner S, Hompesch M, Pohl R, et al. A novel insulin formulation with a more rapid onset of action. Diabetologia 2008;51:1602–6.
165. Hompesch M, McManus L, Pohl R, et al. Intra-individual variability of the metabolic effect of a novel rapid-acting insulin (VIAject) in comparison to regular human insulin. J Diabetes Sci Technol 2008;2:568–71.
166. Heinemann L, Nosek L, Flacke F, et al. U-100, pH-Neutral formulation of VIAject((R)): faster onset of action than insulin lispro in patients with type 1 diabetes. Diabetes Obes Metab 2012;14(3):222–7. DOI: 10.1111/j.1463-1326.2011.01516.x. [Epub 2011 Nov 13].
167. Owens DR. Insulin preparations with prolonged effect. Diabetes Technol Ther 2011;13(Suppl 1):S5–14.
168. Simon AC, DeVries JH. The future of basal insulin supplementation. Diabetes Technol Ther 2011;13(Suppl 1):S103–8.
169. Chacra AR, Kipnes M, Ilag LL, et al. Comparison of insulin lispro protamine suspension and insulin detemir in basal-bolus therapy in patients with Type 1 diabetes. Diabet Med 2010;27:563–9.
170. Fogelfeld L, Dharmalingam M, Robling K, et al. A randomized, treat-to-target trial comparing insulin lispro protamine suspension and insulin detemir in insulin-naive patients with Type 2 diabetes. Diabet Med 2010;27:181–8.

171. Hinds KD, Kim SW. Effects of PEG conjugation on insulin properties. Adv Drug Deliv Rev 2002;54:505–30.
172. Chan YP, Meyrueix R, Kravtzoff R, et al. Review on Medusa: a polymer-based sustained release technology for protein and peptide drugs. Expert Opin Drug Deliv 2007;4:441–51.
173. Jonassen I, Havelund S, Ribel U, et al. Insulin degludec is a new generation ultra-long acting basal insulin with a unique mechanism of protraction based on multihexamer formation [abstract]. Diabetes 2010;59:A11.
174. Birkeland KI, Home PD, Wendisch U, et al. Insulin degludec in type 1 diabetes: a randomized controlled trial of a new-generation ultra-long-acting insulin compared with insulin glargine. Diabetes Care 2011;34:661–5.
175. Heise T, Tack CJ, Cuddihy R, et al. A new-generation ultra-long-acting basal insulin with a bolus boost compared with insulin glargine in insulin-naive people with type 2 diabetes: a randomized, controlled trial. Diabetes Care 2011;34: 669–74.
176. Zinman B, Fulcher G, Rao PV, et al. Insulin degludec, an ultra-long-acting basal insulin, once a day or three times a week versus insulin glargine once a day in patients with type 2 diabetes: a 16-week, randomised, open-label, phase 2 trial. Lancet 2011;377:924–31.
177. Canadian Diabetes Association 2008 clinical practice guidelines for the prevention and management of diabetes in Canada. Can J Diabetes 2008;32:S1–201.
178. American Diabetes Association. Standards of medical care in diabetes—2011. Diabetes Care 2011;34(Suppl 1):S11–61.
179. Handelsman Y, Mechanick JI, Blonde L, et al. American Association of Clinical Endocrinologists Medical Guidelines for Clinical Practice for developing a diabetes mellitus comprehensive care plan. Endocr Pract 2011;17(Suppl 2):1–53.
180. Rydén L, Standl E, Bartnik M, et al. Guidelines on diabetes, pre-diabetes, and cardiovascular diseases: executive summary. The Task Force on Diabetes and Cardiovascular Diseases of the European Society of Cardiology (ESC) and of the European Association for the Study of Diabetes (EASD). Eur Heart J 2007;28:88–136.
181. International Diabetes Federation. Guideline for the management of post-meal blood glucose. Diabetes Voice 2007;52:9–11.

Physiology of Glucose Homeostasis and Insulin Therapy in Type 1 and Type 2 Diabetes

Ele Ferrannini, MD

KEYWORDS

• Type 2 diabetes • Type 1 diabetes • Glucose homeostasis
• Insulin therapy

Glucose homeostasis is the maintenance of plasma glucose concentrations within a very narrow band under most circumstances. In normal subjects, plasma glucose oscillations rarely exceed 3 mmol/L (54 mg/dL), whereas lipid substrates, for example, free fatty acids (FFA), can range up to 20-fold between a prolonged fast and the postcibal period. A tightly homeostatic variable, such as eg, tissue perfusion pressure, requires a multiple, redundant set of controls, and a coordinated deployment of primary and subsidiary mechanisms. In the hierarchy, insulin is by far the chief regulating element of plasma glucose in both the short and long time frames. Several other factors play a secondary role, glucagon being next in charge.

A preliminary consideration is the unique organization of the insulin/glucagon system. For many protein and nonprotein hormones, action is modulated by at least 1, and often 2, hierarchical hormonal feedback pathways (eg, corticotropin-releasing hormone and corticotropin for cortisol, gonadotropin-releasing hormone and gonadotropins for sex steroids). In these cases sensitivity is provided by the circulating hormone concentrations, which act on specific receptors located on target tissues as well as on the master gland of the feedback loop (eg, the pituitary). In the case of insulin and glucagon, there is no pituitary or hypothalamic relay; target tissues control secretion directly. Thus, the circulating concentrations of substrates (mostly glucose but also amino acids, FFA, and ketone bodies), which result from insulin action on intermediary metabolism in different tissues, feed signals back to the β-cell and the α-cell. Sensitivity gating is provided by insulin and glucagon receptors on target tissues.

The author has nothing to disclose.
Department of Internal Medicine, University of Pisa School of Medicine, Via Roma 67, 56100 Pisa, Italy
E-mail address: ferranni@ifc.cnr.it

Endocrinol Metab Clin N Am 41 (2012) 25–39
doi:10.1016/j.ecl.2012.01.003
0889-8529/12/$ – see front matter © 2012 Elsevier Inc. All rights reserved.
endo.theclinics.com

An additional level of regulation is autocrine/paracrine in nature, that is, insulin receptors on the β-cell and α-cell, respectively. β-Cells are richly endowed with insulin receptors and their intracellular signaling machinery. Historically, insulin has been thought to exert a negative feedback on β-cells. However, more recent in vitro and animal data provide evidence for a positive role of insulin in transcription, translation, ion flux, insulin secretion, proliferation, and β-cell survival (see Ref.[1] for a comprehensive review). In healthy nondiabetic subjects, both insulin exposure and insulin sensitivity modulate the β-cell secretory response under normoglycemic conditions.[2] Thus, a higher degree of preinsulinization and better insulin sensitivity translate into a stimulatory action of insulin on its own secretion, whereas insulin resistance and antecedent relative hypoinsulinemia determine an inhibitory effect of insulin on β-cell secretion. Likewise, under hyperglycemic conditions a higher degree of antecedent insulin exposure causes a higher endogenous insulin response to glucose stimulation.[3] α-Cells also carry insulin receptors, which transduce an inhibitory action of insulin on glucagon release.[4] This response too is modulated by insulin sensitivity, as fasting glucagon levels are inversely related to insulin sensitivity independently of other factors.[5]

GLUCOSE HOMEOSTASIS: THE FASTING STATE

Glucose control can be simplified to an input-output problem (**Fig. 1**). At any given time, the glucose concentration in the glucose space (which averages 250 mL/kg of body weight, of which 70 mL/kg is the intravascular space) represents the balance

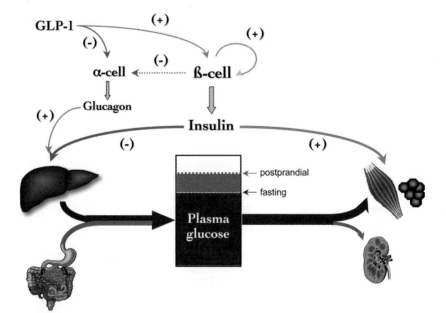

Plasma glucose: primary hormonal control

Fig. 1. Diagram of the primary hormonal control of plasma glucose concentrations organized as an input-output system centered on plasma glucose level. (+) stimulation; (−) inhibition. GLP-1, glucagon-like peptide 1.

between entry of glucose into, and exit from, the circulation via cellular metabolism or excretion: excessive release or defective removal (or combinations of the two) will result in rising glucose levels. After an overnight fast (or in interprandial states), the liver contributes greater than 90% of endogenous glucose release (the remainder being released by the kidney), derived in equal parts from breakdown of glycogen and de novo glucose synthesis from 3-carbon precursors.[6] An endogenous glucose input of 11 μmol/min/kg (extrapolating to 1.1 mmol [= 200 g] per day in a 70-kg adult) maintains a fasting plasma concentration of approximately 5 mmol/L (90 mg/dL) in the glucose space as the same amount of glucose is disposed of by all body tissues. Glucose output is directly related to fat-free mass (FFM), that is, to the mass of metabolically active tissues, indicating that the metabolic need is the main factor driving hepatic glucose release.[7] Independently of FFM, glucose output is also directly related to fasting plasma glucose concentrations even within the nondiabetic range (ie, 4–7 mmol/L) (**Fig. 2**).

The dominant hormonal control of the fasting rate of glucose release is the insulin/glucagon ratio in the prehepatic venous plasma, with insulin inhibiting, and glucagon stimulating, both glycogenolysis and gluconeogenesis (see **Fig. 1**).[8–11] Eighty percent of the blood supply to the liver comes from the portal vein, which carries pancreatic endocrine secretions, while 20% flows from the hepatic artery. Because of this double vascular connection, in parallel to the left heart and in series with the endocrine pancreas, the liver is exposed to higher hormone concentrations than are peripheral tissues.[12] Fasting insulin secretion rates can be calculated from fasting C-peptide concentrations using the deconvolution method.[13] In nondiabetic subjects (with a body mass index [BMI] from lean to very obese), fasting insulin secretion ranges from 50 to 120 pmol/min/m²; extrapolated over 24 hours, basal insulin output ranges from 0.35 to 0.56 U/kg per day. The corresponding fasting plasma insulin concentrations also are progressively higher as a function of the degree of obesity (**Fig. 3**). Assuming a portal plasma flow of 12 L/min/kg, prehepatic insulin concentrations

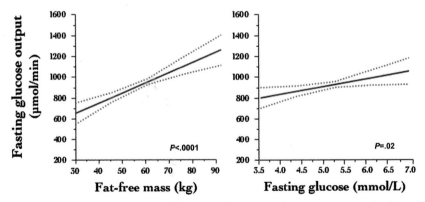

Fig. 2. Simultaneous dependence of fasting endogenous glucose output on fat-free mass and fasting plasma glucose concentrations. The P values refer to the significance of the partial correlation coefficients of the lines of best fit (*blue lines*) and their 95% confidence intervals (*dotted red lines*) from a general linear regression model also adjusting for sex, age, and body mass index. Data (Ferrannini E, unpublished data, 2012) from 330 nondiabetic subjects in the RISC study. (*Data from* Ferrannini E, Balkau B, Coppack SW, et al. RISC Investigators. Insulin resistance, insulin response, and obesity as indicators of metabolic risk. J Clin Endocrinol Metab 2007;92:2885–92.)

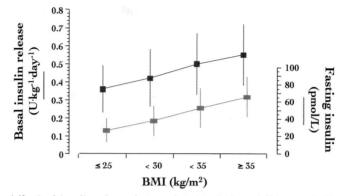

Fig. 3. Basal (fasting) insulin release (extrapolated to 24 hours) (*blue symbols*) and fasting plasma insulin concentrations (*red symbols*) by body mass index (BMI). Data (Ferrannini E, unpublished data, 2012) from 1151 nondiabetic subjects from the RISC Study. Plots are mean ± SD. (*Data from* Ferrannini E, Balkau B, Coppack SW, et al. RISC Investigators. Insulin resistance, insulin response, and obesity as indicators of metabolic risk. J Clin Endocrinol Metab 2007;92:2885–92.)

can be estimated from the insulin secretion rate and the relative contribution of hepatic arterial flow. As shown in **Fig. 4**, in nondiabetic subjects prehepatic insulin levels are 2- to 4-fold higher than peripheral insulin concentrations. This portosystemic gradient is due to insulin being abundantly degraded by the liver, for the most part by receptor-mediated processes; because its first-pass extraction exceeds 50%, in normal subjects approximately 80% of the hormone is eventually metabolized in liver tissues, the remainder being degraded by the kidney.[14]

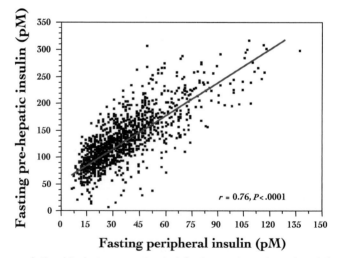

Fig. 4. Linear relationship between estimated fasting prehepatic and peripheral plasma insulin concentrations in the nondiabetic subjects in **Fig. 3**. The r and P values refer to the significance of the line of best fit (*red line*). Data (Ferrannini E, unpublished data, 2012) from 1151 nondiabetic subjects from the RISC Study. (*Data from* Ferrannini E, Balkau B, Coppack SW, et al. RISC Investigators. Insulin resistance, insulin response, and obesity as indicators of metabolic risk. J Clin Endocrinol Metab 2007;92:2885–92.)

In contrast to insulin, glucagon is minimally, if at all, degraded by hepatocytes (most of its catabolism taking place in the kidney); therefore, the portosystemic glucagon gradient is roughly equal to the ratio of portal blood flow to cardiac output.[15] In the nondiabetic cohort in **Fig. 4**, the prehepatic insulin/glucagon ratio has a median value of 5 ng/ng (or a molar ratio of 3). As expected, the higher this ratio, the lower the rate of fasting glucose release (**Fig. 5**). The fact that this relationship is somewhat weak even in a relatively large group of subjects certainly depends on the variability of the measures and the uncertainty of the estimates, but may also signal the involvement of additional control mechanisms (such as portal glucose sensing[16] and brain insulin action[17]).

An empiric index of hepatic insulin resistance can be constructed by multiplying fasting endogenous glucose output by the estimated fasting prehepatic insulin concentration.[18] In lean individuals with normal glucose tolerance, this index has a median value of 1760 μmol/min/kg$_{FFM}$/pM (with an interquartile range of 1200–2300), gradually increasing in obese or otherwise insulin-resistant subjects. In fact, hepatic insulin resistance is generally coherent with peripheral insulin resistance (as measured by a euglycemic hyperinsulinemic clamp) throughout the range of these variables seen in humans (**Fig. 6**).

Fasting glucose disposal occurs in both insulin-dependent (skeletal muscle, adipose tissue, myocardium) and insulin-independent tissues; among the latter, the brain, an obligate glucose consumer, alone accounts for half the amount of hepatic glucose output. Of note is that in all body tissues, glucose uptake, whether insulin sensitive or not, also occurs by mass action, that is, in proportion to the glucose concentration itself.[19]

In practical terms, the physiologic organization of the insulin system is such that if fasting insulin secretion were totally absent (as in C-peptide–negative type 1 diabetes), one would have to infuse between 0.35 and 0.56 U/kg per day intraportally to reproduce the peripheral fasting plasma insulin concentrations observed in nondiabetic subjects over a wide BMI range. By contrast, if the same peripheral plasma insulin levels were to be maintained by peripheral insulin administration, the insulin infusion

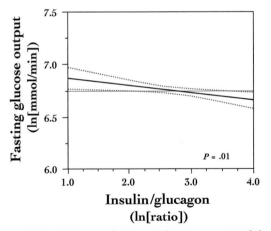

Fig. 5. Power function linking fasting endogenous glucose output and the estimated prehepatic insulin-to-glucagon ratio in the nondiabetic subjects in **Fig. 2**. The P value refers to the significance of the partial correlation coefficient of the line of best fit (*blue line*) and its 95% confidence intervals (*dotted red lines*) from a general linear regression model also adjusting for sex, age, and body mass index. Note the log transformation of both axes.

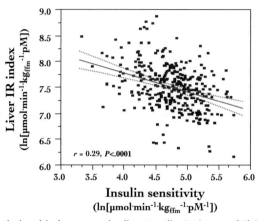

Fig. 6. Reciprocal relationship between the liver Insulin Resistance (IR) index (calculated as the product of fasting endogenous glucose output and estimated prehepatic plasma insulin concentration) and whole-body insulin sensitivity (M/I, calculated as the M value from the euglycemic insulin clamp normalized by the steady-state plasma insulin concentrations during the clamp) in the nondiabetic subjects in **Fig. 2**. The *r* and *P* values refer to the significance of the partial correlation coefficient of the line of best fit (*red line*) and its 95% confidence intervals (*dotted red lines*) from a general linear regression model also adjusting for sex, age, and body mass index. Note the log transformation of both axes.

rate would have to range between 0.08 and 0.11 U/kg per day. In the latter case, however, peripheral tissues would be normally insulinized, whereas the liver would be exposed to hypoinsulinemia; hepatic glucose output would be insufficiently restrained by insulin, thereby contributing to hyperglycemia. Conversely, adequate insulinization of the liver by peripheral insulin administration would create peripheral hyperinsulinemia, with the attendant risk of hypoglycemia. The difficulty in achieving and maintaining normoglycemia in insulin-treated type 1 diabetes largely originates from the obligate peripheral route of insulin administration. Because of erratic absorption and bioavailability, delivery of oral insulin is not feasible at present.

In summary, short-term control of glucose homeostasis in the fasting or interprandial state is delegated mostly to the liver, with a marginal contribution of peripheral tissues, in which glucose uptake is either independent of insulin or only slightly stimulated by fasting insulin levels. It is nevertheless important to consider that in the longer term the setpoint of fasting glucose release is dictated by the tissue metabolic requirements (see the strong relation of fasting glucose output to FFM in **Fig. 2**).[7] This fact implies that signals expressing the energy status of bodily tissues reach the liver and modulate its delivery of glucose to the periphery. Although the nature of these signals is incompletely understood, it is clear that glucose occupies a dominant position among energy-rich substrates in metabolic control.

The pharmacokinetics of insulin outlined here do not readily translate into an insulin effect because of the different dose-response relationships of insulin action on the liver (inhibition of glucose release) and peripheral tissues (enhancement of glucose disposal), and the sizeable activation and deactivation times of the hormone. In fact, the dose-response curve for hepatic insulin action is shifted to the left relative to the dose-response curve of peripheral insulin action (**Fig. 7**).[19] Thus, the half-maximal portal insulin concentration for glucose output is approximately 300 pmol/L (~50 µU/mL), whereas the half-maximal peripheral insulin concentration for glucose

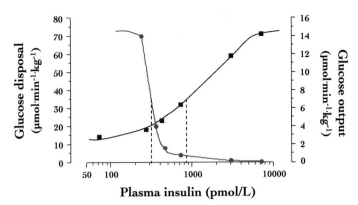

Fig. 7. Dose-response curves for the effect of insulin on fasting endogenous glucose output (*red line*) and clamp-derived whole-body glucose disposal (*blue line*) in normal individuals. The plasma insulin concentrations on the horizontal axis are peripheral insulin levels for glucose disposal and estimated prehepatic plasma insulin concentrations for glucose output. The dashed vertical lines plot to the respective half-maximal plasma insulin concentrations of glucose output and disposal. (*Data from* DeFronzo RA, Ferrannini E, Hendler R, et al. Regulation of splanchnic and peripheral glucose uptake by insulin and hyperglycemia in man. Diabetes 1983;32:35–45.)

disposal is approximately 860 pmol/L (∼150 μU/mL), 3 times higher. For example, at plasma insulin levels at which glucose output is halved, peripheral glucose disposal is hardly enhanced at all. As a consequence, dose and route of delivery determine which tissues, in what order, will respond to insulin. In addition, the activation times of insulin action are much shorter for liver than for peripheral tissues, both being inversely related to the insulin dose (**Fig. 8**).[20] Significantly longer activation times at the level of both liver and peripheral tissues characterize insulin action in obese, insulin-resistant subjects. Conversely, deactivation times are longer for liver than for peripheral tissues, and progressively longer with increasing insulin dose. Moreover, deactivation is faster in obese, insulin-resistant subjects than in lean individuals. Thus, progressively higher levels of insulin engage the intracellular glucose effector pathway more rapidly than do lower levels, particularly in the liver and peripheral tissues, but action persists longer at both sites. These pharmacodynamic characteristics account for the clinical observations of a delay in insulin action when levels are raised (by stimulation of β-cell release or exogenous administration) and the protracted hypoglycemic action when secretion is turned off (or exogenous administration stopped). Such characteristics also highlight the role of the liver in whole-body insulin action, and predict that a strong insulinization enhances the risk of prolonged hypoglycemia, predominantly on account of a protracted inability of the liver to respond to falling glucose levels. In insulin-resistant individuals, activation is delayed and liver deactivation is anticipated; thus not only do insulin-resistant subjects need more insulin than do insulin-sensitive subjects to attain a given glucose-lowering effect, but the effect itself is manifested in a time pattern that suggests reduced efficacy.

THE FASTING STATE IN DIABETES

In patients with type 2 diabetes, fasting insulin secretion rates are generally normal or higher, because of the persistent stimulus of fasting hyperglycemia, and glucose

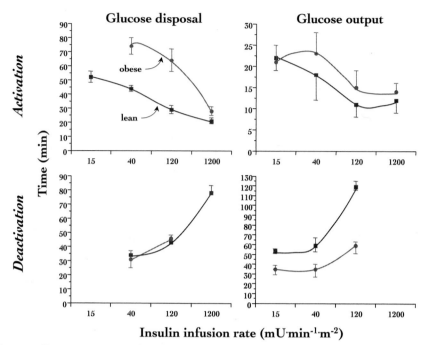

Fig. 8. Half-maximum times of activation (*top panels*) and deactivation (*bottom panels*) for glucose disposal and glucose output as a function of exogenous insulin infusion rates during euglycemic clamps in lean subjects (*blue lines*) and obese subjects (*red lines*). Data are mean ± SEM. (*Data from* Prager R, Wallace P, Olefsky JM. In vivo kinetics of insulin action on peripheral glucose disposal and hepatic glucose output in normal and obese subjects. J Clin Invest 1986;78:472–81.)

output is not elevated in absolute terms until fasting glucose exceeds 10 to 15 mmol/L (180–270 mg/dL).[18,21] Plasma glucagon concentrations are generally higher than normal.[15] When the maximal absorptive capacity for glucose of the proximal renal tubule is exceeded, glycosuria provides an additional sink for plasma glucose. As shown by numerous studies,[22] marked insulin resistance is typically present both at the level of peripheral tissues (ie, the M value on an insulin clamp) and in the liver (eg, the hepatic insulin resistance index). Subjects with impaired fasting glycemia and/or impaired glucose tolerance exhibit intermediate patterns between those of normotolerant subjects and type 2 patients for all the parameters of the input-output system shown in **Fig. 1**. In other words, for all the quantitative relationships described so far, subjects with preserved glucose tolerance and individuals with various degrees of dysglycemia/hyperglycemia are essentially part of the same continuum.[23]

In type 1 diabetes, fasting insulin secretion is absent or profoundly decreased, glucagon is elevated, and endogenous glucose output may be elevated in absolute terms.[24] A similar, if less severe, picture may also be found in patients with advanced, decompensated type 2 diabetes.

GLUCOSE HOMEOSTASIS: THE FED STATE

As exogenous glucose is absorbed (from an oral glucose load or a mixed meal), the splanchnic area retains a quota for its own metabolic use (in humans, a small extraction fraction, mostly insulin independent[25,26]), and passes the remainder to the post-hepatic veins and on to the arterial circulation. Intestinal glucose absorption is a rapid and high-capacity phenomenon[27]; therefore, arterial plasma glucose concentrations (**Fig. 9**) and the appearance of oral glucose (**Fig. 10**) rise and fall over a time course that is dictated essentially by the rate of gastric emptying. Typically an early peak in glucose absorption and plasma glucose occurs 30 to 40 minutes following ingestion, and a second, flatter peak is frequently evident at 120 to 150 minutes (see **Fig. 10**). Of note is that at the time when plasma glucose levels have returned to baseline, the metabolic perturbation is far from extinguished (eg, absorption of oral glucose is still ongoing 5 hours after ingesting a mixed meal at rates different from zero) (see **Fig. 10**).

The increments in plasma glucose and, in the case of a mixed meal, also in circulating amino acids, signal to β-cells to augment insulin release. In normal subjects, insulin secretion rises promptly, and tailgates glucose levels closely (see **Fig. 9**). The portosystemic insulin gradient is maintained at the levels obtained during the fasting state, but starts to attenuate at prehepatic insulin concentrations of 800 to 1000 pmol/L (130–170 µU/mL) because of the saturation of hepatic clearance capacity.[14]

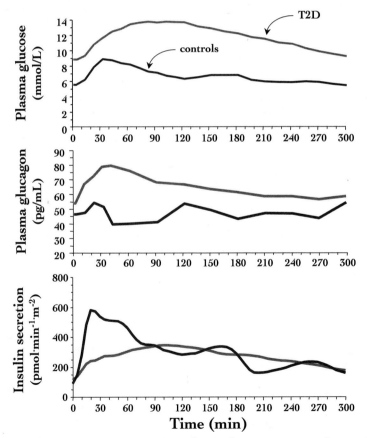

Fig. 9. Mean plasma glucose concentration, plasma glucagon concentration, and insulin secretion profiles in patients with type 2 diabetes (T2D) and age- and weight-matched nondiabetic controls following the ingestion of a mixed meal (Ferrannini E, unpublished data, 2012).

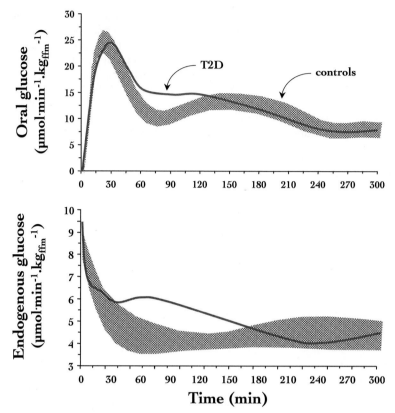

Fig. 10. Time course of appearance of oral and endogenous glucose in patients with type 2 diabetes (T2D) and age- and weight-matched nondiabetic controls (shaded areas are mean ± SEM) following the ingestion of a mixed meal (Ferrannini E, unpublished data, 2012).

At peak postglucose insulinemia, the portosystemic gradient typically falls below 1.5 (**Fig. 11**), indicating that more pancreatic insulin bypasses the liver onto the systemic circulation. In liver cirrhosis, saturation of hepatic insulin degradation occurs at lower insulin levels, because of both parenchymal insufficiency and portosystemic shunts.[28] Plasma glucagon concentrations, though suppressed when glucose alone is ingested, increase in small and brief bursts in response to a mixed meal (see **Fig. 9**).

A standard oral glucose load (75 g) releases an average 0.12 U/kg of insulin above basal output over 2 hours. A mixed meal will release more insulin over a longer period of time, depending on caloric content and composition. Thus, a 70-kg nonobese adult consuming 3 mixed meals over 24 hours needs a total of 40 to 50 units of insulin to maintain normoglycemia (with a rather large scatter around this value[29]).

Passage of glucose through the gastrointestinal tract triggers an increased release of hormones by endocrine cells of the intestinal mucosa. Prominent among these hormones is glucagon-like peptide 1 (GLP-1), which potentiates glucose-induced insulin release by a direct action on β-cells and simultaneously restrains glucagon release (see **Fig. 1**).[30] Thus, following glucose ingestion the prehepatic insulin-to-glucagon ratio increases to higher than in the fasting state. As a result, endogenous glucose output is suppressed by an average of 50%, thereby keeping some 20 g of endogenous glucose from appearing in the systemic circulation throughout 5 hours

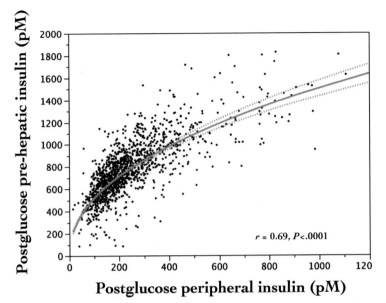

Fig. 11. Nonlinear relationship between estimated prehepatic and peripheral plasma insulin concentrations in the nondiabetic subjects in **Fig. 3**. The r and P values refer to the significance of the partial correlation coefficient of the line of best fit (*green line*) and its 95% confidence intervals (*dotted green lines*). Data (Ferrannini E, unpublished data, 2012) from 1151 nondiabetic subjects from the RISC Study. (*Data from* Ferrannini E, Balkau B, Coppack SW, et al. RISC Investigators. Insulin resistance, insulin response, and obesity as indicators of metabolic risk. J Clin Endocrinol Metab 2007;92:2885–92.)

of postcibal period. As approximately 55 g of oral glucose enters the circulation over the same time period, total glucose disposal (75 g) takes place under the combined effect of hyperglycemia (mass action) and insulin stimulation. Because total insulin output averages 25 U over 5 hours, it can be calculated that the net metabolic efficiency of the hormone is approximately 0.3 units per gram of glucose disposed. Postprandial glucose homeostasis is therefore imposed on both the liver, to curtail its glucose release, and peripheral tissues, to stimulate their glucose uptake, in an approximate proportion of 1:3.

Of note is that if similar plasma glucose and insulin levels to those achieved with glucose or mixed-meal ingestion were created by an intravenous glucose infusion, endogenous glucose output would be fully suppressed.[19] This conspicuous difference clearly speaks for the activation of neuroendocrine processes specific to the physiologic route of nutrient entry. Examples are increases in splanchnic blood flow,[31–33] splanchnic adrenergic activation,[33] release of multiple peptides exerting both local and systemic effects, and excitation of autonomic neural arches eventually firing back to liver and other peripheral tissues.[34]

THE FED STATE IN DIABETES

In typical type 2 diabetes, the response to a mixed meal features higher plasma glucose and glucagon concentrations (see **Fig. 9**). The meal GLP-1 response may be sluggish,[35] but potentiation of glucose-induced insulin secretion and inhibition of glucagon release are definitely impaired.[36,37] However, rates of oral glucose appearance, endogenous glucose output, and whole-body glucose disposal are similar to those of nondiabetic individuals (see **Fig. 10**). Thus, overall glucose flux balance and metabolic insulin efficiency are apparently unaltered, except that the glucose area is double the normal value and the incremental glucose area is triple the normal value. Higher glucose in the face of normal or high insulin level is the definition of insulin resistance: at the level of the liver, hyperglycemia fails to fully inhibit glucose release (which it normally does with a very sensitive dose-response relationship[19]), in peripheral tissue glucose clearance is reduced, and hyperglycemia promotes glucose uptake by mass action. One can then recalculate metabolic insulin efficiency as the ratio of secreted insulin to plasma glucose clearance: in the representative subjects in **Figs. 9** and **10**, this value is 32 U/L (of plasma cleared of glucose) in controls and 56 U/L in diabetic patients. Given the logarithmic relationship between peripheral plasma insulin concentrations and glucose disposal rates (see **Fig. 7**), to normalize metabolic insulin efficiency requires raising plasma insulin levels 3- to 4-fold.

In decompensated type 2 diabetes[38] and in type 1 diabetes,[39] feeding may not suppress, and may actually enhance, endogenous glucose output and fail to stimulate total glucose disposal because of marked insulin deficiency. Postabsorptive glycemic excursions will be exacerbated, and the disposal of meal-derived glucose will be protracted for several hours, such that the patient will be rarely, if at all, in a state of metabolic fast.

It should be mentioned that in vitro insulin secretion occurs in discrete bursts that are synchronous with 4-minute oscillations of cytoplasmic calcium concentrations.[40] In vivo, both high-frequency (5–10 minutes) and ultradian (~2 hours) oscillations can be demonstrated by combining frequent blood sampling with C-peptide deconvolution (to reconstruct insulin secretion rate). At least part of these oscillations can be entrained by high-frequency plasma glucose pulses, a typical feature of feedback systems.[41] By exposing the liver to peaks of insulin concentration, secretory oscillations in portal blood enhance the ability of insulin to suppress glucose output.[42] The oscillatory pattern is altered early in the course of type 2 diabetes,[43] and may have pathogenetic significance.[44] However, whether abnormal pulsatility is a cause or effect of the β-cell defect at the root of type 2 diabetes has not been determined.

SUMMARY

Insulin resistance and β-cell dysfunction are the main defects of type 2 diabetes; they also predict[45] and precede overt hyperglycemia in individuals at risk.[46,47] β-Cell mass is likely to be variably reduced[48] (and α-cell mass relatively increased[49]) in longstanding type 2 diabetes, and is virtually lost at onset in type 1 diabetes. Regardless of the pathophysiological basis of these abnormalities, an input-output schematization of plasma glucose homeostasis provides quantitative information on glucose fluxes and their control by insulin. In a nutshell, insulin action is dependent on target tissue (liver vs peripheral tissues), dose-response characteristics, route of delivery (intraportal vs peripheral), and kinetics of activation and deactivation. Under normal conditions, the closed-loop control of minute-by-minute insulin release by arterial glucose levels protects against both hyperglycemia and hypoglycemia. Open-loop insulin therapy faces the complexities of insulin pharmacokinetics and pharmacodynamics outlined in this article. Thus, despite the science of the glucose-insulin system being arguably the most precisely known in physiology, insulin therapy remains defiantly empiric, and an engrossing challenge to both the patient and physician.

REFERENCES

1. Leibiger IB, Leibiger B, Berggren PO. Insulin signaling in the pancreatic beta-cell. Annu Rev Nutr 2008;28:233–51.
2. Mari A, Tura A, Natali A, et al. Influence of hyperinsulinemia and insulin resistance on in vivo β-cell function: their role in human β-cell dysfunction. Diabetes 2011; 60(12):3141–7.
3. Bouche C, Lopez X, Fleischman A, et al. Insulin enhances glucose-stimulated insulin secretion in healthy humans. Proc Natl Acad Sci U S A 2010;107:4770–5.
4. Kawamori D, Kurpad AJ, Liew CW, et al. Insulin signaling in alpha cells modulates glucagon secretion in vivo. Cell Metab 2009;9:350–61.
5. Ferrannini E, Muscelli E, Natali A, et al. Association of fasting glucagon and proinsulin concentrations with insulin resistance. Diabetologia 2007;50:2342–7.
6. Gastaldelli A, Baldi S, Pettiti M, et al. Influence of obesity and type 2 diabetes on gluconeogenesis and glucose output in humans: a quantitative study. Diabetes 2000;49:1367–73.
7. Natali A, Toschi E, Camastra S, et al. Determinants of postabsorptive endogenous glucose output in non-diabetic subjects. Diabetologia 2000;43:1266–72.
8. Cherrington AD, Chiasson JL, Liljenquist JE, et al. Control of hepatic glucose output by glucagon and insulin in the intact dog. Biochem Soc Symp 1978;43: 31–45.
9. Cherrington AD, Edgerton D, Sindelar DK. The direct and indirect effects of insulin on hepatic glucose production in vivo. Diabetologia 1998;41:987–96.
10. Cherrington AD. Banting Lecture 1997. Control of glucose uptake and release by the liver in vivo. Diabetes 1999;48:1198–214.
11. Cherrington AD, Moore MC, Sindelar DK, et al. Insulin action on the liver in vivo. Biochem Soc Trans 2007;35:1171–4.
12. Ferrannini E, Wahren J, Faber OK, et al. Splanchnic and renal metabolism of insulin in human subjects: a dose-response study. Am J Physiol 1983;244: E517–27.
13. Byrne MM, Sturis J, Polonsky KS. Insulin secretion and clearance during low-dose graded glucose infusion. Am J Physiol 1995;268:E21–7.
14. Ferrannini E, Cobelli C. The kinetics of insulin in man. II. Role of the liver. Diabetes Metab Rev 1987;3:365–97.
15. Lefèbvre PJ. Glucagon and its family revisited. Diabetes Care 1995;18:715–30.
16. Cherrington AD. Central versus peripheral glucose sensing and the response to hypoglycemia. Diabetes 2008;57:1158–9.
17. Ramnanan CJ, Saraswathi V, Smith MS, et al. Brain insulin action augments hepatic glycogen synthesis without suppressing glucose production or gluconeogenesis in dogs. J Clin Invest 2011;121:3713–23.
18. Ferrannini E, Groop LC. Hepatic glucose production in insulin-resistant states. Diabetes Metab Rev 1989;5:711–26.
19. DeFronzo RA, Ferrannini E, Hendler R, et al. Regulation of splanchnic and peripheral glucose uptake by insulin and hyperglycemia in man. Diabetes 1983;32: 35–45.
20. Prager R, Wallace P, Olefsky JM. In vivo kinetics of insulin action on peripheral glucose disposal and hepatic glucose output in normal and obese subjects. J Clin Invest 1986;78:472–81.
21. DeFronzo RA, Ferrannini E, Simonson DC. Fasting hyperglycemia in non-insulin-dependent diabetes mellitus: contributions of excessive hepatic glucose production and impaired tissue glucose uptake. Metabolism 1989;38:387–95.

22. DeFronzo RA, Ferrannini E. Insulin resistance. A multifaceted syndrome responsible for NIDDM, obesity, hypertension, dyslipidemia, and atherosclerotic cardiovascular disease. Diabetes Care 1991;14:173–94.
23. Ferrannini E, Gastaldelli A, Iozzo P. Pathophysiology of prediabetes. Med Clin North Am 2011;95:327–39.
24. DeFronzo RA, Simonson D, Ferrannini E. Hepatic and peripheral insulin resistance: a common feature of type 2 (non-insulin-dependent) and type 1 (insulin-dependent) diabetes mellitus. Diabetologia 1982;23:313–9.
25. Ferrannini E, Wahren J, Felig P, et al. The role of fractional glucose extraction in the regulation of splanchnic glucose metabolism in normal and diabetic man. Metabolism 1980;29:28–35.
26. Iozzo P, Hallsten K, Oikonen V, et al. Insulin-mediated hepatic glucose uptake is impaired in type 2 diabetes: evidence for a relationship with glycemic control. J Clin Endocrinol Metab 2003;88:2055–60.
27. Modigliani R, Bernier JJ. Absorption of glucose, sodium, and water by the human jejunum studied by intestinal perfusion with a proximal occluding balloon and at variable flow rates. Gut 1971;12:184–93.
28. Petrides AS, Vogt C, Schulze-Berge D, et al. Pathogenesis of glucose intolerance and diabetes mellitus in cirrhosis. Hepatology 1994;19:616–27.
29. Polonsky KS, Given BD, Hirsch LJ, et al. Abnormal patterns of insulin secretion in non-insulin-dependent diabetes mellitus. N Engl J Med 1988;318:1231–9.
30. Holst JJ. The physiology of glucagon-like peptide 1. Physiol Rev 2007;87:1409–39.
31. Waldhäusl WK, Gasic S, Bratusch-Marrain P, et al. The 75-g oral glucose tolerance test: effect on splanchnic metabolism of substrates and pancreatic hormone release in healthy man. Diabetologia 1983;25:489–95.
32. Ferrannini E, Bjorkman O, Reichard GA Jr, et al. The disposal of an oral glucose load in healthy subjects. A quantitative study. Diabetes 1985;34:580–8.
33. Waldhäusl WK, Gasic S, Bratusch-Marrain P, et al. Effect of stress hormones on splanchnic substrate and insulin disposal after glucose ingestion in healthy humans. Diabetes 1987;36:127–35.
34. Burcelin R. The gut-brain axis: a major glucoregulatory player. Diabetes Metab 2010;36(Suppl 3):S54–8.
35. Nauck MA, Vardarli I, Deacon CF, et al. Secretion of glucagon-like peptide-1 (GLP-1) in type 2 diabetes: what is up, what is down? Diabetologia 2011;54:10–8.
36. Nauck M, Stöckmann F, Ebert R, et al. Reduced incretin effect in type 2 (non-insulin-dependent) diabetes. Diabetologia 1986;29:46–52.
37. Muscelli E, Mari A, Casolaro A, et al. Separate impact of obesity and glucose tolerance on the incretin effect in normal subjects and type 2 diabetic patients. Diabetes 2008;57:1340–8.
38. Firth RG, Bell PM, Marsh HM, et al. Postprandial hyperglycemia in patients with noninsulin-dependent diabetes mellitus. Role of hepatic and extrahepatic tissues. J Clin Invest 1986;77:1525–32.
39. Vella A, Shah P, Basu A, et al. Prandial insulin and the systemic appearance of meal-derived glucose in people with type 1 diabetes. Diabetes Care 2008;31:2230–1.
40. Tengholm A, Gylfe E. Oscillatory control of insulin secretion. Mol Cell Endocrinol 2009;297:58–72.
41. Polonsky KS, Sturis J, Van Cauter E. Temporal profiles and clinical significance of pulsatile insulin secretion. Horm Res 1998;49:178–84.
42. Caumo A, Luzi L. First-phase insulin secretion: does it exist in real life? Considerations on shape and function. Am J Physiol Endocrinol Metab 2004;287:E371–85.

43. O'Rahilly S, Turner RC, Matthews DR. Impaired pulsatile secretion of insulin in relatives of patients with non-insulin-dependent diabetes. N Engl J Med 1988; 318:1225–30.

44. Pørksen N, Hollingdal M, Juhl C, et al. Pulsatile insulin secretion: detection, regulation, and role in diabetes. Diabetes 2002;51(Suppl 1):S245–54.

45. Ferrannini E, Massari M, Nannipieri M, et al. Plasma glucose levels as predictors of diabetes: the Mexico City diabetes study. Diabetologia 2009;52:818–24.

46. Walker M, Mari A, Jayapaul MK, et al. Impaired beta cell glucose sensitivity and whole-body insulin sensitivity as predictors of hyperglycaemia in non-diabetic subjects. Diabetologia 2005;48:2470–6.

47. Ferrannini E, Natali A, Muscelli E, et al. on behalf of the RISC Investigators. Natural history and physiological determinants of changes in glucose tolerance in a non-diabetic population: the RISC Study. Diabetologia 2011;54:1507–16.

48. Rahier J, Guiot Y, Goebbels RM, et al. Pancreatic beta-cell mass in European subjects with type 2 diabetes. Diabetes Obes Metab 2008;10(Suppl 4):32–42.

49. Henquin JC, Rahier J. Pancreatic alpha cell mass in European subjects with type 2 diabetes. Diabetologia 2011;54:1720–5.

Reevaluating Goals of Insulin Therapy: Perspectives from Large Clinical Trials

Matthew C. Riddle, MD*, Kevin C.J. Yuen, MD

KEYWORDS

- Diabetes • Insulin • Microvascular • Macrovascular
- Cardiovascular risk • Tactics • Goals • Glycemic control

The modern era of clinical research on treatments for diabetes dates back to the report of the University Group Diabetes Program (UGDP) published in 1970.[1] Although the UGDP yielded controversial and inconclusive results, it provided a stimulus for the design of several subsequent long-term clinical trials. The results of these trials have shown that improved glycemic control can reduce the microvascular complications of diabetes (eye, nerve, and kidney disease) and have led to treatment guidelines that are, at least in part, based on good evidence. However, a major question remains unanswered: what is the appropriate and safe target for glycemic control to minimize cardiovascular risks in patients with type 2 diabetes? This article surveys recent epidemiologic studies and interventional trials, examines current understanding of the natural history of type 2 diabetes, and proposes possible new goals and tactics for optimizing insulin therapy. The opinions expressed are our own and should not be taken as the views of any commercial entity or professional organization.

EPIDEMIOLOGIC ASSOCIATION OF HYPERGLYCEMIA WITH DIABETIC COMPLICATIONS

Hyperglycemia is the defining feature of diabetes and a key determinant of diabetic complications. Thus, the diagnosis of diabetes has been based on specific levels of hyperglycemia as advised by a group of experts assembled by the American Diabetes Association in 1997. This group examined the epidemiologic findings then available,

This work was supported in part by the Rose Hastings and Russell Standley Memorial Trusts. The authors have nothing to disclose.
Division of Endocrinology, Diabetes and Clinical Nutrition, Department of Medicine, Oregon Health and Science University, 3181 Southwest Sam Jackson Park Road, Mailcode L345, Portland, OR 97239, USA
* Corresponding author.
E-mail address: riddlem@ohsu.edu

Endocrinol Metab Clin N Am 41 (2012) 41–56
doi:10.1016/j.ecl.2012.03.003
0889-8529/12/$ – see front matter © 2012 Elsevier Inc. All rights reserved.

endo.theclinics.com

and proposed a rational basis for diagnosis and treatment.[2] **Fig. 1A** displays cross-sectional data that were cited in that report. In a population of persons not known to have diabetes, diabetic retinopathy found on fundoscopy was limited to the highest decile of the distribution of levels of fasting plasma glucose (FPG), glucose 2 hours after an oral glucose challenge (2-hour PG), and hemoglobin A1c (A1c). The upper boundary of the highest decile of values not associated with retinopathy was 109 mg/dL (6.1 mmol/L) for FPG, 154 mg/dL for 2-hour PG (8.6 mmol/L), and 5.9% for A1c. Thus, levels of hyperglycemia associated with retinopathy have provided the basis for defining diabetes. At present, the American Diabetes Association considers FPG greater than 126 mg/dL (7 mmol/L), 2-hour PG greater than 200 mg/dL (>11.1 mmol/L), and A1c greater than or equal to 6.5% to suggest the presence of diabetes, pending confirmation by a second test.[3]

More recently, other large epidemiologic studies have examined relationships between levels of hyperglycemia and cardiovascular disease.[4–7] Examples of these are presented in **Fig. 1B** and **C**. **Fig. 1B** shows data prospectively collected from more than 4500 participants in the United Kingdom Prospective Diabetes Study (UKPDS) and analyzed epidemiologically. The risk of myocardial infarction was lowest at A1c less than 6.0%, and increased steadily at higher levels of A1c.[6] **Fig. 1C** shows a meta-analysis including FPG samples from ~700,000 individuals with the lowest risk of coronary heart disease evident at values near 90 mg/dL (5 mmol/L) and increased risk at more than 100 mg/dL (5.6 mmol/L) either in the presence of known diabetes or

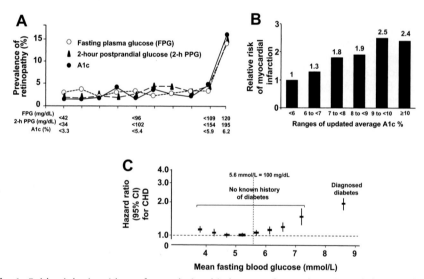

Fig. 1. Epidemiologic evidence for a relationship between hyperglycemia and the complications of diabetes. (*A*) The prevalence of retinopathy detected by fundoscopy in a cross-sectional population in the United States (NHANES III), displayed by deciles of fasting plasma glucose, glucose 2 hours after an oral glucose challenge, and A1c.[2] (*B*) Relative risk of myocardial infarction (adjusted for age, sex, and duration of diabetes) by ranges of updated average A1c over 10 years in the United Kingdom Prospective Diabetes Study (UKPDS) population, referenced to A1c less than 6.0%.[6] (*C*) Hazard ratio for incident coronary heart disease (CHD) in a meta-analysis of 102 prospective studies (adjusted for age, sex, systolic blood pressure, and body mass index) by mean fasting blood glucose, referenced to 5.0 to 5.5 mmol/L (90–100 mg/dL).[6]

not.[8] Such evidence continues to strengthen the case that increasing hyperglycemia is associated with increasing risk of both microvascular and cardiovascular disease starting from low levels of A1c or FPG.

EARLY IN DIABETES: INSULIN-AUGMENTING TREATMENT REDUCES MICROVASCULAR COMPLICATIONS

Despite epidemiologic evidence linking hyperglycemia with diabetic complications, skepticism that treating hyperglycemia might limit these complications persisted until the presentation of favorable results from the Diabetes Control and Complications Trial (DCCT)[9] in 1993 and the UKPDS[10,11] in 1997. Arguments against potential benefits of antihyperglycemic treatment included the view that diabetic complications could be mediated by means other than hyperglycemia[12,13] and that adverse effects accompanying treatment, such as hypoglycemia, might lead to more harm than benefit.[14,15] Findings of the DCCT and the UKPDS, which verified that the benefits of intensive treatment of hyperglycemia can outweigh the risks, are summarized in **Table 1**.

Despite studying different populations of patients (young adults with type 1 diabetes in the DCCT and middle-aged persons with type 2 in the UKPDS), these trials had several similarities. Both trials used insulin as an important part of the intervention. In the DCCT, multiple doses of insulin by injection or by pump delivery were used by all participants.[9] In the UKPDS, the main randomized comparison was between a conventional regimen based on lifestyle therapy alone at the outset and more intensive treatment with basal (ultralente) insulin or a sulfonylurea.[11] An important substudy of the UKPDS mandated early addition of basal insulin to a sulfonylurea in one treatment group.[16] Another similarity between the DCCT and the UKPDS was that intervention began early in the natural history of diabetes. Participants in the DCCT were known to have type 1 diabetes for an average of 6 years, presumably with only a short interval of hyperglycemia before diagnosis. Those in the UKPDS were treated within a year after diagnosis but, because of the known delay between onset of type 2 diabetes and diagnosis,[17] were likely to have had an onset of diabetes for at least 4 years

Table 1
Microvascular end points and cardiovascular events in the DCCT and UKPDS

	Number of Participants	Known Diabetes Duration (y)	Time of Randomized Treatment (y)	A1c (%) Difference Between Treatments	Reduction of Microvascular End Points	Reduction of Cardiovascular Events
DCCT[9]	1441	6	6.5	~2.0 9.0 vs 7.1	Retinopathy 3-step progression 63% (P<.002) Albuminuria Micro 39% (P<.002) Macro 54% (P = .04)	CV composite 41% (NS)
UKPDS[10,11]	3867	<1	10	0.9 7.9 vs 7.0	Aggregate microvascular 25% (P<.001)	Myocardial infarction 16% (P = .052)

before randomization. Hence, the duration of hyperglycemia consistent with diabetes may have averaged about 6 years before entry to each trial.

The effect of intensive treatment on microvascular outcomes was also similar in the 2 trials. The difference of mean A1c levels between standard and intensive treatment in the DCCT ranged from 1.7% to 2.0% during the randomized comparison. In the UKPDS, both main treatment groups (lifestyle alone vs insulin or sulfonylurea) showed steady increases of A1c levels over time, but the median difference between the 2 groups over 10 years was 0.9%. The microvascular end points shown in **Table 1** were reduced by 39% to 63% in the DCCT, and the aggregate microvascular outcome in the UKPDS was reduced by 25% in the UKPDS. Despite the limitations of comparing trials with different designs, the findings in each suggest approximately 25% reduction of microvascular end points accompanying a 1% reduction of A1c. In contrast, effects on cardiovascular end points were not convincing. Neither a 41% reduction of a cardiovascular composite in the DCCT nor a 16% reduction of myocardial infarction in the UKPDS achieved statistical significance.

LATER IN TYPE 2 DIABETES: INTENSIVE TREATMENT OF HYPERGLYCEMIA YIELDS MIXED RESULTS

In addition to confirming the ability of glycemic intervention to reduce microvascular complications in both type 1 and type 2 diabetes, the DCCT and UKPDS results supported an A1c level of 7%, a level of control commonly achieved in each trial, as an appropriate goal for treatment. However, whether cardiovascular risk could be reduced by intensive glycemic control remained an open question. This finding prompted the design of 3 large clinical trials testing strategies targeting different levels of A1c in type 2 diabetes. The Veterans Affairs Diabetes Trial (VADT) began in 2000, and the Action in Diabetes and Vascular Disease: Preterax and Diamacron MR Controlled Evaluation (ADVANCE) and the Action to Control Cardiovascular Risk (ACCORD) trials both began in 2001. Initial reports from these trials first appeared in 2008 and 2009,[18–20] and further reports followed.[21–23]

The VADT, ACCORD, and ADVANCE trials were designed to avoid some limitations of the earlier ones. The limitations included the small numbers of participants and low cardiovascular risk in the DCCT and UKPDS populations, and the suboptimal levels of glycemic control achieved. By enrolling more participants with evidence of cardiovascular risk and targeting nearly normal glycemic control, the power to show potential cardiovascular benefits of intensive glycemic treatment was thought to be increased. In ADVANCE, the intensive treatment strategy was based on treatment with a sulfonylurea (gliclazide), and, in ACCORD and VADT, all available types of treatments were used, including extensive use of both basal and prandial insulins. Some of the main results are shown in **Table 2**.

All of these trials achieved a significant and sustained reduction of A1c levels in the intensive compared with the conventional treatment group. The average A1c level achieved with intensive therapy ranged from 6.4% in ACCORD to 6.9% in VADT; lower than in the DCCT and UKPDS. Intensive intervention in all 3 trials reduced at least 1 microvascular end point to a degree that, relative to the between-treatment differences of A1c levels, was comparable with the benefit shown in the DCCT and UKPDS. In contrast, none of the 3 trials showed an improvement of its main cardiovascular end point. In the case of ACCORD, an increase of total and cardiovascular mortality accompanying intensive therapy offset a 24% reduction of nonfatal myocardial infarction, leading to a small but nonsignificant reduction of the cardiovascular composite. A subsequent meta-analysis of data from these 3 trials and also from the UKPDS

Table 2
Microvascular end points and cardiovascular outcomes in Action in Diabetes and Vascular Disease: Preterax and Diamacron MR Controlled Evaluation (ADVANCE), Action to Control Cardiovascular Risk (ACCORD), and the Veterans Affairs Diabetes Trial (VADT)

	Number of Participants	Known Diabetes Duration (y)	Time of Randomized Treatment (y)	A1c (%) Difference Between Treatments	Reduction of Microvascular End Points	Reduction of Cardiovascular Events
ADVANCE[19]	11,140	8	5.0	0.7 7.3 vs 6.5	Retinopathy 5% (P = .50) Nephropathy composite 21% (P = .006)	CV composite 6% (P = .32)
ACCORD[18]	10,251	10	3.7	1.1 7.5 vs 6.4	Retinopathy 33% (P = .003) Microalbuminuria 21% (P = .0005)	CV composite 10% (NS) Nonfatal MI 24% (P = .004)
VADT[20]	1791	11.5	5.6	1.5 8.4 vs 6.9	Retinopathy 2-step progression 23% (P = .07) Albuminuria Any increase 33% (P = .01)	CV composite 12% (P = .14)

showed no significant effect of intensive glycemic treatment on overall cardiovascular events or mortality,[24] but a significant 15% decrease of fatal or nonfatal myocardial infarction and ~2.5-fold increased risk of major hypoglycemic events. An exploratory subgroup analysis from this data-set showed greater potential for reduction of cardiovascular risk with intensive treatment in persons with diabetes without known prior cardiovascular events than in those with such a history (hazard ratio 0.84, confidence interval [CI] 0.74–0.94] vs hazard ratio 1.00, CI 0.89–1.13; for interaction, $P = .04$).[24]

TEN YEARS AFTER CESSATION OF RANDOMIZED TREATMENT IN DCCT AND UKPDS: MICROVASCULAR BENEFITS PERSIST AND CARDIOVASCULAR BENEFITS ARE EVIDENT

The disappointing findings of the large intervention trials that enrolled high-risk participants later in the natural history of type 2 diabetes have provoked much discussion. To some extent, this ongoing debate has obscured further important reports from the DCCT and UKPDS populations. Key findings from these reports are shown in **Table 3**.

In 2005, the investigators of the DCCT and its Epidemiology of Diabetes Interventions and Complications (EDIC) follow-up study reported cardiovascular results from 10 years of observation after cessation of the randomized treatment comparison.[25] Participants in EDIC were not assigned to different regimens and maintained similar levels of glycemic control, with mean A1c levels that were slightly less than 8%. This observational study showed that the group previously using intensive insulin therapy had a statistically significant 42% reduction ($P = .02$) of risk of the broad cardiovascular composite end point used in the prior analysis. The commonly used composite of cardiovascular death, nonfatal myocardial infarction, or nonfatal stroke was reduced by 56% ($P = .02$) in the prior intensive group. A later report from EDIC showed that large reductions (53%–59%) of retinopathy progression in the prior intensive group persisted after 10 years of follow-up.[26]

Similarly, in 2008, the UKPDS investigators reported their 10-year follow-up findings.[27] The participants previously randomized to different therapies in the main UKPDS study had mean A1c levels that converged at approximately 8.0% during the period of follow-up. The risk ratio for various end points was lower in the prior insulin or sulfonylurea-treated group than in the conventionally treated group: 13% lower ($P = .007$) for all-cause mortality, 15% for myocardial infarction ($P = .01$), and

	Age at Entry (y)	Age After Randomized Treatment (y)	Age at 10 More Years of Follow-up (y)	Reduction of Microvascular End Points More than 17 y (%)	Reduction of Cardiovascular Events Over 17 y (%)
DCCT and EDIC[25]	27	34	44	Retinopathy 3-step progression 53–59 (P<.0001)	CV composite 42 (P = .02) CV death, MI, or CVA 57 (P = .02)
UKPDS[10,11] and UKPDS follow-up[27]	54	63	73	Aggregate microvascular 24 (P<.001)	Myocardial infarction 15 (P = .01) All-cause death 27 (P = .002)

Table 3
Effect of treatments on microvascular end points and cardiovascular events at the end of randomized treatment and 10 years later in the DCCT and UKPDS

24% for a microvascular composite ($P = .001$). In contrast with the end of randomized treatment, the mortality and myocardial infarction differences became statistically significant during the observational follow-up period because of the accrual of more events, whereas the relative differences between treatment groups were almost unchanged.

CONCEPTS DERIVED FROM EXPERIENCE WITH LARGE MEDICAL END POINT TRIALS TO DATE

The information obtained by long-term observation of participants in DCCT/EDIC and UKPDS sheds light on the findings from randomized treatment in ADVANCE, ACCORD, and VADT. Consider the following conclusions suggested by the 17-year to 20-year follow-up of the earlier trials together with short-term data from the more recent ones.

Early Treatment Reduces Complications

Glycemic intervention early in the natural history of diabetes, achieving A1c levels close to 7%, can (as hypothesized from epidemiologic data) reduce long-term risks of both microvascular and macrovascular events. However, the ~50% reduction of cardiovascular complications observed in DCCT/EDIC 10 years after cessation of 6.5 years of intensive therapy must be confirmed by further follow-up studies, especially because the mean age of participants at the time of this finding was only about 45 years. The UKPDS follow-up found quantitatively smaller reductions of cardiovascular events but also verified significant reduction of mortality.

Beneficial Effects of Treatment Persist for Years

Intensive glycemic treatment early in diabetes has a beneficial momentum that can persist for a decade or more, even when later treatment is less intensive. The DCCT/EDIC investigators suggested the term metabolic memory,[25,28] whereas the UKPDS investigators proposed the term legacy effect for this phenomenon.[27]

Harmful Effects of Preceding Poor Metabolic Control also Persist

A reverse legacy effect may also exist. Intensive glycemic intervention started late in the natural course of diabetes seems disappointingly ineffective in limiting cardiovascular events. That is, established cardiovascular disease that includes structural abnormalities (complex atheromatous plaques, diffusely sclerotic blood vessels) may no longer be reversible. Ineffective management of hyperglycemia, dyslipidemia, and hypertension may have caused or accelerated the development of these lesions, but improving metabolic control once these lesions are established may have little ability to reduce subsequent risk of clinically apparent cardiovascular events.

Intensive Intervention has Risks as well as Benefits

Vigorous treatment of hyperglycemia, like most forms of treatment, has risks and these may be more apparent in some individuals than others. Long duration of diabetes, which is often accompanied by significant injury to myocardial, neural, renal, and cognitive function, may expose patients to increased risk in addition to reduced benefit from treatment. The hazards include severe hypoglycemia and increased risk of unexplained cardiovascular death, as found in the ACCORD trial. Intensive glycemic treatment late in the course of type 2 diabetes, especially in individuals selected for high cardiovascular risk, may lead to some benefits but these may be offset by adverse effects. Thus, individualization of treatment aiming to improve the benefit/risk ratio seems necessary in this setting, and new forms of treatment may facilitate this.

A1c LEVELS DURING THE NATURAL HISTORY OF TYPE 2 DIABETES: EVOLVING PATTERNS

The observations summarized earlier and the hypotheses derived from them have clinical implications. Among these are the potential for identifying high-risk subgroups and for developing safer and more effective therapies; these are beyond the scope of this article. Another application of these findings might be a new way of defining glycemic goals for insulin therapy.

Fig. 2 shows 3 possible patterns of glycemic control as reflected by A1c levels during the natural history of type 2 diabetes in a typical patient. The first pattern (see Fig. 2A) is adapted from an earlier review[29] and depicts experience that is consistent with clinical reports published up to around 2000,[30] an interval of time mostly preceding the application of epidemiologic findings and the results of the DCCT and UKPDS to specific goals for A1c. The figure illustrates vulnerability to developing gestational diabetes in young adulthood. In the hypothetical person shown, the diagnosis of diabetes was made at age 50 years but was preceded by a period of unrecognized hyperglycemia during which diabetic complications may have begun.[17] This possibility is supported by data from patients recruited for the UKPDS at the time of diagnosis of type 2 diabetes at mean age 52 years.[31] Of these newly diagnosed patients, 21% had retinopathy detected by fundoscopy, 18% an abnormal electrocardiogram, and 13% absent foot pulses. The mean level of A1c at diagnosis and entry into the run-in period that determined eligibility for randomization in the UKPDS was 11.6%.[31] As in the UKPDS, initial treatment with lifestyle and an oral agent usually causes a good therapeutic response but, in many individuals, intensification of

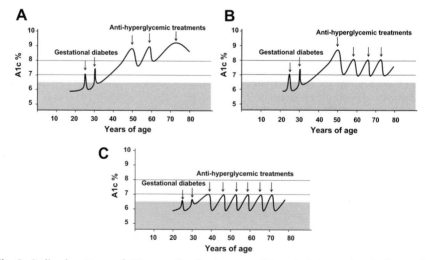

Fig. 2. Stylized patterns of A1c over the time course of type 2 diabetes, in relation to the time of diagnosis and therapeutic interventions. (*A*) A pattern typical of clinical experience before 1990. (*B*) A pattern typical of experience in the interval between 1990 and 2012. (*C*) A hypothetical pattern that might reflect future alteration of the natural history of type 2 diabetes, with timely diagnosis and early intensification of treatment.

treatment has been delayed until A1c levels had again risen to more than 8.0%. This delay has been termed clinical inertia.[32] Hence, before 2000, the diagnosis of diabetes was frequently made years after the onset of overt diabetes, complications were often present at the time of diagnosis, improvements of A1c levels by treatment were seldom sustained, and patients often had A1c levels between 8% and 9% for much of the time after the onset of diabetes.

The second pattern (see **Fig. 2**B) depicts the A1c levels that have been sought during the last decade. The DCCT and UKPDS findings strongly influenced the recommendations of expert groups, with an A1c level of 7.0% being most often identified as the goal of treatment.[3] Concurrently, cross-sectional studies of adults with known diabetes (including some treated with diet only) showed that mean levels of A1c decreased from nearly 8% in 2000 to 7.1% to 7.2% in 2006 and about half of these persons were maintaining A1c levels at 7.0% or less.[33–35] This trend suggests that efforts to achieve an A1c level of 7% have frequently led to the intensification of therapy when the A1c level was around 8.0%. How much of the observed improvement of mean A1c levels has been caused by successful use of this therapeutic approach and how much to earlier diagnosis of diabetes is less clear. Information is limited about the period of time before diagnosis of diabetes or the frequency of complications that are already present at diagnosis.

The third pattern (see **Fig. 2**C) suggests A1c levels that might possibly be achieved if at-risk persons were routinely screened to diagnose diabetes soon after the onset of hyperglycemia. In this speculative scenario, therapy is started before A1c levels have risen to more than 7.0%, or soon after that, with the intention of preventing the earliest accrual of tissue injury. In this setting, an A1c level of 7.0% might be viewed not as a goal of treatment started at much higher levels, but as a threshold at which intensification of treatment should be considered. Hypothetically, for recently diagnosed patients, this strategy would produce a high ratio of benefit to risk and would be easy to implement.

INDIVIDUALIZATION OF INSULIN THERAPY FOR TYPE 2 DIABETES: NEW GOALS, NEW TACTICS

Both the reality of managing persons with well-established diabetes and the potential for earlier and more consistently effective treatment require further attention. The pattern of glycemic control over time shown in **Fig. 2**A should be relegated to history, but that in **Fig. 2**B continues to be appropriate for many patients. The demonstration of excess mortality accompanying more intensive glycemic management in a subgroup of participants in ACCORD calls for caution in further intensifying glycemic therapy using currently available methods of treatment once A1c levels between 7.0% and 8.0% have been established. Such individuals are presumably common among groups with long duration of diabetes,[20,36] known prior cardiovascular events,[24,36] and a history of prior A1c levels in excess of 8.5%.[37] Intensifying treatment of these persons when A1c levels are greater than 8.0%, using insulin when necessary, with the aim of maintaining glycemic control between 7.0% and 8.0% is consistent with the method used in the standard treatment group in ACCORD.[22,38] Using this method, the ACCORD standard therapy participants achieved a median A1c level of 7.5%.[22]

However, failing to seek near-normal glycemic control in the large number of lower-risk persons with type 2 diabetes is difficult to justify. Experience in the DCCT and the UKPDS suggests that patients with recently diagnosed diabetes and without other significant illnesses deserve treatment to prevent increases in A1c levels to more than 7.0%, with the aim of maintaining the pattern shown in **Fig. 2**C. The median level of A1c in the insulin and sulfonylurea group of the UKPDS during randomized treatment was 7.0%, but the level in the first year after randomization was near 6.0% and the level 10 years later was nearer to 8.0%. However, this pattern of control resulted from initial allocation to monotherapy with agents that are now outdated (ultralente insulin, glyburide, and chlorpropamide), and progression to combination therapy regimens occurred only later in the study. With appropriate use of newer agents such as GLP-1 receptor agonists,[39–42] DPP-4 inhibitors,[39,43,44] or amylin receptor agonists[45,46] in complementary combinations with other agents, including insulin, long-term maintenance of A1c levels between 6.0% and 7.0% without excessive risks may be achievable, especially when treatment is started when A1c levels have not yet risen to more than 7.0%. At the least, this is a testable hypothesis.

However, the difficulties are in the details of such proposals. How can high-risk individuals who have less potential for benefit and perhaps higher risk from targeting A1c levels lower than 7.0% be reliably identified, and how can these persons be matched to current and future forms of therapy that are best suited to them? What therapies are appropriate for lower-risk persons with newly diagnosed adult-onset diabetes, and, specifically, what may be the role of insulin? The first of these questions has been addressed in part already, but the second deserves further comment here. Insulin therapy is relevant in 3 common clinical scenarios early in type 2 diabetes.

Late-onset Type 1 Diabetes

There is an extensive literature on the significant population of persons who develop insulin-deficient diabetes in adulthood.[47] Type 1 diabetes with onset before age 20 years accounts for about 10% of all cases of diabetes in North America, but an approximately equal number of older persons develop a similar disorder, commonly termed latent autoimmune diabetes in adulthood (LADA).[48–50] How the adult-onset version differs from typical type 1 diabetes is debatable, but its tendency to progress more rapidly to insulin dependency than type 2 diabetes is well documented. In the UKPDS, 12% of participants had glutamic acid decarboxylase (GAD) or other anti-islet antibodies at study entry, and the presence of these antibodies was a strong predictor of requirement for insulin therapy both immediately and over the course of 10 years of follow-up.[51] Moreover, a subset of participants in the DCCT had residual β-cell function, and ~90% of these were older than 18 years at diagnosis.[52] These patients with adult-onset type 1 with residual β-cell function retained endogenous insulin secretion longer when assigned to intensive, compared with standard, insulin therapy. Patients diagnosed with diabetes in adulthood can be identified as having LADA by measurement of islet cell or anti-GAD antibodies, and the need for testing may be suggested by clinical features common to this type of diabetes. These features include a family history of type 1 diabetes or other autoimmune syndromes, lack of family history of type 2 diabetes, lack of history of gestational diabetes, and rapid onset before age 40 years in nonobese persons. Such patients may not respond well to early treatment with regimens designed for type 2 diabetes, and, when insulin therapy is needed, it should not be delayed. Attention to sustained early increases of A1c levels to more than 7.0% despite conventional oral therapies would do much to address this need.

Symptomatic Hyperglycemia at Diagnosis

Patients are often diagnosed with type 2 diabetes because of symptoms associated with marked hyperglycemia. Textbooks often refer to excessive urination, thirst, and hunger as cardinal features, but probably just as common are fatigue, mental sluggishness, and skin infections. A1c levels greater than 10% accompanied by symptoms at diagnosis suggest possible late-onset type 1 diabetes, but typical type 2 diabetes can present this way as well. In these patients, treatment with diet and oral therapies may be ineffective because of insulin resistance and reduced β-cell function caused by poor metabolic control (glucolipotoxicity).[53,54] Short-term intensive insulin therapy has long been known to produce prompt symptomatic relief and to reduce many physiologic abnormalities, leading in some cases to a sustained remission of diabetes.[55–57] Recent reports have verified this possibility in larger populations.[58,59] Some evidence suggests that β-cell function may be better retained after early intensive insulin therapy for type 2 diabetes followed by oral therapy compared with oral therapy alone.[59]

Diagnosis at the Time of a Cardiovascular Event

Because obesity and related metabolic disorders predispose both to diabetes and to cardiovascular disease, diabetes is frequently diagnosed at the time of a cardiovascular event.[60,61] Intravenous insulin therapy is usually advised for treatment of hyperglycemia at such times. Physiologic and clinical studies provide a strong rationale for this, including evidence that the severity of myocardial injury and other complications may be reduced by timely administration of insulin.[62–65] One early study suggested that intensive insulin treatment at the time of a myocardial infarction in persons with known diabetes reduces short-term mortality, and possibly also the risk of death from a subsequent infarction (case fatality). However, other studies have not confirmed these observations.[66,67]

A large, ongoing clinical trial based partly on the foregoing rationale is studying the effects of basal insulin treatment early in type 2 diabetes in patients with high cardiovascular risk, most of whom have already had a cardiovascular event. The Outcome Reduction with an Initial Glargine Intervention (ORIGIN) trial has enrolled more than 12,500 participants with either type 2 diabetes treated with lifestyle with or without 1 oral agent.[68] Of the participants enrolled, 82% had previously known diabetes with a mean duration of 6 years, whereas the remaining 18% had either newly diagnosed diabetes, impaired glucose tolerance, or impaired fasting glucose levels. The mean A1c level in the whole population at study entry was 6.5%. High risk of cardiovascular events was required for study entry, and two-thirds of the population had a previous cardiovascular event. Participants were randomized to treatment with glargine targeting FPG levels of less than 95 mg/dL (5.3 mmol/L) or to standard step therapy with oral agents targeting A1c levels as considered customary at each site, generally less than 7.0%. The primary end point of the glycemic treatment comparison in ORIGIN is the composite of cardiovascular death, nonfatal myocardial infarction, or nonfatal stroke, but proteinuria, hypoglycemia, and progression of dysglycemic participants to overt diabetes will be studied as well. This trial ended in late 2011 after 7 years of randomized treatment, and the results have the potential to define both the risks and benefits of early use of basal insulin in the setting of high cardiovascular risk. A favorable balance of benefits versus risks in ORIGIN might support the early use of insulin in type 2 diabetes to prevent A1c levels from increasing to more than 7.0%, even for patients with established cardiovascular disease.

SUMMARY

The views of the last 2 decades are changing to a new approach to type 2 diabetes. The most compelling finding of long-term observations from the DCCT and UKPDS is that intensive glycemic control established early in the natural history of diabetes has a favorable benefit/risk ratio, but that 10 or more years are required to see the full effects. The more recent clinical trials (ADVANCE, ACCORD, and VADT) showed that vigorous therapeutic efforts applied too late may yield limited short-term benefit, and may even cause more harm than benefit. That is, achieving near-normal glucose control in high-risk individuals may lead to increased cardiovascular mortality, the result that these trials were designed to prevent. Although the cause of increased cardiovascular risk accompanying intensive treatment remains uncertain, weight gain and hypoglycemia, both known consequences of insulin therapy, are obvious candidates. Thus, both glycemic treatment goals and the tactics used to achieve them require closer evaluation. For the present, while awaiting further evidence from analyses of completed studies and new findings from studies that are underway or in planning, we propose 3 courses of action.

First, for patients with 10 or more years' duration of suboptimally controlled type 2 diabetes and known microvascular or macrovascular complications, achieving A1c levels less than 7.0% may not be an appropriate goal. For such patients, similar to those who participated in ACCORD and the VADT, A1c levels between 7.0% and 8.0% may be appropriate as the target range in most cases, with 8.0% serving as the level at which to intensify treatment.

Second, for patients with newly recognized type 2 diabetes or A1c values known to be less than 8.0% most of the time since diagnosis, a usual target range between 6.0% and 7.0% may be appropriate, with intensification of treatment at any level more than 7.0%. How to treat patients with intermediate duration of diabetes and mild complications, or with long duration but with no apparent complications, is less clear and calls for further study.

Third, more information about the risks and benefits of all forms of therapy, including insulin, is urgently needed. Improved methods of epidemiologic analysis are now being brought to bear on this question, and several large studies longer than 3 years in duration are now underway testing various agents and their roles in the management of diabetes. Categories of patients for whom each of the main classes of agents (metformin, glucagonlike-peptide-1 agonists, insulins, and others) are preferred may soon be identified. Evidence is accumulating to suggest that use of insulin earlier in the natural history of adult-onset diabetes may be desirable, as in cases of LADA and diabetes presenting with acute illness or after a cardiovascular event. An increased level of detail, describing goals and tactics specific to different groups of patients, may soon be provided in clinical practice recommendations by professional advisory groups.

No one promised that the management of complex chronic diseases like diabetes would be straightforward. Hippocrates was right: "Life is short, and the Art long; the crisis fleeting, experiment perilous, and decision difficult."[69] However, efforts to better manage patients with diabetes continue to progress.

REFERENCES

1. Meinert CL, Knatterud GL, Prout TE, et al. A study of the effects of hypoglycemic agents on vascular complications in patients with adult-onset diabetes. II. Mortality results. Diabetes 1970;19(Suppl):789–830.
2. American Diabetes Association. Report of the expert committee on the diagnosis and classification of diabetes mellitus. Diabetes Care 1997;20:1183–97.
3. American Diabetes Association. Standards of medical care in diabetes–2012. Diabetes Care 2012;35(Suppl 1):S11–63.
4. Milicevic Z, Raz I, Beattie SD, et al. Natural history of cardiovascular disease in patients with diabetes: role of hyperglycemia. Diabetes Care 2008;31(Suppl 2): S155–60.

5. Saydah S, Tao M, Imperatore G, et al. GHb level and subsequent mortality among adults in the U.S. Diabetes Care 2009;32:1440–6.
6. Stratton IM, Adler AI, Neil HA, et al. Association of glycaemia with macrovascular and microvascular complications of type 2 diabetes (UKPDS 35): prospective observational study. BMJ 2000;321:405–12.
7. Sung J, Song YM, Ebrahim S, et al. Fasting blood glucose and the risk of stroke and myocardial infarction. Circulation 2009;119:812–9.
8. Sarwar N, Gao P, Seshasai SR, et al. Diabetes mellitus, fasting blood glucose concentration, and risk of vascular disease: a collaborative meta-analysis of 102 prospective studies. Lancet 2010;375:2215–22.
9. The Diabetes Control and Complications Trial Research Group. The effect of intensive treatment of diabetes on the development and progression of long-term complications in insulin-dependent diabetes mellitus. The Diabetes Control and Complications Trial Research Group. N Engl J Med 1993;329:977–86.
10. United Kingdom Prospective Study Group. Effect of intensive blood-glucose control with metformin on complications in overweight patients with type 2 diabetes (UKPDS 34). UK Prospective Diabetes Study (UKPDS) Group. Lancet 1998;352:854–65.
11. United Kingdom Prospective Study Group. Intensive blood-glucose control with sulphonylureas or insulin compared with conventional treatment and risk of complications in patients with type 2 diabetes (UKPDS 33). UK Prospective Diabetes Study (UKPDS) Group. Lancet 1998;352:837–53.
12. Feingold KR, Browner WS, Siperstein MD. Prospective studies of muscle capillary basement membrane width in prediabetics. J Clin Endocrinol Metab 1989;69:784–9.
13. Williamson JR, Kilo C. Vascular complications in diabetes mellitus. N Engl J Med 1980;302:399–400.
14. The Diabetes Control and Complications Trial Research Group. Epidemiology of severe hypoglycemia in the Diabetes Control and Complications Trial. The DCCT Research Group. Am J Med 1991;90:450–9.
15. Wredling R, Levander S, Adamson U, et al. Permanent neuropsychological impairment after recurrent episodes of severe hypoglycaemia in man. Diabetologia 1990;33:152–7.
16. Wright A, Burden AC, Paisey RB, et al. Sulfonylurea inadequacy: efficacy of addition of insulin over 6 years in patients with type 2 diabetes in the U.K. Prospective Diabetes Study (UKPDS 57). Diabetes Care 2002;25:330–6.
17. Harris MI, Klein R, Welborn TA, et al. Onset of NIDDM occurs at least 4-7 yr before clinical diagnosis. Diabetes Care 1992;15:815–9.
18. Gerstein HC, Miller ME, Byington RP, et al. Effects of intensive glucose lowering in type 2 diabetes. N Engl J Med 2008;358:2545–59.
19. Patel A, MacMahon S, Chalmers J, et al. Intensive blood glucose control and vascular outcomes in patients with type 2 diabetes. N Engl J Med 2008;358:2560–72.
20. Duckworth W, Abraira C, Moritz T, et al. Glucose control and vascular complications in veterans with type 2 diabetes. N Engl J Med 2009;360:129–39.
21. Chew EY, Ambrosius WT, Davis MD, et al. Effects of medical therapies on retinopathy progression in type 2 diabetes. N Engl J Med 2010;363:233–44.
22. Gerstein HC, Miller ME, Genuth S, et al. Long-term effects of intensive glucose lowering on cardiovascular outcomes. N Engl J Med 2011;364:818–28.
23. Zoungas S, Patel A, Chalmers J, et al. Severe hypoglycemia and risks of vascular events and death. N Engl J Med 2010;363:1410–8.

24. Turnbull FM, Abraira C, Anderson RJ, et al. Intensive glucose control and macrovascular outcomes in type 2 diabetes. Diabetologia 2009;52:2288–98.
25. Nathan DM, Cleary PA, Backlund JY, et al. Intensive diabetes treatment and cardiovascular disease in patients with type 1 diabetes. N Engl J Med 2005; 353:2643–53.
26. White NH, Sun W, Cleary PA, et al. Prolonged effect of intensive therapy on the risk of retinopathy complications in patients with type 1 diabetes mellitus: 10 years after the Diabetes Control and Complications Trial. Arch Ophthalmol 2008;126:1707–15.
27. Holman RR, Paul SK, Bethel MA, et al. 10-year follow-up of intensive glucose control in type 2 diabetes. N Engl J Med 2008;359:1577–89.
28. Lind M, Oden A, Fahlen M, et al. The shape of the metabolic memory of HbA1c: re-analysing the DCCT with respect to time-dependent effects. Diabetologia 2010;53:1093–8.
29. Riddle MC. Tactics for type II diabetes. Endocrinol Metab Clin North Am 1997;26: 659–77.
30. Koro CE, Bowlin SJ, Bourgeois N, et al. Glycemic control from 1988 to 2000 among U.S. adults diagnosed with type 2 diabetes: a preliminary report. Diabetes Care 2004;27:17–20.
31. United Kingdom Prospective Study Group. UK Prospective Diabetes Study 7: response of fasting plasma glucose to diet therapy in newly presenting type II diabetic patients, UKPDS Group. Metabolism 1990;39:905–12.
32. Brown JB, Nichols GA, Perry A. The burden of treatment failure in type 2 diabetes. Diabetes Care 2004;27:1535–40.
33. Cheung BM, Ong KL, Cherny SS, et al. Diabetes prevalence and therapeutic target achievement in the United States, 1999 to 2006. Am J Med 2009;122:443–53.
34. Mann DM, Woodward M, Ye F, et al. Trends in medication use among US adults with diabetes mellitus: glycemic control at the expense of controlling cardiovascular risk factors. Arch Intern Med 2009;169:1718–20.
35. McWilliams JM, Meara E, Zaslavsky AM, et al. Differences in control of cardiovascular disease and diabetes by race, ethnicity, and education: U.S. trends from 1999 to 2006 and effects of Medicare coverage. Ann Intern Med 2009;150:505–15.
36. Ismail-Beigi F, Moghissi E, Tiktin M, et al. Individualizing glycemic targets in type 2 diabetes mellitus: implications of recent clinical trials. Ann Intern Med 2011;154: 554–9.
37. Calles-Escandon J, Lovato LC, Simons-Morton DG, et al. Effect of intensive compared with standard glycemia treatment strategies on mortality by baseline subgroup characteristics: the Action to Control Cardiovascular Risk in Diabetes (ACCORD) trial. Diabetes Care 2010;33:721–7.
38. Gerstein HC, Riddle MC, Kendall DM, et al. Glycemia treatment strategies in the Action to Control Cardiovascular Risk in Diabetes (ACCORD) trial. Am J Cardiol 2007;99:34i–43i.
39. Arnolds S, Dellweg S, Clair J, et al. Further improvement in postprandial glucose control with addition of exenatide or sitagliptin to combination therapy with insulin glargine and metformin: a proof-of-concept study. Diabetes Care 2010;33:1509–15.
40. Buse JB, Bergenstal RM, Glass LC, et al. Use of twice-daily exenatide in Basal insulin-treated patients with type 2 diabetes: a randomized, controlled trial. Ann Intern Med 2011;154:103–12.
41. Kendall DM, Riddle MC, Rosenstock J, et al. Effects of exenatide (exendin-4) on glycemic control over 30 weeks in patients with type 2 diabetes treated with metformin and a sulfonylurea. Diabetes Care 2005;28:1083–91.

42. Russell-Jones D, Vaag A, Schmitz O, et al. Liraglutide vs insulin glargine and placebo in combination with metformin and sulfonylurea therapy in type 2 diabetes mellitus (LEAD-5 met+SU): a randomised controlled trial. Diabetologia 2009;52:2046–55.

43. DeFronzo RA, Hissa MN, Garber AJ, et al. The efficacy and safety of saxagliptin when added to metformin therapy in patients with inadequately controlled type 2 diabetes with metformin alone. Diabetes Care 2009;32:1649–55.

44. Vilsboll T, Rosenstock J, Yki-Jarvinen H, et al. Efficacy and safety of sitagliptin when added to insulin therapy in patients with type 2 diabetes. Diabetes Obes Metab 2010;12:167–77.

45. Riddle M, Frias J, Zhang B, et al. Pramlintide improved glycemic control and reduced weight in patients with type 2 diabetes using basal insulin. Diabetes Care 2007;30:2794–9.

46. Riddle M, Pencek R, Charenkavanich S, et al. Randomized comparison of pramlintide or mealtime insulin added to basal insulin treatment for patients with type 2 diabetes. Diabetes Care 2009;32:1577–82.

47. Fourlanos S, Dotta F, Greenbaum CJ, et al. Latent autoimmune diabetes in adults (LADA) should be less latent. Diabetologia 2005;48:2206–12.

48. Borg H, Gottsater A, Landin-Olsson M, et al. High levels of antigen-specific islet antibodies predict future beta-cell failure in patients with onset of diabetes in adult age. J Clin Endocrinol Metab 2001;86:3032–8.

49. Gottsater A, Landin-Olsson M, Fernlund P, et al. Beta-cell function in relation to islet cell antibodies during the first 3 yr after clinical diagnosis of diabetes in type II diabetic patients. Diabetes Care 1993;16:902–10.

50. Zimmet P. Antibodies to glutamic acid decarboxylase in the prediction of insulin dependency. Diabetes Res Clin Pract 1996;34(Suppl):S125–31.

51. Davis TM, Wright AD, Mehta ZM, et al. Islet autoantibodies in clinically diagnosed type 2 diabetes: prevalence and relationship with metabolic control (UKPDS 70). Diabetologia 2005;48:695–702.

52. The Diabetes Control and Complications Trial Research Group. Effect of intensive therapy on residual beta-cell function in patients with type 1 diabetes in the Diabetes Control and Complications Trial. A randomized, controlled trial. The Diabetes Control and Complications Trial Research Group. Ann Intern Med 1998; 128:517–23.

53. Poitout V, Robertson RP. Glucolipotoxicity: fuel excess and beta-cell dysfunction. Endocr Rev 2008;29:351–66.

54. Yki-Jarvinen H. Glucose toxicity. Endocr Rev 1992;13:415–31.

55. Garvey WT, Olefsky JM, Griffin J, et al. The effect of insulin treatment on insulin secretion and insulin action in type II diabetes mellitus. Diabetes 1985;34: 222–34.

56. Ilkova H, Glaser B, Tunckale A, et al. Induction of long-term glycemic control in newly diagnosed type 2 diabetic patients by transient intensive insulin treatment. Diabetes Care 1997;20:1353–6.

57. Ryan EA, Imes S, Wallace C. Short-term intensive insulin therapy in newly diagnosed type 2 diabetes. Diabetes Care 2004;27:1028–32.

58. Li Y, Xu W, Liao Z, et al. Induction of long-term glycemic control in newly diagnosed type 2 diabetic patients is associated with improvement of beta-cell function. Diabetes Care 2004;27:2597–602.

59. Weng J, Li Y, Xu W, et al. Effect of intensive insulin therapy on beta-cell function and glycaemic control in patients with newly diagnosed type 2 diabetes: a multicentre randomised parallel-group trial. Lancet 2008;371:1753–60.

60. Bartnik M, Ryden L, Ferrari R, et al. The prevalence of abnormal glucose regulation in patients with coronary artery disease across Europe. The Euro Heart Survey on Diabetes and the Heart. Eur Heart J 2004;25:1880–90.
61. Norhammar A, Tenerz A, Nilsson G, et al. Glucose metabolism in patients with acute myocardial infarction and no previous diagnosis of diabetes mellitus: a prospective study. Lancet 2002;359:2140–4.
62. Chaudhuri A, Janicke D, Wilson MF, et al. Anti-inflammatory and profibrinolytic effect of insulin in acute ST-segment-elevation myocardial infarction. Circulation 2004;109:849–54.
63. Malmberg K, Ryden L, Efendic S, et al. Randomized trial of insulin-glucose infusion followed by subcutaneous insulin treatment in diabetic patients with acute myocardial infarction (DIGAMI study): effects on mortality at 1 year. J Am Coll Cardiol 1995;26:57–65.
64. Malmberg K, Ryden L, Hamsten A, et al. Effects of insulin treatment on cause-specific one-year mortality and morbidity in diabetic patients with acute myocardial infarction. DIGAMI Study Group. Diabetes Insulin-Glucose in Acute Myocardial Infarction. Eur Heart J 1996;17:1337–44.
65. Szabo Z, Arnqvist H, Hakanson E, et al. Effects of high-dose glucose-insulin-potassium on myocardial metabolism after coronary surgery in patients with type II diabetes. Clin Sci (Lond) 2001;101:37–43.
66. Ceremuzynski L, Budaj A, Czepiel A, et al. Low-dose glucose-insulin-potassium is ineffective in acute myocardial infarction: results of a randomized multicenter Pol-GIK trial. Cardiovasc Drugs Ther 1999;13:191–200.
67. Mehta SR, Yusuf S, Diaz R, et al. Effect of glucose-insulin-potassium infusion on mortality in patients with acute ST-segment elevation myocardial infarction: the CREATE-ECLA randomized controlled trial. JAMA 2005;293:437–46.
68. Gerstein H, Yusuf S, Riddle MC, et al. Rationale, design, and baseline characteristics for a large international trial of cardiovascular disease prevention in people with dysglycemia: the ORIGIN Trial (Outcome Reduction with an Initial Glargine Intervention). Am Heart J 2008;155:26–32, 32.e21–6.
69. Hippocrates. Aphorisms. In: Lloyd GER, editor. Hippocratic writings. Middlesex (England): Pelican Books Ltd.; 1978. p. 206.

Insulin Therapy and Hypoglycemia

Anthony L. McCall, MD, PhD

KEYWORDS

- Hypoglycemia • Diabetes type 1 • Diabetes type 2
- Insulin therapy

Hypoglycemia impedes safe achievement of optimal glycemia. The benefits of nearly normal glycemia in reducing microvascular diabetes complications are clear, although the benefits and risk-to-benefit ratio for macrovascular disease is contentious and complex. Overall achievement of excellent glycemia seems beneficial to cardiovascular risk when implemented early in the course of both type 1 and type 2 diabetes. Despite strong evidence of likely benefit, those trying to decrease the risk of microvascular complications through intensive glycemic control inevitably face a 3-fold increased risk of severe hypoglycemia, often without warning symptoms and potentially with severe consequences, especially to heart and brain. This is especially true for those with type 1 diabetes mellitus (DM) but also for insulin-deficient patients with type 2 DM (**Fig. 1**).

Studies of glycemic control and diabetes complications before ACCORD (Action to Control Cardiovascular Risk in Diabetes),[1] ADVANCE (Action in Diabetes to Prevent Vascular Disease),[2] and VADT (Veterans Administration Diabetes Trial)[3] indicate that severe hypoglycemia is less common with tight glycemic control in type 2 (see **Fig. 1**, left) when compared with type 1 DM (see **Fig. 1**, right). Studies of type 1, such as the DCCT (Diabetes Control and Complications Trial), show that severe insulin reactions occur up to severalfold more than 60 per 100 patient-years and have a three-fold increased risk relative to those of control groups with less intensive glucose control. Studies of type 2 diabetes, by contrast, found a risk of severe hypoglycemia with tight glycemic control that was substantially less. It is noteworthy, however, that some studies found an overlap in frequency indicating that some type 2 DM[4–12] patients have a risk comparable with that seen with intensive control in type 1 DM.[13–18]

Optimal glycemia goals must be individualized, but may be generally defined as hemoglobin A_{1c} (HgbA$_{1c}$) of less than 7% (**Table 1**) as recommended by the American Diabetes Association (ADA).[19] A simplified summary is to achieve the best possible control by trying to achieve control that is as tight as possible, as early as possible, as safely as possible, for as long as possible. This goal and this strategy are based

Division of Endocrinology, University of Virginia School of Medicine, 450 Ray C. Hunt Drive, Charlottesville, VA 22903, USA
E-mail address: alm3j@virginia.edu

Endocrinol Metab Clin N Am 41 (2012) 57–87
doi:10.1016/j.ecl.2012.03.001
0889-8529/12/$ – see front matter © 2012 Elsevier Inc. All rights reserved.

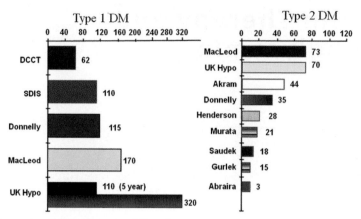

Fig. 1. Severe insulin reactions per 100 patient years.

on evidence from studies in both type 1 and type 2 DM, such as the DCCT and the UKPDS (United Kingdom Prospective Diabetes Study) and their long-term follow-up.[20–22] Moreover, this level of control is more achievable than ever with the panoply of therapies available. Because of negative results from 3 studies of tight control and cardiovascular end points in type 2 diabetes,[1–3] caution is urged in application of tight glycemic control for those with long diabetes duration, advanced complications, or multiple comorbidities. Newer insulins and strategies, such as insulin pumps and continuous glucose monitoring in type 1 DM, and use of drugs combined with insulin that enhances glycemic control for type 2 DM with low hypoglycemia risk, make excellent control usually achievable.

The pathophysiology of hypoglycemia unawareness (inability to recognize hypoglycemia) and defective insulin counterregulation (weakened hormone defenses against hypoglycemia) remains under active investigation. The importance of hypoglycemia as

Table 1
American Diabetes Association 2011 summary of glycemic recommendations for many nonpregnant adults with diabetes

A_{1c} $\longrightarrow$	< 7.0%
Pre-prandial capillary BG $\longrightarrow$	70-130 mg/dl
Peak Post-prandial capillary BG $\longrightarrow$	< 180 mg/dl

Individualization	ALSO

Individualize goals based on:
    Duration of diabetes
    Age/life expectancy
    Comorbid conditions
    Known cardiovascular disease or
      advanced microvascular
      complications
    Hypoglycemia unawareness
    Individual patient considerations
	More or less stringent glycemic goals may be
	    appropriate for individual patients
	Postprandial glucose may be despite
	    reaching preprandial glucose goals

Adapted from American Diabetes Association. Standards of medical care in diabetes mellitus. Diabetes Care 2011;34(Suppl 1):S19.

a barrier to safe therapy has been confirmed in recent studies. Risk factors for severe hypoglycemia include: (1) prior severe hypoglycemia; (2) hypoglycemia unawareness; (3) defective insulin counterregulation; (4) age under 5 years and (5) being elderly; and (6) certain comorbid conditions such as renal disease, malnutrition, coronary heart disease, and liver disease. New minimally invasive continuous monitoring of glycemia, in addition to self-monitoring of blood glucose (SMBG) with finger-stick testing, shows promise in attaining better control with enhanced safety.[23–25] One hopes ongoing research can create an artificial pancreas that will emerge as a clinical therapeutic modality.[26] Providers and patients increasingly strive for excellent glycemic control while recognizing the dangers of hypoglycemia. Thus, continued emphasis on treatment strategies to reduce the frequency of hypoglycemia in practice is needed. Such emphasis and reduced glycemic variability permits safer achievement of optimal glycemia. This article reviews the risks of hypoglycemia and discusses how to use insulin alone or in combination to reduce that risk. Readers wishing more information on these subjects are referred to 2 excellent books.[27,28]

THE IMPORTANCE OF HYPOGLYCEMIA IN TYPE 1 DM

Hypoglycemia is a major backlash of insulin therapy and is the primary barrier to safe attainment of optimal glycemia in both type 1 and type 2 DM. There is an important Endocrine Society clinical practice guidelines statement about hypoglycemia that provides information on a variety of diagnostic and management issues.[29] Untold numbers of mild to moderate and sometimes asymptomatic hypoglycemic reactions occur in most patients with good control. As reviewed by Frier,[30] type 1 DM patients average severe hypoglycemic reactions 1 to 1.7 times per year. In unselected patients 30% to 40% have severe hypoglycemia, defined as requiring external help to treat, in a year compared with the DCCT, in which there were only 0.6 episodes per year, but DCCT patients were screened to rule history of severe hypoglycemia.[17] Hypoglycemia may also be related to weight gain and consequently increased cardiometabolic risk with intensive treatment.[31] In the DCCT a 2-point improvement in percent $HgbA_{1c}$ for 6.5 years reduced chronic diabetes microvascular and neuropathic complications by 50% or more. The increase or decrease in risk for intensive insulin therapy is given in **Table 2** for several parameters based on data from the DCCT.[17,20,31,32]

The DCCT

In the DCCT, despite dramatic benefits of tight control there was a 3-fold excess of severe hypoglycemia.[32] During follow-up of the 1441 patients, there were 3788 episodes of severe hypoglycemia. Of these, 1027 were associated with coma and/or seizure. Overall, 65% of patients in the intensive group and 35% of patients in the conventional group had at least one episode of severe hypoglycemia during the study. Several subgroups had a particularly high risk of severe hypoglycemia irrespective of their treatment group: (1) males, (2) adolescents, (3) those without residual C-peptide, and (4) those with prior severe hypoglycemia. These subgroups initially defined those at high risk for hypoglycemia with intensive therapy. Glycemic goals need adjustment upward for safety in such high-risk patients. Of note, $HgbA_{1c}$ was not a good predictor of hypoglycemia, predicting only about 8% of severe hypoglycemia over a 6-month period. This finding emphasizes a general principle that measures of central tendency in glycemia (means, medians, A_{1c}) are poor predictors of extremes of hypoglycemia and hyperglycemia.

Severe hypoglycemia in the DCCT and elsewhere is defined as requiring external assistance to recover. Similar to the DCCT, the Stockholm Diabetes Intervention

Table 2
Benefits and risks of glycemic control in the DCCT and EDIC trials

Reduction of Risk[17]	Increased Risk[32]
Primary prevention	Hypoglycemia
Retinopathy 76% (62%–85% CI)	Serious hypoglycemia RR of 3.28
Secondary prevention	Coma and seizures
Retinopathy 54% (39%–66% CI)	RR of 3.02
Combined cohorts	Hospitalization for hypoglycemia
Severe retinopathy 47% (14%–67% CI)	RR 1.5 (54 vs 36 hospitalizations)
Microalbuminuria (>40 mg/d)	Weight gain (4.6 kg > controls at 5 y)
39% (21%–52% CI)	RR of 1.33 for >120% of ideal BW
Albuminuria (>300 mg/d)	Weight-related metabolic abnormalities[30]
54% (19%–74% CI)	
Clinical neuropathy by 60% (38%–74% CI)	
Reduced risk of major cardiovascular events by 57% (EDIC)[20]	

Abbreviations: BW, body weight; CI, confidence interval; DCCT, Diabetes Control and Complications Trial; EDIC, Epidemiology of Diabetes Interventions and Complications trial; RR, relative risk.

Study (SDIS)[16] reported reduced risk for microvascular complications and increased risk of hypoglycemia with intensive glycemic control. There were 1.1 episodes of serious hypoglycemia with intensive treatment versus 0.4 episodes per patient per year.[16] Studies such as the DCCT[32] and SDIS[16] delineate the increased risk of hypoglycemia in tightly treated type 1 diabetic patients. The clinical question raised is how to recognize and reduce that risk. **Fig. 1** shows the frequency of severe hypoglycemia in several studies of type 1 diabetes.

Recognizing Hypoglycemia: Common Clinical Manifestations

Symptoms of hypoglycemia are usually divided into 2 main categories: (1) autonomic (sometimes called neurogenic or sympathoadrenal) and (2) neuroglycopenic, which means related to deprivation of brain fuel (**Box 1**). Normally, autonomic symptoms precede neuroglycopenic symptoms, that is, patients become shaky and sweaty before confusion sets in. A reversal of symptom order or loss of autonomic symptoms occurs in hypoglycemia unaware patients (part of the syndrome known as hypoglycemia-associated autonomic failure [HAAF]).[29] For example, some patients will perspire when markedly hypoglycemic only after an hour or more of mental slowing. **Box 1** shows the 2 major types of hypoglycemia symptoms; the autonomic symptoms (associated with hypoglycemia awareness) usually permit early warning and allow self-treatment, whereas neuroglycopenic symptoms (related to fuel deprivation of the brain) may result in inability to self treat. Retraining patients and families to recognize changing symptoms (blood glucose awareness training[33,34]) is a focus for research and shows promise as treatment for patients with problematic hypoglycemia. This educational approach is available over the Internet.

Common symptoms are divided into autonomic (associated with hypoglycemia awareness) and neuroglycopenic (related to fuel deprivation of the brain) symptoms.

Potential to harm the brain exists with repeated or severe hypoglycemia. Acute hypoglycemia has many clinical manifestations, not all of which are commonly

Box 1
Common symptoms of hypoglycemia
Autonomic
Cold sweats
Paresthesias
Fine tremor
Hunger
Palpitations
Anxiety
Neuroglycopenic
Confusion or slow mentation
Blurred vision or diplopia
General fatigue or weakness
Faint or dizzy feeling
Mood disturbance
Feeling of warmth

appreciated clinically, such as acute hemiparesis. A summary of some acute neurologic manifestations of severe hypoglycemia is given in **Table 3**.

Brain Vulnerability to Hypoglycemia

Repeated bouts of severe hypoglycemia may impair cognitive function or damage the brain. Deary and colleagues[35] found that of patients with type 1 DM and a history of severe hypoglycemia a slight but significant decline in IQ scores occurred in comparison with a matched control group. Perros and colleagues[36] compared magnetic resonance imaging (MRI) in 11 subjects with type 1 DM with no history of severe hypoglycemia with 11 type 1 DM patients with a history of 5 or more episodes of severe hypoglycemia, and found cortical atrophy in nearly half of those with a history of severe hypoglycemia ($P<.05$). Computed tomography and MRI have been used to show that the basal ganglia, cerebral cortex, substantia nigra, and hippocampus are vulnerable brain areas after profound, but sublethal hypoglycemia.[37] Hypoglycemia with seizures predicts cognitive dysfunction in diabetic children,[38,39] and early onset (<5 years old) of diabetes also portends cognitive problems.[40] One clinical concern raised by such findings is that repeated hypoglycemia may interfere with the complex

Table 3	
Neurologic manifestations of acute hypoglycemia	
Decortication	**Locked-In Syndrome**
Decerebration	Amnesia
Hemiplegia (transient)	Stroke
Choreoathetosis	Cortical atrophy
Ataxia	Peripheral neuropathy
Convulsions (generalized or focal)	Other focal neurologic abnormalities (pons, visual pathways)

task of managing insulin therapy in type 1 DM. This interference may result in a vicious cycle during which subtle neurocognitive dysfunction increases the risk of subsequent hypoglycemia. Recent work suggests that both uncontrolled hyperglycemia and repeated hypoglycemia may be risk factors for dementia in patients with DM.[41–43]

Hypoglycemia Unawareness

Hypoglycemia unawareness is associated with more profound cognitive dysfunction during hypoglycemia, as shown by Gold and colleagues.[44] Moreover, recovery of intellectual function was delayed significantly in those with hypoglycemia unawareness. Full neurocognitive recovery after severe hypoglycemia may take as long as a few days.[45]

Hypoglycemia and Sudden Death

While it has been emphasized that the brain is at risk from hypoglycemia, other organs, particularly the heart, may be affected, perhaps to a greater degree in type 2 DM.[46] Consequences of hypoglycemia include possible alterations in cardiac ventricular repolarization that could underlie sudden death.[47,48] Hypoglycemia creates a pro-thrombotic state[49] and may predispose to acute cardiac ischemia, as exemplified in the dual assessment of continuous glucose monitoring system and Holter monitors in the study of Desouza and colleagues[50]; ischemia may occur either in the coronary or cerebral circulation. Ischemic events may be more common in patients with type 2 diabetes or those with long-standing type 1 diabetes because of underlying athero-sclerosis. Surprisingly few reports of such events occur in the literature,[51,52] although they do occasionally occur in practice, with an acute hypoglycemic event appearing to trigger a myocardial infarction or a thrombotic stroke. One of the most feared conse-quences of hypoglycemia is the dead-in-bed syndrome.[53,54] A focus on both the potentially atherogenic effect of hypoglycemia[46] and abnormalities in the Q-T interval[48] after severe hypoglycemia are clear concerns raised by several investiga-tors, the latter perhaps important in light of the 22% increased mortality observed in the ACCORD trial.[1]

HYPOGLYCEMIA IN TYPE 2 DM

In general, hypoglycemia is thought to be less frequent and less severe in type 2 DM[29] than in type 1 DM (see **Fig. 1**). In part this might reflect a relative resistance to insulin action in type 2 DM, greater endogenous insulin secretion, and better-preserved counterregulation with protective responses at higher glucose levels.[55] For example, in the DCCT-like Kumamoto study of glycemic control and complications,[11] no severe hypoglycemia occurred and mild hypoglycemia was only slightly increased after inten-sive insulin therapy in type 2 DM patients. In the UKPDS,[12] symptomatic hypoglycemia occurred in about 30%, but severe hypoglycemia in only about 2%. **Fig. 1** shows that rates of severe hypoglycemia in studies of type 1 DM (left panel) are much greater than in type 2 DM (right panel), although overlap clearly occurs.

Three recent studies in type 2 diabetes, The VADT,[3] the ACCORD,[1] and the ADVANCE[2] trials (**Fig. 2** and **Table 4**), have influenced thoughts about type 2 DM and cardiac risk. The latter 2 have both found what seems to be a favorable adapta-tion[56,57] to tighter glycemic control, likely due to episodic moderate hypoglycemia. Although with intensive glycemic control the absolute risk of severe hypoglycemia is 2-fold to 3-fold greater, especially in the ACCORD trial, the relative risk of a poor outcome appears to be proportionately higher in those with poor rather than with tight control. Also, it should be noted that the severe hypoglycemia appears to be a marker

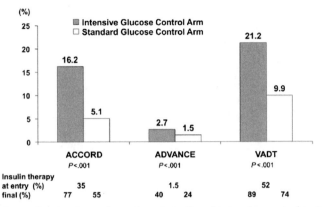

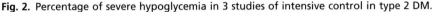

Fig. 2. Percentage of severe hypoglycemia in 3 studies of intensive control in type 2 DM.

of risk generally for numerous adverse outcomes, and has at least the potential to be a cause of severe outcomes especially in those who have overall poor glycemic control.

The high rates of hypoglycemia observed in the ACCORD and in the VADT remain a concern, with intensive therapy especially at a later stage of type 2 diabetes in comparison with the ADVANCE trial. It is noteworthy that there were much higher rates of insulin usage in the ACCORD and VADT studies.

Table 4 shows the clinical characteristics and the effects of intensive glucose lowering compared with standard therapy on a primary cardiovascular composite end point, total mortality, and cardiovascular mortality in the ACCORD, ADVANCE, and VADT studies. The bottom 3 rows of **Table 4** emphasize the absence of proven benefit to end points of cardiovascular disease, the worrisome increase in mortality observed in the ACCORD trial, and the equally worrisome increase in cardiovascular mortality in ACCORD. A concerning trend was also observed in the VADT trial, but this was not statistically significant.

Table 4 Summary of 3 major studies of intensive control in type 2 DM			
	ACCORD	**ADVANCE**	**VADT**
N	10,251	11,140	1791
Age (y)	62	66	60
Men/women (%)	61/39	58/42	97/3
Duration of study (y)	3.5	5.0	5.6
BMI (kg/m²)	32.2 ± 5.5	28.0 ± 5.0	31.3 ± 3.5
Duration of diabetes (y)	10	8	11.5
CVD (%)	35	32	40
Primary CVD end point (%)	↓10 (P = .16)	↓6 (P = .37)	↓13 (P = .12)
Mortality (overall) (%)	↑22 (P = .04)	↓7 (P = NS)	↑6.5 (P = NS)
CV mortality (%)	↑35 (P = .02)	↓12 (P = NS)	↑25 (P = NS)

Abbreviations: BMI, body mass index; CV, cardiovascular; CVD, cardiovascular disease; NS, not significant.

Adapted from Frier BM, Schernthaner G, Heller SR. Hypoglycemia and cardiovascular risks. Diabetes Care 2011:34(Suppl 1):S132–7.

Hypoglycemia and the Elderly

Despite the apparent favorable adaptation to hypoglycemia in tight control, hypoglycemia in the elderly and certain others with type 2 DM may be a serious concern. Matyka and colleagues[58] tested hormone and symptom responses to controlled hypoglycemia in young versus older subjects. Hormonal responses were similar, but hypoglycemia symptoms began at higher glucose levels in the younger men and were more intense, permitting recognition and self-treatment. Neurologic function, such as reaction time, deteriorated earlier and to a greater degree in the older men. Most importantly, the difference between the glucose level for awareness of hypoglycemia and the onset of cognitive dysfunction was lost in the older men, meaning that older subjects were less likely to experience prior autonomic warning symptoms. Thus, reduced hypoglycemia warning or awareness may characterize normal aging. The prevalence of diabetes after age 65 years in the United States is 10.9 million or 26.9% in 2010; many eventually need insulin therapy and thus may risk significant hypoglycemia. It is noteworthy that 50% of those older than 65 have prediabetes based on fasting plasma glucose or $HgbA_{1c}$.

Risk Factors for Serious Hypoglycemia in Type 2 DM

Certain factors may predispose to serious hypoglycemia in type 2 DM. In a large study of Medicaid enrollees, aged 65 years or older, who used insulin or sulfonylureas from 1985 through 1989, Shorr and colleagues[59] found that the rates of serious hypoglycemia were 2.76 per 100 person-years among insulin users. Predictors of subsequent hypoglycemia included: (1) recent discharge (the strongest predictor)—relative risk of serious hypoglycemia was 4.5 from 1 to 30 days after discharge; (2) advanced age (relative risk 1.8); (3) black race (relative risk 2.0); and (4) use of 5 or more concomitant medications (relative risk 1.3).

Awareness and Defenses in Type 2 DM

Counterregulation and hypoglycemia unawareness have been studied in type 2 DM.[60] Bolli and colleagues[61] reported deficient glucagon, growth hormone, and cortisol responses, but normal epinephrine responses and increased norepinephrine release characterize counterregulation in type 2 DM. Enhanced suppression of glucose use more than increased hepatic glucose production accounts for euglycemia restoration. Shamoon and colleagues[62] similarly found decreased glucagon responses but increased epinephrine responses to hypoglycemia in type 2 DM. Spyer and colleagues[55] reported that counterregulation occurs at higher glucose levels in well-controlled ($HgbA_{1c}$ 7.4%) type 2 DM than in nondiabetic individuals. Heller[54] found that when type 1 and type 2 DM patients are matched for insulin therapy and glycemic control there is not a significant difference in hypoglycemia frequency. In a study comparing those with and without hypoglycemia unawareness and type 2 DM, Ohno and colleagues[63] found indirect evidence to suggest autonomic neuropathy in those with hypoglycemia unawareness. Segel and colleagues[64] found that type 2 diabetes patients with a 5-year or greater duration of insulin treatment also had evidence to suggest defective counterregulation (**Box 2**).

Box 2 lists the common factors implicated in impairment of hypoglycemia defenses. Antecedent hypoglycemia itself is perhaps the most important precursor to significant later hypoglycemia. Prior hypoglycemia may occur during the daytime and often occurs at night. It need not be very severe to be important in reducing hypoglycemia defenses. A history of severe hypoglycemia, however, is a most important predictor of recurring severe hypoglycemia. It is also important to realize that patients have often

---

Box 2
Factors impairing hypoglycemia defenses

Antecedent hypoglycemia

Diabetic autonomic neuropathy

Defective insulin counterregulation

Hypoglycemia unawareness

Nutritional factors

    Gastroparesis

    Alcohol intake

    Fasting and skipped meals

    Low-carbohydrate fad diets

    Malnutrition

Hormonal environment

    Adrenocortical insufficiency

    Hypopituitarism

    Pregnancy

    Hypothyroidism

    ?Glucocorticoid excess

Extremes of age (young and old)

Renal and hepatic insufficiency

Sliding-scale insulin therapy

Erratic schedules

Exercise

---

extreme variability in glycemia, with marked highs and lows in the 48 hours before and after a severe hypoglycemic episode. This variation indicates a need for prompt action when seeing a patient with increasing glycemic variability. It also can be confusing about which aspect of glycemia to address, but the answer is clear: first address the lows.

CLINICAL DETERMINATION OF RISK FACTORS FOR HYPOGLYCEMIA

What are the risk factors for hypoglycemia in insulin-treated diabetes patients? Depicted in **Box 2** are a variety of the known factors. Most of these are apparent on routine history and physical examination, or with simple laboratory testing (eg, thyroid-stimulating hormone). Diabetic autonomic neuropathy (DAN) clearly is important, but is poorly reversible when autonomic neuropathy is established.[64,65] Most of the time, however, it is not fixed autonomic neuropathy that predisposes to severe hypoglycemia. Glycemic goals in such patients should be adjusted to minimize the risk of severe hypoglycemia. Drugs such as nonselective β-blockers may best be avoided unless there is compelling indication for their use, because of the potential to minimize hypoglycemia recovery.

The HAAF Syndromes

Cryer has coined the term hypoglycemia-associated autonomic failure (HAAF) to indicate a constellation of abnormalities that are largely reversible, specifically induced by prior hypoglycemia, and affect protective body responses to hypoglycemia.[29] Reduced glucagon and epinephrine responses to hypoglycemia appear to be especially important losses. The etiology of this syndrome, which includes hypoglycemia unawareness and defective insulin counterregulation, is incompletely understood. There seem to be numerous adaptations, many in the brain, that may underlie aspects of HAAF.[66] The recent focus has been especially on adaptation of the ventromedial hypothalamus and several signaling pathways including adenosine monophosphate kinase (AMPK),[67] a fuel sensor signaling enzyme. Many areas of the brain and also the liver may adapt through redundant and complementary mechanisms that indicate the potential severity of hypoglycemia as a condition and the many ways in which the body tries to adjust. Altered transport of glucose into the brain may be a part of ineffective hypoglycemia defenses.[68–70] Excessive glucocorticoid secretion in response to hypoglycemia has been implicated as an aspect of defective awareness and counterregulation.[71,72] Whether these mechanisms are complementary, overlapping, or independent is unknown. One of the most important aspects of the HAAF syndromes and hypoglycemia unawareness is that they appear to be directly linked to prior episodes of hypoglycemia and their reversal within days to weeks (**Box 3**) with strict avoidance of all hypoglycemia. Thus, the clinical take-home point from what is known of the pathophysiology for most patients with hypoglycemia is first to do whatever is necessary to prevent recurrence of hypoglycemia. By doing so, the problem will rapidly resolve itself. What is less clear, however, is whether the poor glucagon responses to hypoglycemia, which do not necessarily reverse as part of the HAAF syndrome, can be repaired by some other mechanism than simple avoidance of hypoglycemia. There are promising animal data, but as yet no convincing proof in humans that this may occur.[73,74]

Reversibility of HAAF Syndromes

Recovery from hypoglycemia unawareness (often coupled with defective insulin counterregulation) may start to occur within as few as 2 to 3 days (see **Box 3**) in people with diabetes if hypoglycemia is strictly avoided.[75] It is not necessary to have severely uncontrolled diabetes,[76] but patients initially often resist dose reduction for fear of (long-term) consequences of hyperglycemia and intolerance of symptoms related to hyperglycemia. Within 2 to 3 weeks, recovery of symptom awareness and insulin

---

Box 3
Management of patients with hypoglycemia unawareness

Mnemonic: Rule of Threes

- Test SMBG more than 3 times a day (typically 4–7 needed)

- May need up to 3 times usual regimen to go over 100 mg/dL (ie, usual 15 g may be increased temporarily up to 30–45 g of dextrose)

- First goal is to avoid all hypoglycemia for 3 days; this is when a pattern begins to emerge with therapy response (reduction of insulin resistance from prior hypoglycemia)

- Next goal is to avoid hypoglycemia for 3 weeks, which is associated with recovery of hypoglycemia awareness and/or counterregulation for those without DAN

- 3 to 6 months needed to improve awareness in DAN patients

counterregulation may be substantial in type 1 DM patients without autonomic neuropathy.[77,78] It may take up to 6 months for recovery in patients with severe neuropathy, and recovery is typically less complete.

Nocturnal Hypoglycemia

The importance of nocturnal hypoglycemia is difficult to overemphasize. Awareness of hypoglycemia is normally reduced during sleep. Nocturnal hypoglycemia can induce hypoglycemia unawareness and reduced insulin counterregulatory defenses.[79] Routine bedtime snacks poorly protect against nocturnal hypoglycemia.[80] Children were found in one study to have nocturnal hypoglycemia half of the time, and half of the events were asymptomatic.[81] Matyka and colleagues[82] have suggested that children with nocturnal hypoglycemia have prolonged episodes as a result of defective insulin counterregulation. Recent studies suggest that continuous glucose monitoring (CGM) may help detect such events, and can signal an alarm that assists patients in avoiding and reducing overnight hypoglycemia.[83]

MANAGING PATIENTS WITH HYPOGLYCEMIA ON INSULIN THERAPY

How can one address the issue and prevent serious hypoglycemia in patients taking insulin? One important first step is to start with setting appropriate glycemic goals for patients and individualize them according to risk of hypoglycemia. The ADA[22] suggests the glycemic goals summarized in **Table 1**. The key point is that while there are general guidelines for control, individualization of goals for glycemia is crucial to the safe achievement of those goals.

Glycemic Goal Adjustments

In practice it is necessary to adjust these glucose goals upwards, at least temporarily, until reversible hypoglycemia unawareness recovers, in patients at clearly increased risk of serious hypoglycemia. Goal adjustment is not only HgbA$_{1c}$ adjustment, as averages reflect very little and inconsistently the extremes of glycemia. It is the author's standard approach to start by increasing the recommended targets by about 20 to 30 mg/dL or more in elderly, chronically ill, or debilitated patients including those with severe ischemia or other known risk factors for severe adverse consequences of hypoglycemia. It is very important to focus on SMBG to ensure it is of adequate frequency. It is also critical to understand the pattern of eating and its consistency in patients to safely prescribe insulin therapy. An increase in HgbA$_{1c}$ of about 1% is all that is required to reverse hypoglycemia unawareness and defective insulin counterregulation.[77] That increase should correlate with an average increase in blood glucose of about 30 to 35 mg/dL. Because average blood sugars are not predictive of glycemic extremes, it is very important to pay attention to the lowest blood sugars of the day in profiles. This monitoring can be done with frequent SMBG, with less frequent SMBG done over different times on different days,[84] or diagnostic CGM can be performed to identify periods of high risk, such as overnight. It should be noted that CGM sensors still have about a 10% failure rate and that the trends and patterns are more reliable than are the individual values in CGM. Moreover, CGM has to be validated, preferably at times when blood glucose values are relatively stable.

Certain patterns of glycemia are important to note. For example, a common observation is overuse of basal insulin and/or underutilization of meal insulin. The pattern of glycemia that results is depicted schematically in **Fig. 3**, whereby there is a progressive rise of glucose values during the day after each meal or snack (daytime staircase) and a large drop of values from after dinner to early morning (overnight cliff), a phenomenon

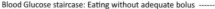

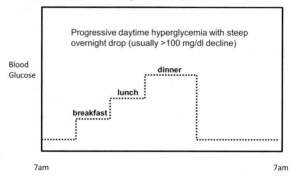

Fig. 3. Glucose staircase with steep drop: signature of basal > meal imbalance.

known as the glucose staircase. This pattern may be seen in either type 1 or type 2 diabetes. The clinical importance relates to the need for better control at meals but also to the importance of recognizing that undertreatment at meals and overtreatment with basal insulin both need to be dealt with in sequence. If more insulin is added just at meals, especially dinner, one can markedly increase the risk of overnight lows. Reducing basal insulin doses before raising meal insulin doses are usually needed. Such reciprocal adjustments in basal and meal insulin achieve better control and reduce the risk of hypoglycemia risk by anticipating that risk based on the recognition of this pattern. What also should be noted is that the fasting values are influenced by poor mealtime control the prior evening and may carry over.[85] Because meals vary considerably, when patients eat less, or lighter meals (a desirable thing normally), it also may increase the risk of overnight lows. Similarly, exercise late in the day may increase overnight lows (see **Fig. 3**).

A glycemic pattern can often be observed in those who are on either basal insulin therapy only or basal bolus therapy, with an imbalance between basal (too much) and meal insulin. The clinical message is that meal insulin will be needed or used in higher doses but that to safely do so, it is necessary to reduce the basal insulin as meal control improves, especially with dinner insulin. A reciprocal decrease in basal insulin and an increase in meal insulin is usually needed to avoid overnight hypoglycemia when correcting this pattern. Patients may state that they cannot take much meal insulin as it tends to precipitate hypoglycemia. No increase in overall insulin with a gradual stepwise redistribution from basal to meal insulin usually will improve overall hyperglycemia while reducing the risk of overnight hypoglycemia.

Elsewhere in this issue are articles dealing with other aspects of insulin therapy. Some unavoidable overlap will occur; strategies presented herein are particularly tied to reducing the hypoglycemic risk in patients with problematic hypoglycemia. The major strategies for reducing hypoglycemic risk in the treatment of diabetes are listed in **Boxes 4** and **5**.

Thinking like a pancreas entails adjusting short-acting insulins at meals, reductions for recent increased activity, and accurate correction doses. For basal insulin, dose must be adjusted based largely on the best fasting glucose in recent times. Further adjustments are needed for stress and pain. Flexible insulin therapy is the primary strategy for adjusting insulin to lifestyle. Ultimately this may mean insulin-pump therapy in appropriate patients. A supply of rapid consumable dextrose is the best remedy, but it should be measured and not out of immediate reach because hypoglycemia is usually unexpected. Patients with frequent hypoglycemia need specific

---

Box 4
Overview of strategies to reduce hypoglycemia risk

- Think like a pancreas: copy normal β-cell physiologic responses with insulin therapy (basal/bolus or pump).
- Always be careful to balance meal insulin and basal insulin; watch out for overtreatment with basal insulin.
- Provide all patients (and family or colleagues) with adequate remedies and training for hypoglycemia therapy including glucagon.
- Set appropriate SMBG glycemic goals (not just A_{1c}); it is necessary to focus often on the lowest blood glucose when adjusting therapy.
- Modify glucose goals with severe hypoglycemia, hypoglycemia unawareness, or defective counterregulation, or other factors increasing severe hypoglycemia or severe consequences.
- Recognize signs of overtreatment early, including nocturnal hypoglycemia, to minimize the risk of severe hypoglycemia.
- Provide alternative insulin strategies for patients not doing well on current strategies (see **Box 5**).
- If current strategies do not work, refer to a diabetes specialist.
- The patient should always carry identification and treatment for hypoglycemia.

---

targets for premeal and bedtime, and in addition often need to have a middle-of-night target. Troubled sleep, sweating at night, and waking lethargic may be signs of overnight hypoglycemia. **Box 5** briefly summarizes several potential strategies to be adopted to reduce the risk of hypoglycemia.

β-CELL MIMICRY AS AN INSULIN STRATEGY TO REDUCE HYPOGLYCEMIA

Mimicking the pancreatic β cell increasingly accounts for successful and safe management of insulin-treated diabetes. Evidence for this is the increasing use of insulin pumps in the management of type 1 and even type 2 DM. Physiologically, the β cell essentially has 2 components of insulin output (**Fig. 4**). The first is a relatively constant level of insulin secreted between feeding periods to maintain euglycemia; this is the basal insulin and represents half or a little less of normal insulin secretion. There is a diurnal rhythm in basal insulin concentrations with a greater degree of insulin resistance in the early hours of the morning (dawn phenomenon) requiring increased insulin in some patients, especially younger ones. The second component of insulin replacement is adequate meal-related insulin secretion; this is the bolus insulin.

Analogue Insulins Mimic Basal and Meal Bolus Insulins Better than NPH and Regular Insulin

These 2 components are matched better with some insulin strategies than with others. Many physicians still use primarily NPH and Regular in their insulin strategies, not uncommonly in a fixed-ratio preparation. These 2 types of insulin are less expensive and may often be successfully combined to achieve excellent control, but they are somewhat less likely to provide a physiologic mimicry than alternative strategies and have a greater risk of hypoglycemia, especially overnight. Because analogue insulins better mimic pancreatic basal and bolus insulin replacement as injection therapy (although less well than insulin pumps), they play an increasingly important role in

---

Box 5
Strategies to reduce hypoglycemia risk with insulin therapy

- Switch from sliding-scale insulin to carbohydrate counting and/or pattern management
- Change fixed-ratio insulins to individual doses or basal bolus therapy
- Move NPH insulin to bedtime but leave meal insulin at dinner time
- Use a correction bolus (1500 rule for Regular; 1700/1800 rule for rapid analogues) but avoid insulin stacking with "insulin on board" given in the last 4 to 6 hours
- Avoid or reduce (no more than one-half) the dose of correction insulin near bedtime (bolus wizard can help here)
- Reduce hypoglycemia before addressing hyperglycemia
- Ensure hypoglycemia recovers to greater than 100 by checking SMBG 15 minutes after therapy
- Provide adequate carbohydrate snacks for increased activity
- If patient varies dose, check total daily dose to ensure there is not too much variation
- Make sure basal therapy is not more than ~50% of total daily dose of insulin
- Overreliance on basal insulin causes late delayed hypoglycemia
- Overreliance on short-acting insulin causes postprandial hypoglycemia
- Manipulate the timing of short-acting insulin (Regular or analogues) relative to meals (lag time)
- Decrease lag time with hypoglycemia or take insulin shortly after the meal; increase with hyperglycemia.
- Switch from NPH or fixed-ratio insulins to basal bolus therapy (Basal Plus 1, 2, or 3)
- Switch from Regular insulin to rapid analogues with meals
- Dose short-acting insulin primarily based on carbohydrate counting and meal composition
- Add a noontime meal dose if not being used
- Reduce overall insulin doses by ~10% to 20% when going from a simple to more complex regimen (basal bolus, insulin pumps) if adequate overall control exists
- Use insulin pumps in appropriate trained and motivated patients

---

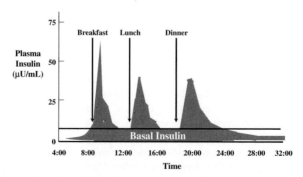

Fig. 4. Insulin levels throughout the day.

successful physiologic insulin replacement strategies and thereby reduce hypogly-cemic risk with intensive therapy (**Fig. 5**).

Reducing Insulin with Exercise

An issue commonly arising in physiologic replacement of insulin, particularly in younger or more active patients, is the adjustment of therapy for increased physical activity. Exercise alters insulin sensitivity often in a biphasic manner by first decreasing it, then increasing it during exercise and for hours afterward (causing delayed hypogly-cemia), while repletion of depleted glycogen content in muscle occurs. Practically speaking, physical activity of moderate intensity (50% Vo_{2max}) for half an hour usually determines need for a reduction in the meal insulin at the nearest (before or after) meal of about 50%. With greater intensity of exercise, reductions of meal insulin may be 75% or more.[86] Both intensity and duration seem to be important. Each individual is somewhat different, and with repeated similar exercise one learns through self-monitoring to gauge the appropriate reductions and/or the need for snacks. For those who use insulin pumps in addition to adjustment of meal insulin, use of a temporary base rate that is reduced from 25% to 90% may be needed, with the reduction based largely on the duration and intensity of the exercise with adjustment based on prior experience. The duration of the temporary basal rate usually extends for hours beyond the activity itself into the postmeal exercise period to avoid hypoglycemia, which is especially important in avoiding nocturnal hypoglycemia with later afternoon or evening exercise. Less often, with injected insulin one has to reduce the basal insulin, although occasionally it is needed with prolonged activity (eg, an all-day hike or city tour).

MONITORING OF DIABETES TO ADJUST INSULIN THERAPY

SMBG is crucial to successful and safe insulin therapy. The frequency required should be individualized, but generally should be increased in those with an increased risk of hypoglycemia, particularly with hypoglycemia unawareness. In general, one should test routinely before meals and at bedtime. Occasional tests in the middle of the night (typically 2–3 AM) are required to rule out nocturnal hypoglycemia. Testing before driving and when working with dangerous machinery is also indicated. Testing at times of anticipated peak insulin action (eg, ~2 hours postprandial with rapid analogues such as lispro, aspart, or glulisine) is helpful to learn how to determine the glucose nadir effect of the meal insulin. With hypoglycemia unawareness, patients may be

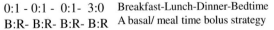

0:1 - 0:1 - 0:1- 3:0   Breakfast-Lunch-Dinner-Bedtime
B:R- B:R- B:R- B:R   A basal/ meal time bolus strategy

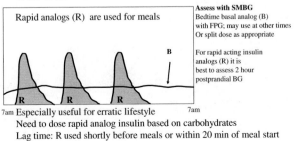

Rapid analogs (R) are used for meals

Assess with SMBG
Bedtime basal analog (B) with FPG; may use at other times Or split dose as appropriate

For rapid acting insulin analogs (R) it is best to assess 2 hour postprandial BG

B

7am Especially useful for erratic lifestyle   7am
Need to dose rapid analog insulin based on carbohydrates
Lag time: R used shortly before meals or within 20 min of meal start

Fig. 5. Insulin regimens for type 1 DM (late type 2).

surprised that they are hypoglycemic much more frequently than they suspect. Similarly, CGM may reveal periods of either undertreatment or overtreatment, often overnight, that were not suspected. **Fig. 6** illustrates basal insulin overtreatment at night, which was masked at times because of persistent hyperglycemia from prior meals.

The area contained within the square in **Fig. 6** shows 2 nights with marked hypoglycemia. Other nights the tendency to hypoglycemia may be masked by the tendency to prolonged hyperglycemia after the last meal or snack of the day, as depicted in traces from several other nights.

Problems with Sliding Scales

Adjusting insulin therapy based on monitoring can be done in several ways. Part of the adjustment involves the art of diabetic medicine. Many patients primarily base their insulin adjustments (including sometimes their long-acting basal doses, a significant error) primarily on the current blood glucose concentrations. This approach is similar to the use of sliding-scale insulin therapy often used in the hospital setting (sometimes referred to in teaching hospitals as 2, 4, 6, 8, call H.O.). As with hospitalized patients,[87] however, it usually is a relatively poor choice, often resulting in both poor and erratic control with unpredictable hypoglycemia.[88,89] Although this approach is nowhere near as effective as carbohydrate counting as the primary basis for meal administration of insulin, so-called correction dosing with refinement of the dose or the timing (adjustment of lag time) are legitimate and useful for short-acting insulin adjustment, especially at meals. **Box 6** lists some of the problems with sliding-scale insulin.

Sliding-scale insulin works poorly in matching insulin needs and timing. It removes context from interpretation of SMBG testing (eg, rebound hyperglycemia), although supplemental correction doses of insulin may be important, particularly on sick days. As a primary strategy, however, it leads to erratic control, with alternating hyperglycemia and hypoglycemia.

Pattern Management

A preferable basis for adjusting insulin therapy for patients is sometimes called pattern management.[90] Pattern management typically examines the pattern and consistency of therapy response (SMBG values) over several days or longer. Selection of 1 or 2 changes in insulin administration to bring the most consistently abnormal values into better control is performed with a subsequent period of observation to see if an improved pattern emerges. Bergenstal and colleagues[25,91] have shown that adjusting

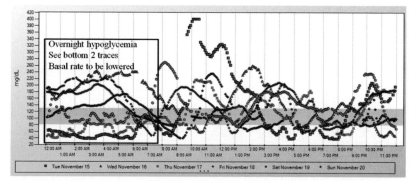

Fig. 6. Detection of overnight hypoglycemia with continuous glucose monitoring.

Box 6
Problems with sliding-scale insulin

- Never to be done for long-acting insulin
- Attempts to make insulin work backward in time
- Uses insulin based on a single glucose value
- Ignores pattern of therapy response
- Ignores what the patient is going to eat
- Does not lead to stability of regimen
- Requires hyperglycemia to initiate therapy especially if given without basal insulin

---

to target (ie, pattern of glycemia) on a weekly basis is as effective as carbohydrate counting.

Four things are required to make pattern management work in insulin-treated patients. First, pattern management needs sufficient monitoring frequency to be able to determine a pattern. Second, it requires clear communication of appropriate glycemic goals and their adjustment upwards in patients at high risk of hypoglycemia. Third, it requires a time interval (typically either 3 or 7 days), after which patterns of glycemia are reevaluated and changes made if glycemic targets are not met. Fourth, it requires an increment or decrement size (commonly 10%–20% of the dose) for the dosage adjustment.

New Monitoring Strategies

Recent innovations in monitoring may eventually permit safer attainment of excellent glycemia. The use of subcutaneous insulin sensors (currently available from 3 manufacturers) is showing considerable improvement from earlier models, although the sensor technology needs further refinement. **Fig. 5** is an example of unsuspected hypoglycemia detected by using a CGM subcutaneous glucose sensor in a patient. There are 3 available systems: the Real Time Guardian, the Abbott Navigator, and the DexCom CGM system. The first can be directly linked to some of the Medtronic Minimed insulin pumps, whereas the other 2 are stand-alone systems. Physicians interested in details of these systems may visit the Web sites of these companies. It must be noted that the absolute values of the monitoring data do not have a perfect correspondence to SMBG for both physiologic reasons (sensor lag) and technical reasons (sensor error). The trend and speed of change and use of appropriately set alarms can, however, help patients improve control and may reduce overnight hypoglycemia.

Carbohydrate Counting

The standard method that is taught to adjust meal insulin to cover food is carbohydrate counting. In type 2 diabetes, it seems that pattern therapy is generally as good. Carbohydrate counting does depend on the assumption that all carbohydrates are about equal in causing hyperglycemia, which is clearly not so as evidenced by extensive literature on glycemic index and glycemic load. In the future it may be helpful to adjust meal insulin based on the physiologic effects of different foods, as has been suggested by a recent study.[92] It is also clear that carbohydrate counting does not take into account the lack of precision in estimation of carbohydrates and the rather significant amount of guessing that is often required, even in those who may use standard sources for carbohydrate content in booklets or with smartphone applications for adults and children that are available.

TREATMENT OF HYPOGLYCEMIA (A TREATMENT, NOT A TREAT)

Urgent situations dictate use of any available sugar source to remedy acute hypoglycemia. However, it is preferable to use a measured, standard amount of pure dextrose when possible. This action has several advantages. It avoids using hypoglycemia as an excuse for ill-considered treats, such as a candy bar. Such sugar sources contain unwanted saturated fat, which slows sugar absorption and delays hypoglycemic recovery as well as potentially adversely affecting hyperlipidemia and caloric balance. Hypoglycemia-unaware patients commonly undertreat themselves, probably because hypoglycemia is less aversive when there are no or few distressing autonomic symptoms. Approximately 15 to 20 g of dextrose typically will restore euglycemia in adults; children should base doses on weight. Examples of treatment for hypoglycemia are given in **Box 7**.

Treatments are listed in suggested order of preference (ie, increase SMBG to 100 mg/dL or more). It is important to remember that one treatment may not reverse hypoglycemia. All patients, particularly those who are hypoglycemic unaware, should retest

---

Box 7
Therapies to reverse hypoglycemia

First choice (marked for hypoglycemia, glucose-based, 15 g carbohydrate, easy dosing)

> Glucose gel: 1 tube (eg, Dex4 gel, Glucoburst gel, Insta-glucose, MonoJel, Glutose 15, ReliOn gel), GlucoPouch 15; glucose liquid: 2 oz (eg, De4liquid blast ReliOn glucose drink)

Second choice (marked as treatment source for hypoglycemia, glucose-based)

> Glucose tablets: 15 to 16 g carbohydrate (eg, 4 Dex4 tablets, 3 Glucoburst tablets, 4 ReliOn glucose tablets), best taken with water; dextrose "Bits" easy to chew, 1 g carbohydrate each

Third choice (common beverage choices; containing 15 to 20 g carbohydrate, quickly absorbed)

> 1/2 cup (4 oz) fruit juice, 1/2 cup (4 oz) sugar-containing (regular) soft drink, 1/2 cup (4 oz) Kool-Aid or lemonade, 1 cup (8 oz) skim milk, 1 cup (8 oz) of a sports drink

Fourth choice (common food choices; all contain 15 to 20 g carbohydrate, readily available)

> 1 small tube Cakemate gel (not cake frosting): 19 g carbohydrate

> 2 tablespoons raisins, 1 tablespoon table sugar, 9 Sweet Tarts

> 1 heaped tablespoon (3–4 teaspoons) table sugar, 9 Sweet Tarts

> 7 Lifesavers, 7 Gummy Bears, 6 large jelly beans, 4 gum drops, 10 Candy Corn

> 3 pieces of butterscotch or peppermint hard candy, 2 Jolly Rancher hard candies

If patient cannot swallow and is combative and/or incoherent

> Injection of glucagon: 0.5 (kids <20 kg) to 1 mg subcutaneously (just like with insulin) or intramuscularly

Other safety issues

> Identification bracelet or necklace needed for any person with prior severe hypoglycemia or hypoglycemia unawareness

> Glucagon instruction of friends, relatives, or coworkers may be needed

> Difficulty reversing hypoglycemia or need for glucagon: refer for emergency room evaluation

in 15 minutes after 15 g of dextrose treatment and re-treat if SMBG is not greater than 100 mg/dL (The 15/15 rule for hypoglycemia treatment). Patients also can be asked to read food labels if these choices are not available, and look for 15 g of carbohydrate with foods that are free of protein, fat, and fiber.

Retest and Re-Treat

It is very important to have HAAF patients (it should be recommended for most patients) retest glucose values 15 minutes after dextrose; some patients with hypoglycemia unawareness and defective counterregulation require 2 or 3 15-g dextrose treatments to raise plasma glucose to greater than 100 mg/dL, the minimum goal. For safety, all patients with increased hypoglycemia risk need a Medic Alert or other identification bracelet, and glucagon kits with instructions given to friends and relatives on its use. **Box 3** suggests some approaches to dealing with hypoglycemia in the setting of reduced or absent hypoglycemia awareness which, as part of the HAAF syndrome, is also usually associated with somewhat reduced or delayed counter-insulin hormonal defenses.

EVOLUTION OF INSULIN THERAPY AND HYPOGLYCEMIA

Initially insulin therapy was historically available only as Regular insulin. The result was inconvenience of multiple injections, poor growth, frequent hyperglycemia and hypoglycemia, and difficulty providing adequate basal insulin replacement. The addition of protamine to insulin, first as PZI insulin (now not used) and later NPH insulin (introduced by Hagedorn), reduced the rate of absorption of insulin and provided the first attempts at a basal insulin strategy, but often led to late, unpredictable hypoglycemia. Human insulins have now replaced animal insulins. Initially it was suspected that human insulins were more likely to predispose to serious hypoglycemia, but this has been proved not to be correct.[93]

NPH-Based Regimens

Many primary care providers continue to prescribe NPH and Regular insulin, typically given together as a predinner and prebreakfast strategy (sometimes referred to a split-mix insulin), although a nonpeaking basal insulin strategy based on the Treat-to-Target Trial in type 2 diabetes with either insulin glargine or insulin detemir is increasingly recognized as valuable. Nonetheless, fixed-ratio insulin preparations, for example, 70/30 insulin (NPH/Regular), are also popular because of their convenience and presumed greater dosing accuracy. Both the NPH and short-acting Regular insulin have problems. Regular insulin needs dosing 30 to 40 minutes before eating and lasts longer than most meals, thus it risks late postmeal hypoglycemia. NPH insulin given at dinnertime works reasonably well for many patients with type 2 DM, especially the more obese patients. However, dinnertime NPH insulin use with lean type 2 DM patients and those with insulin deficiency from type 1 DM or pancreatic diabetes is notoriously problematic because of nocturnal hypoglycemia. Nocturnal hypoglycemia is expected when the peak action of NPH insulin in glucose lowering occurs within 8 hours of administration, sometimes earlier. If dinnertime is 6 PM then peak insulin action occurs often after midnight, when patients are asleep and less able to recognize and effectively treat hypoglycemia. For type 1 diabetes, basal/bolus regimens are considered the standard of care.

Preventing nocturnal hypoglycemia on NPH and NPH-like insulin regimens

The remedy for nocturnal hypoglycemia from dinnertime NPH is to move the NPH (but not the short-acting meal insulin) to near bedtime. If the patient is on fixed-ratio insulin preparation (eg, 70/30), this means individual dosing of intermediate-acting and short-acting insulins (eg, NPH and Regular) and NPH-like effects of analogue insulin mixes should be similarly separated, in the case of nocturnal hypoglycemia due to neutral protamine aspart or lispro. To determine the correct starting dose the total dose is multiplied by 0.7 to determine NPH amount and by 0.3 to determine the Regular insulin dose. The need to separate evening NPH and Regular applies to type 1 DM patients not on basal bolus therapy and to leaner type 2 DM patients (see **Box 5**).

Timing mismatch with fixed-ratio insulins

Similarly, patients on fixed-ratio insulin preparations (eg, 50/50 NPH and Regular) may have poor control or hypoglycemia with tighter control because the ratio does not permit flexible dosing that corrects for the meal being eaten. A high-carbohydrate low-fat meal may have mismatch in postprandial glycemia or nocturnal hypoglycemia if the ratio is wrong for the meal composition (see later discussion). As already mentioned, the remedy to this kind of problem is individual dosing and proper timing of the insulins. It has been suggested that preprandial combinations of short-acting and intermediate-acting insulin at each meal will provide adequate basal insulin and bolus insulin, but in the author's experience this is too complex a strategy for most patients or providers to adequately assess pattern management adjustments. Although fixed-ratio insulins (NPH and regular combinations as well as analogue mixes) have convenience in avoiding mixing of insulin and separately drawing them up, the fixed-ratio insulins in several studies, although more effective in glucose and HgbA$_{1c}$ lowering overall, have a greater propensity to produce hypoglycemia. Although it seems likely that it is the NPH-like effect that is often responsible for middle-of-the-night peaks, there are also problems with patients who use such fixed-ratio insulin if they miss or delay meals.

Erratic Schedules and Intermediate Insulins

Patients with erratic schedules, such as erratic mealtimes or activity, changing work shifts, and so forth, often do poorly on NPH-based (or neutral protamine aspart/lispro) insulin regimens, paying the price of frequent hypoglycemia or poor glycemic control to avoid hypoglycemia. Switching to a basal bolus regimen may remedy this kind of problem with hypoglycemia. The use of insulin glargine and insulin detemir, so-called designer basal insulins, may help patients reduce the frequency of hypoglycemia, especially at night,[94,95] and may be a superior basal insulin strategy, in part due to greater reproducibility. Some trade-offs occur, however, because neither glargine nor detemir can be mixed with other insulins. Moreover, there is some increased discomfort with subcutaneous glargine injection. The efficacy in treat-to-target trials is equal to that of NPH, but consistently the risk of hypoglycemia, largely overnight, is reduced in frequency.

Basal Insulin Strategies

For most patients with erratic schedules or who have profound hypoglycemia when on NPH and Regular or other short-acting insulin, a switch to better basal insulin may reduce hypoglycemia frequency and severity. Basal insulin normally comprises about half of the total daily insulin dose. Overreliance on basal insulin, however, risks delayed hypoglycemia usually overnight; this may be seen when basal insulin far exceeds 50% of total daily dosage. Basal bolus therapy now usually means once or twice daily dosing of insulin glargine or insulin detemir while rapid-acting analogue insulin is used for meal coverage. Although bolus insulin in theory could be Regular or any of the 3 rapid analogues, lispro, aspart, or glulisine (see **Fig. 5**), in practice it is most common to use the rapid analogues. This strategy has been shown to be effective and flexible. In outpatient practice, long-acting basal insulin doses are usually adjusted once a week to minimize risk of overinsulinization as doses are adjusted upwards.

The Treat-to-Target Trial by Riddle and colleagues[94] with a forced basal insulin dose titration of NPH and insulin glargine is illustrated in **Figs. 7** and **8**). Equally good efficacy in glycemic control is exhibited by both study arms, NPH and glargine, titrated at bedtime when aiming for a fasting glucose of less than 100 mg/dL. HgbA$_{1c}$ was similarly lowered to values in the 110 to 120 range in fasting plasma glucose and in HbgA$_{1c}$. Although glycemic efficacy was equal, there was clearly an increased risk of hypoglycemia in the study shown in **Fig. 8**, with a risk that was highest in the early hours of the morning. A similar strategy has been published by Hermansen and colleagues[95] (**Fig. 9**) with comparison of insulin detemir and NPH insulin, with very similar results.

Presumably the increase in peak effects of NPH insulin in comparison with those for insulin glargine explains this difference. These data emphasize that the middle of the night through early morning remains a time of high risk of hypoglycemia with any basal insulin if it is improperly dosed in excess of needs. One additional aspect that needs emphasis is that basal insulin titration based on fasting plasma glucose may lead to inadvertent increased risk of hypoglycemia, particularly if there is considerable variability in postsupper hyperglycemia. Poor postsupper glycemic control may mask this tendency toward overnight hypoglycemia, but improved control with titration of suppertime meal insulin may unmask basal insulin overtreatment.

Inadvertent overdose of basal insulin is actually a common occurrence and usually produces overnight or early-morning hypoglycemia. **Fig. 10** illustrates the risk periods for basal insulin overtreatment in type 2 diabetes, as in the Treat-to-Target Trial. The

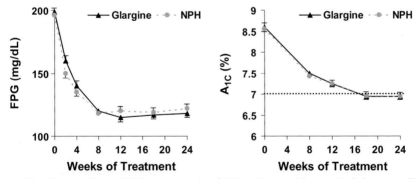

Fig. 7. The Treat-to-Target Trial was a study of 756 patients with type 2 diabetes mellitus previously treated with 1 or 2 oral agents but inadequately controlled as judged by HgbA1c of >7.5 %. Subjects were randomized to either NPH or insulin glargine at bedtime and underwent a forced weekly titration until they achieved the target fasting plasma glucose (based on self monitored blood glucose; SMBG) of <100 mg/dL or were prevented from further titration by occurrence of hypoglycemia. As this figure shows, average fasting plasma glucose (*FPG on the left*) did not achieve the goal but averaged 117 mg/dL in the glargine group and 130 mg/dL in the NPH group at 24 weeks with baseline of 194 mg/dL in the glargine group and 198 mg/dL in the NPH group. The HgbA1c was initially 8.6% in both groups and declined in both to 6.9% on average and the data were not statistically different for either treatment arm.

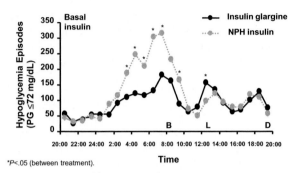

*P<.05 (between treatment).

Fig. 8. In the Treat-to-Target Trial,[94] although the treatment efficacy was similar with both basal insulin glargine and NPH insulin, increased risk of hypoglycemia (here defined as plasma glucose [PG] ≤72 mg/dL) occurred in both groups starting in the middle of the night (although less with glargine) and continuing on through early morning. Increased risk of hypoglycemia was prominent by 3 AM and continued until before breakfast to a greater degree in the NPH treatment group.

pattern of hypoglycemia risk with basal insulin overdose is given against a background of normal peripheral plasma insulin levels.

To avoid hypoglycemia with basal insulin overtreatment, patients must snack frequently or graze during the day, eat a large meal, and snack at bedtime. Even so, basal insulin overdose usually shows up in the early morning, with timing somewhat similar to that observed in the Treat-to-Target study. If a meal is skipped, such as lunch, then a long risk period without food in the middle of the day is also likely to risk hypoglycemia.

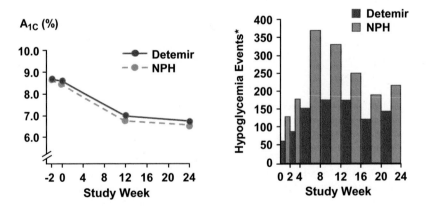

*All reported events, including symptoms only.

Fig. 9. Hermansen and colleagues[95] performed a basal insulin titration (with oral agent failure) comparison over one half year with insulin detemir versus NPH insulin. As seen here and similar to results in the **Figs. 7** and **8** for the Treat-to-Target trial with insulin glargine, there was equal efficacy in glycemic lowering (*left hand panel*) based on HgbA1c. Likewise, as shown in the right hand panel, there was substantially reduced incidence overall in all hypoglycemic events (including those only with symptoms).

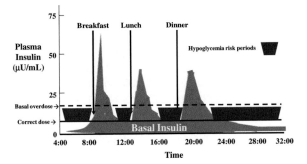

Fig. 10. Basal insulin overtreatment.

Bolus Insulin Strategies

Matching bolus insulin to meals represents an ongoing challenge for many patients with DM, particularly those who are markedly insulin deficient. Important variables often not attended to include those factors mentioned in **Box 4**. It is clear from older studies that the timing of insulin can be as important as the dose of insulin (**Fig. 11**). In this study, the investigators examined the glycemic response to meal regular (R) insulin (doses from 11 to 13 units) in well controlled type 1 DM patients at varying lag times, 0 minutes, 30 minutes, and 60 minutes before a mixed meal (10 kcal/kg, 45% carbohydrate, 35% fat, 20% protein). One may conclude from this study that timing of insulin may be as important as dose in determining postprandial hypoglycemia or hyperglycemia. Similarly, rapid-acting analogues may have their timing manipulated to reduce hypoglycemia risk (postmeal dosing or negative lag time) or to enhance glycemic control without increasing dose for premeal hyperglycemia (eg, administer bolus 30–45 minutes before eating).

Manipulation of the lag time to avoid hypoglycemia
As **Fig. 11** illustrates, altering the lag time, defined here as the time between insulin injection and meal ingestion, could be used as a successful strategy to achieve good postprandial glycemic control with avoidance of hypoglycemia. Patients who are hypoglycemic are understandably concerned about injection of short-acting concentrated insulin preparations when they have hypoglycemia, yet the omission or reduction of bolus insulin dose may still risk extension of hypoglycemia because of rebound hyperglycemia and, typically, subsequent overcorrection. The remedy for bolus dosing in the face of hypoglycemia is to reduce the lag time (for Regular

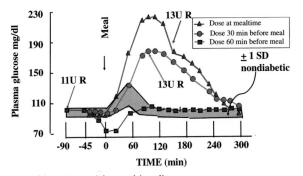

Fig. 11. Importance of lag time with meal insulin.

insulin) or make it a negative (ie, take a rapid analogue, lispro, glulisine, or aspart) shortly after the meal to minimize hypoglycemia. This action avoids the excessive rebound that undertreatment of the meal insulin would permit. On the other hand, one can also help avoid delayed hypoglycemia from excessive insulin bolus (prandial) doses by simply allowing increased time for the insulin to work instead of a taking a large increase in insulin to catch up (see **Box 5**). In practice, the lag time for Regular may be from 1 hour before to a half hour after meals (the latter usually in patients with gastroparesis), with that for the rapid analogues being from a half hour before to half an hour after meals.

Inconsistency of bolus timing

It is important to inquire specifically about the timing and consistency of the interval between insulin administration and meals. Many patients do not time their insulin therapy consistently before meals. Rather than the recommended lag time (30–45 minutes) for Regular insulin, it is commonly taken within 5 to 10 minutes before meals, with a resultant degree of hyperglycemia (see **Fig. 11**). This timing also may differ when patients eat out. If the dose is increased to prevent postprandial hyperglycemia, the result sometimes is late postprandial hypoglycemia as there is a mismatch between timing of insulin and food absorption. In patients who consume a very high-fat meal, however, the usual lag time for Regular insulin may not need to be attended to so assiduously, because a high-fat meal slows carbohydrate absorption and better matches insulin to meal absorption–related hyperglycemia.

Rapid-acting insulin analogues

Use of rapid analogues such as lispro, aspart, or glulisine requires little or no lag time as a standard recommendation, although taking them up to 20 minutes or more before a meal can be a useful strategy for a low-fat meal. However, for a high-fat meal these very fast-acting insulins may both come on too soon and wear off too soon. Increasing the dose to prevent late postprandial hyperglycemia may give too concentrated an effect with early postprandial hypoglycemia. To rectify such a problem, some practitioners will combine Regular with rapid analogue insulin in a 1:1 proportion with a high-carbohydrate, high-fat meal (typically dinner). People who use insulin pumps have the option with higher-fat meals of using a square-wave or dual-wave bolus to accomplish a similar objective of more physiologic matching of bolus insulin to meal composition.

Carbohydrate counting

The total carbohydrate content of a meal is still probably the best guide currently to the amount of insulin needed as a bolus to cover the meal. Less sophisticated patients can be introduced to this concept, but may not be able to count grams of carbohydrate formally at each meal with sufficient precision. A simple strategy is to ask patients to assess their meal-related insulin's effects 2 or 4 hours postprandially (lispro or Regular, respectively) and observe patterns of glycemic response. When hypoglycemia occurs with meals containing lower carbohydrate, the patient can reduce standard bolus doses to prevent postprandial hypoglycemia. Insulin/carbohydrate ratios can be estimated in most patients based on standard ranges (1:10–1:20, ie, 1 unit of bolus insulin for every 10–20 g of total carbohydrate in the meal) for insulin-sensitive patients and a lower ratio for those who are more insulin resistant. Use of a 450 rule (450/total daily dose of insulin) can help estimate the insulin/carbohydrate ratio.

Strategies for carbohydrate counting come to a large degree from insulin-pump therapy. Teaching "carb counting" requires motivation and attention to detail. Several visits with a registered dietician skilled in dealing with bolus insulin adjustments for diabetes are usually required. In general, most patients with type 1 DM require about 1 unit of short-acting insulin for every 10 to 15 g of carbohydrate. The individual range, however, is wide. Although relative consistency is observed in individuals, insulin/carbohydrate ratios can also change according to circumstances. For example, they may be markedly increased after exercise or may be reduced as a result of the dawn phenomenon. Some patients carry books on carbohydrates with them and, increasingly, patients use a variety of smartphone applications for use with diabetes to aid in carbohydrate counting and to estimate accurate carbohydrate content in meals. In general, the use of an 1800 (older rule and slightly more conservative) or 1700 rule to calculate insulin sensitivity is done based on the total daily dose (TDD) of insulin. The author's preference is to use the 1800 rule, which means dividing TDD of insulin into 1800 to estimate the drop in glucose from the premeal time to the 2-hour postmeal glucose level. With patients who have frequent hypoglycemia and unawareness, it is often best to be conservative because they are more likely to have a TDD that is in excess of their needs. It is sometimes quite remarkable that a patient with repeated hypoglycemia may be required on several occasions to reduce their dose of insulin to find out the actual need. Correction dosing at bedtime is discouraged.

High-fat meals and postprandial insulin–food absorption mismatch

Another potentially important variable in successful matching of bolus insulin to meals is the fat content of a meal. While meal carbohydrate is expected to influence the total postprandial glycemic response, the fat content will potentially modify the timing of carbohydrate absorption. High-fat meals slow carbohydrate absorption whereas low-fat meals produce relatively faster carbohydrate absorption. A high-fat meal is common at dinner and when eating out. Lispro or aspart insulin may not last long enough to prevent late postprandial hyperglycemia. Compensatory increases in dose may lead to early postprandial hypoglycemia. The appropriate remedy is to either double the dose of these short-acting insulins or to combine them, typically in a 1:1 ratio, that is, 1 unit of lispro (or aspart) and 1 unit of Regular insulin. The total number of units of the 2 short-acting insulins combined is based still on carbohydrate counting.

Gastroparesis is a very difficult complication in diabetes. It is a challenge to achieve stable glycemic control and avoid hypoglycemia. It is important to remember that absorption of liquids is much less affected than absorption of solids. Administration of Regular insulin either with no lag time or after meals may be required to avoid early postprandial hypoglycemia. Unfortunately, hyperglycemia itself tends to worsen gastroparesis. A trial of metoclopramide or erythromycin may be warranted in some patients with very erratic control and problematic hypoglycemia to see whether it can improve and stabilize glycemic control. The long-term use of these medications, however, is problematic because of very modest efficacy, central nervous system side effects with metoclopramide (such as tardive dyskinesia) and the P-glycoprotein 3A4 drug interaction effects with erythromycin. For patients who use rapid analogue injections or an insulin pump, manipulation of the lag time can be helpful in dealing with gastroparesis. In addition, pumps allow extended boluses, either dual-wave or square-wave, that may be helpful in achieving control with reduced risk of hypoglycemia. For patients with gastroparesis the use of high-fat, high-fiber meals may also exacerbate symptoms.

Ultimately, for some patients with severe hypoglycemia or extreme variability with marked highs and lows, insulin-pump therapy will be the best solution, with sufficient power and flexibility to achieve more stable glycemic control. In appropriately motivated patients who are willing to monitor frequently and learn carbohydrate counting and its variations, it will be the best solution for avoidance of severe hypoglycemia.

Combination therapy

When combining insulin with tablets, it may be important to recognize that certain combinations result in different hypoglycemia patterns. Certain sulfonylureas such as glyburide seem to have a high propensity to cause hypoglycemia in the daytime.[63] Metformin seems to have less propensity to do so in combination, but certainly may require downward insulin dosage adjustment to avoid hypoglycemia. Thiazolidinediones often cause hypoglycemia if doses of insulin are not reduced. Because this may take a month or more to become clinically manifest, some patients find the hypoglycemia unexpected. Combining insulin therapy with GLP-1 agonists also usually leads to the need to reduce basal insulin doses. Again, dose reductions are often required.

SUMMARY

Hypoglycemia remains the biggest obstacle to safe and excellent control of diabetes with insulin. The largely acquired physiologic defects that create much of the risk of overtreatment, namely hypoglycemia unawareness and defective insulin counterregulation components of the HAAF syndrome, appear to be largely reversible except for deficient glucagon responses. The solution is to avoid moderate hypoglycemia, perhaps especially at night, as a useful strategy in avoiding severe hypoglycemia with little warning and thus no chance to self treat. Identifying patients at risk is crucial because their glucose and HgbA$_{1c}$ goals should be individualized to reduce their risk, and their monitoring frequency done so as to lead to recognition of poorly symptomatic hypoglycemia. Full treatment of hypoglycemia, especially in those with few symptoms, is also crucial for patient safety. Physiologic mimicry with basal bolus injection therapy or insulin pumps are essential for those with marked insulin deficiency. Avoiding peaks of insulin when not needed and adapting the use of monitoring information to aid therapy adjustment can help in the key task of avoiding nocturnal hypoglycemia. Nonetheless, basal insulin overtreatment with analogues can and does occur, and is often not recognized promptly. Its masking by undertreatment at meals can be deduced from patterns of glucose, thus helping to guide the patient to safer therapy. Although frequent adjustments and correction of dosing are important, looking at the big picture, pattern management can enhance safety and exploit the benefit of modern insulins and administration, to reduce glycemic variability and accurately provide safe and effective therapy through copying the body's own physiology of insulin delivery.

REFERENCES

1. The Action to Control Cardiovascular Risk in Diabetes Study Group. Effects of intensive glucose lowering in type 2 diabetes. N Engl J Med 2008;358(24):2545–59.
2. The ADVANCE Collaborative Group. Intensive blood glucose control and vascular outcomes in patients with Type 2 diabetes. N Engl J Med 2008; 358(24):2560–72.
3. Duckworth W, Abraira C, Moritz T, et al. Glucose control and vascular complications in Veterans with Type 2 diabetes. N Engl J Med 2009;360(2):129–39.
4. Akram K, Pedersen-Bjergaard U, Carstensen B, et al. Frequency and risk factors of severe hypoglycaemia in insulin-treated type 2 diabetes: a cross-sectional survey. Diabet Med 2006;23:750–6.

5. Henderson JN, Allen KV, Deary IJ, et al. Hypoglycaemia in insulin-treated type 2 diabetes: frequency, symptoms and impaired awareness. Diabet Med 2003;20: 1016–21.
6. Murata GH, Duckworth WC, Shah JH, et al. Hypoglycemia in stable, insulin-treated veterans with type 2 diabetes: a prospective study of 1662 episodes. J Diabetes Complications 2005;19(1):10–7.
7. Saudek CD, Duckworth WC, Giobbie-Hurder A, et al. Implantable insulin pump vs multiple-dose insulin for non-insulin-dependent diabetes mellitus: a randomized clinical trial. Department of Veterans Affairs Implantable Insulin Pump Study Group. JAMA 1996;276:1322–7.
8. Gurlek A, Erbas T, Gedik O. Frequency of severe hypoglycaemia in type 1 and type 2 diabetes during conventional insulin therapy. Exp Clin Endocrinol Diabetes 1999;107:220–4.
9. Abraira C, Colwell JA, Nuttall FQ, et al. Veterans Affairs Cooperative Study on glycemic control and complications in type II diabetes (VA CSDM). Results of the feasibility trial. Veterans Affairs Cooperative Study in Type II Diabetes. Diabetes Care 1995;18:1113–23.
10. Yki-Jarvinen H, Ryysy L, Nikkila K, et al. Comparison of bedtime insulin regimens in patients with type 2 diabetes mellitus. A randomized, controlled trial. Ann Intern Med 1999;130:389–96.
11. Ohkubo Y, Kishikawa H, Araki E, et al. Intensive insulin therapy prevents the progression of diabetic microvascular complications in Japanese patients with non-insulin-dependent diabetes mellitus: a randomized prospective 6-year study. Diabetes Res Clin Pract 1995;28:103–17.
12. Wright AD, Cull CA, Macleod KM, et al. Hypoglycemia in type 2 diabetic patients randomized to and maintained on monotherapy with diet, sulfonylurea, metformin, or insulin for 6 years from diagnosis: UKPDS73. J Diabetes Complications 2006;20:395–401.
13. UK Hypoglycaemia Study Group. Risk of hypoglycaemia in types 1 and 2 diabetes: effects of treatment modalities and their duration. Diabetologia 2007;50: 1140–7.
14. MacLeod KM, Hepburn DA, Frier BM. Frequency and morbidity of severe hypoglycaemia in insulin-treated diabetic patients. Diabet Med 1993;10:238–45.
15. Donnelly LA, Morris AD, Frier BM, et al. Frequency and predictors of hypoglycaemia in type 1 and insulin-treated type 2 diabetes: a population-based study. Diabet Med 2005;22:749–55.
16. Reichard P, Pihl M. Mortality and treatment side-effects during long-term intensified conventional insulin treatment in the Stockholm Diabetes Intervention Study. Diabetes 1994;43:313–7.
17. The Diabetes Control and Complications Trial Research Group. The effect of intensive treatment of diabetes on the development and progression of long-term complications in insulin-dependent diabetes mellitus. N Engl J Med 1993; 329:977–86.
18. Hepburn DA, MacLeod KM, Pell AC, et al. Frequency and symptoms of hypoglycaemia experienced by patients with type 2 diabetes treated with insulin. Diabet Med 1993;10(3):231–7.
19. UK Prospective Diabetes Study (UKPDS) Group. Effect of intensive blood-glucose control with metformin on complications in overweight patients with type 2 diabetes (UKPDS 34). Lancet 1998;352(9131):854–65.
20. The Diabetes Control and Complications Trial/Epidemiology of Diabetes Interventions and Complications (DCCT/EDIC) Study Research Group. Intensive diabetes

treatment and cardiovascular disease in patients with type 1 diabetes. N Engl J Med 2005;353(25):2643–53.

21. Holman RR, Paul SK, Bethel MA, et al. 10-year follow-up of intensive glucose control in type 2 diabetes. N Engl J Med 2008;359(15):1577–89.

22. American Diabetes Association. Standards of medical care in diabetes mellitus 2011. Diabetes Care 2011;34(Suppl 1):S11–61.

23. Juvenile Diabetes Research Foundation Continuous Glucose Monitoring Study Group. Effectiveness of continuous glucose monitoring in a clinical care environment: evidence from the Juvenile Diabetes Research Foundation Continuous Glucose Monitoring (JDRF-CGM) trial. N Engl J Med 2010;363:311–20.

24. Bergenstal RM, Tamborlane WV, Ahmann A, et al. Effectiveness of sensor-augmented insulin-pump therapy in type 1 diabetes. N Engl J Med 2010;363: 383–4.

25. Battelino T, Phillip M, Bratina N, et al. Effect of continuous glucose monitoring on hypoglycemia in type 1 diabetes. Diabetes Care 2011;34(4):795–800.

26. Cobelli C, Renard E, Kovatchev B. Artificial pancreas: past, present, future. Diabetes 2011;60(11):2672–82.

27. Frier BM, Fisher BM, editors. Hypoglycemia and diabetes. London: Edward Arnold; 1993.

28. Cryer PE. Hypoglycemia: pathophysiology, diagnosis and treatment. New York: Oxford University Press; 1997.

29. Cryer PE, Axelrod L, Grossman AB, et al. Evaluation and management of adult hypoglycemic disorders: an Endocrine Society Clinical Practice Guideline. J Clin Endocrinol Metab 2009;94(3):709–28.

30. Frier BM. How hypoglycaemia can affect the life of a person with diabetes. Diabetes Metab Res Rev 2007;24:87–92, 238–45.

31. Purnell JQ, Hokanson JQ, Marcovina JQ, et al. Effect of excessive weight gain with intensive therapy of type 1 diabetes on lipid levels and blood pressure: results from the DCCT. J Am Med Assoc 1998;280(2):140–6.

32. The Diabetes Control and Complications Trial Research Group. Hypoglycemia in the Diabetes Control and Complications Trial. Diabetes 1997;46(2):271–86.

33. Cox DJ, Gonder-Frederick LA, Kovatchev BP, et al. Biopsychobehavioral model of severe hypoglycemia. II. Understanding the risk of severe hypoglycemia. Diabetes Care 1999;22(12):2018–25.

34. Cox D, Ritterband L, Magee J, et al. Blood glucose awareness training delivered over the internet. Diabetes Care 2008;31(8):1527–8.

35. Deary IJ, Crawford JR, Hepburn DA, et al. Severe hypoglycemia and intelligence in adult patients with insulin-treated diabetes. Diabetes 1993;42(2):341–4.

36. Perros P, Deary IJ, Sellar RJ, et al. Brain abnormalities demonstrated by magnetic resonance imaging in adult IDDM patients with and without a history of recurrent severe hypoglycemia. Diabetes Care 1997;20(6):1013–8.

37. Fujioka M, Okuchi K, Hiramatsu KI, et al. Specific changes in human brain after hypoglycemic injury. Stroke 1997;28(3):584–7.

38. Kaufman FR, Epport K, Engilman R, et al. Neurocognitive functioning in children diagnosed with diabetes before age 10 years. J Diabetes Complications 1999; 13(1):31–8.

39. Rovet JF, Ehrlich RM. The effect of hypoglycemic seizures on cognitive function in children with diabetes: a 7-year prospective study. J Pediatr 1999;134(4): 503–6.

40. Rovet JF, Ehrlich RM, Czuchta D. Intellectual characteristics of diabetic children at diagnosis and one year later. J Pediatr Psychol 1990;15:775–88.

41. Wessels AM, Lane KA, Gao S, et al. Diabetes and cognitive decline in elderly African Americans: a 15-year follow-up study. Alzheimers Dement 2011;7(4):418–24.
42. Daviglus ML, Plassman BL, Pirzada A, et al. Risk factors and preventive interventions for Alzheimer disease: state of the science. Arch Neurol 2011;68(9):1185–90.
43. Strachan MW, Reynolds RM, Marioni RE, et al. Cognitive function, dementia and type 2 diabetes mellitus in the elderly. Nat Rev Endocrinol 2011;7(2):108–14.
44. Gold AE, MacLeod KM, Deary IJ, et al. Hypoglycemia-induced cognitive dysfunction in diabetes mellitus: effect of hypoglycemia unawareness. Physiol Behav 1995;58(3):501–11.
45. Strachan MW, Deary IJ, Ewing FM, et al. Recovery of cognitive function and mood after severe hypoglycemia in adults with insulin-treated diabetes. Diabetes Care 2000;23(3):305–12.
46. Frier BM, Schernthaner G, Heller SR. Hypoglycemia and cardiovascular risks. Diabetes Care 2011;34(Suppl 1):S132–7.
47. Marques JL, George E, Peacey SR, et al. Altered ventricular repolarization during hypoglycaemia in patients with diabetes. Diabet Med 1997;14(8):648–54.
48. Robinson RT, Harris ND, Ireland RH, et al. Mechanisms of abnormal cardiac repolarization during insulin-induced hypoglycemia. Diabetes 2003;52(6):1469–74.
49. Trovati M, Anfossi G, Cavalot F, et al. Studies on mechanisms involved in hypoglycemia-induced platelet activation. Diabetes 1986;35(7):818–25.
50. Desouza C, Salazar H, Cheong B, et al. Association of hypoglycemia and cardiac ischemia: a study based on continuous monitoring. Diabetes Care 2003;26:1485–9.
51. Duh E, Feinglos M. Hypoglycemia-induced angina pectoris in a patient with diabetes mellitus. Ann Intern Med 1996;44(7):751–5.
52. Kamijo Y, Soma K, Aoyama N, et al. Myocardial infarction with acute insulin poisoning—a case report. Angiology 2000;51(8):689–93.
53. Sovik O, Thordarson H. Dead-in-bed syndrome in young diabetic patients. Diabetes Care 1999;22(Suppl 2):B40–2.
54. Heller SR. Diabetic hypoglycaemia. Best Pract Res Clin Endocrinol Metab 1999;13(2):279–94.
55. Spyer G, Hattersley AT, Macdonald IA, et al. Hypoglycaemic counter-regulation at normal blood glucose concentrations in patients with well controlled type-2 diabetes. Lancet 2000;356:1970–4.
56. Riddle MC, Ambrosius WT, Brillon DJ, et al. Epidemiologic relationships between A1C and all-cause mortality during a median 3.4-Year follow-up of glycemic treatment in the ACCORD trial. Diabetes Care 2010;33(5):983–90.
57. Zoungas S, Patel A, Chalmers J, et al. Severe hypoglycemia and risks of vascular events and death. N Engl J Med 2010;363(15):1410–8.
58. Matyka K, Evans M, Lomas J, et al. Altered hierarchy of protective responses against severe hypoglycemia in normal aging in healthy men. Diabetes Care 1997;20(2):135–41.
59. Shorr RI, Ray WA, Daugherty JR, et al. Incidence and risk factors for serious hypoglycemia in older persons using insulin or sulfonylureas. Arch Intern Med 1997;157(15):1681–6.
60. Veneman TF, Erkelens DW. Clinical review: hypoglycemia unawareness in noninsulin-dependent diabetes mellitus. J Clin Endocrinol Metab 1997;82(6):1682–4.
61. Bolli GB, Tsalikian E, Haymond MW, et al. Defective glucose counterregulation after subcutaneous insulin in noninsulin-dependent diabetes mellitus. Paradoxical suppression of glucose utilization and lack of compensatory increase in

glucose production, roles of insulin resistance, abnormal neuroendocrine responses, and islet paracrine interactions. J Clin Invest 1984;73:1532–41.

62. Shamoon H, Friedman S, Canton C, et al. Increased epinephrine and skeletal muscle responses to hypoglycemia in non-insulin-dependent diabetes mellitus. J Clin Invest 1994;93(6):2562–71.

63. Ohno T, Toyama T, Hoshizaki H, et al. Evaluation of cardiac sympathetic nervous function by ^{123}I-metaiodobenzylguanidine scintigraphy in insulin-treated non-insulin dependent diabetics with hypoglycemia unawareness. Intern Med 1996; 35(2):94–9.

64. Segel SA, Paramore DS, Cryer PE. Hypoglycemia-associated autonomic failure in advanced type 2 diabetes. Diabetes 2002;51(3):724–33.

65. Cryer PE. Iatrogenic hypoglycemia as a cause of hypoglycemia-associated autonomic failure in IDDM. A vicious cycle. Diabetes 1992;41(3):255–60.

66. McCrimmon R. The mechanisms that underlie glucose sensing during hypoglycaemia in diabetes. Diabet Med 2008;25(5):513–22.

67. McCrimmon RJ, Shaw M, Fan X, et al. Key role for AMP-activated protein kinase in the ventromedial hypothalamus in regulating counterregulatory hormone responses to acute hypoglycemia. Diabetes 2008;57(2):444–50.

68. McCall AL. IDDM, counterregulation, and the brain. Diabetes Care 1997;20(8): 1228–30.

69. Boyle PJ, Nagy RJ, O'Connor AM, et al. Adaptation in brain glucose uptake following recurrent hypoglycemia. Proc Natl Acad Sci U S A 1994;91(20): 9352–6.

70. Boyle PJ, Kempers SF, O'Connor AM, et al. Brain glucose uptake and unawareness of hypoglycemia in patients with insulin-dependent diabetes mellitus. N Engl J Med 1995;333(26):1726–31.

71. Davis SN, Shavers C, Davis B, et al. Prevention of an increase in plasma cortisol during hypoglycemia preserves subsequent counterregulatory responses. J Clin Invest 1997;100(2):429–38.

72. Davis SN, Shavers C, Costa F, et al. Role of cortisol in the pathogenesis of deficient counterregulation after antecedent hypoglycemia in normal humans. J Clin Invest 1996;98(3):680–91.

73. Farhy LS, McCall AL. Optimizing reduction in basal hyperglucagonaemia to repair defective glucagon counterregulation in insulin deficiency. Diabetes Obes Metab 2011;13(Suppl 1):133–43.

74. Farhy LS, McCall AL. Models of glucagon secretion, their application to the analysis of the defects in glucagon counterregulation and potential extension to approximate glucagon action. J Diabetes Sci Technol 2010;4(6):1345–56.

75. George E, Marques JL, Harris ND, et al. Preservation of physiological responses to hypoglycemia 2 days after antecedent hypoglycemia in patients with IDDM. Diabetes Care 1997;20(8):1293–8.

76. Bolli GB. How to ameliorate the problem of hypoglycemia in intensive as well as nonintensive treatment of type 1 diabetes. Diabetes Care 1999;22(Suppl 2): B43–52.

77. Fanelli CG, Epifano L, Rambotti AM, et al. Meticulous prevention of hypoglycemia normalizes the glycemic thresholds and magnitude of most of neuroendocrine responses to, symptoms of, and cognitive function during hypoglycemia in intensively treated patients with short-term IDDM. Diabetes 1993;42(11):1683–9.

78. Fanelli C, Pampanelli S, Lalli C, et al. Long-term intensive therapy of IDDM patients with clinically overt autonomic neuropathy: effects on hypoglycemia awareness and counterregulation. Diabetes 1997;46(7):1172–81.

79. Veneman T, Mitrakou A, Mokan M, et al. Induction of hypoglycemia unawareness by asymptomatic nocturnal hypoglycemia. Diabetes 1993;42(9):1233–7.
80. Saleh TY, Cryer PE. Alanine and terbutaline in the prevention of nocturnal hypoglycemia in IDDM. Diabetes Care 1997;20(8):1231–6.
81. Beregszaszi M, Tubiana-Rufi M, Benali M, et al. Nocturnal hypoglycemia in children and adolescents with insulin-dependent diabetes mellitus: prevalence and risk factors. J Pediatr 1997;131(1):27–33.
82. Matyka P, Crowne EC, Havel EC, et al. Counterregulation during spontaneous nocturnal hypoglycemia in prepubertal children with type 1 diabetes. Diabetes Care 1999;22(7):1144–50.
83. Scaramuzza AE, Iafusco D, Rabbone I, et al, Diabetes Study Group of the Italian Society of Paediatric Endocrinology and Diabetology. Use of integrated real-time continuous glucose monitoring/insulin pump system in children and adolescents with type 1 diabetes: a 3-year follow-up study. Diabetes Technol Ther 2011;13(2):99–103.
84. Polonsky WH, Fisher L, Schikman CH, et al. Structured self-monitoring of blood glucose significantly reduces A1C levels in poorly controlled, noninsulin-treated type 2 diabetes. Diabetes Care 2011;34(2):262–7.
85. Monnier L, Colette C. Targeting prandial hyperglycemia: how important is it and how best to do this? Curr Diab Rep 2008;8(5):368–74.
86. Rabasa-Lhoret R, Ducros F, Bourque J, et al. Guidelines for premeal insulin dose reduction for postprandial exercise of different intensities and durations in type 1 diabetic subjects treated intensively with a basal-bolus insulin regimen (Ultralente-Lispro). Diabetes Care 2001;24:625–30.
87. Umpierrez GE, Smiley D, Zisman A, et al. Randomized study of basal-bolus insulin therapy in the inpatient management of patients with type 2 diabetes (RABBIT 2 Trial). Diabetes Care 2007;30(9):2181–6.
88. Gearhart JG, Ducan JL 3rd, Replogle JH, et al. Efficacy of sliding-scale insulin therapy: a comparison with prospective regimens. Fam Pract Res J 1994;14(4):313–22.
89. Sawin CT. Action without benefit. The sliding scale of insulin use. Arch Intern Med 1997;157(5):489.
90. Guthrie DW, Guthrie RA. Approach to management. Diabetes Educ 2000;16(5):401–6.
91. Bergenstal RM, Johnson M, Powers MA, et al. Adjust to target in type 2 diabetes. Diabetes Care 2008;31(7):1305–10.
92. Bao J, Gilbertson HR, Gray R, et al. Improving the estimation of mealtime insulin dose in adults with type 1 diabetes. Diabetes Care 2011;34(10):2146–51.
93. Jones TW, Caprio S, Diamond MP, et al. Does insulin species modify counterregulatory hormone response to hypoglycemia? Diabetes Care 1991;14(8):728–31.
94. Riddle MC, Rosenstock J, Gerich J. The Treat-to-Target trial: randomized addition of glargine or human NPH insulin to oral therapy of type 2 diabetic patients. Diabetes Care 2003;26(11):3080–6.
95. Hermansen K, Davies M, Derezinski T, et al. A 26-week, randomized, parallel, treat-to-target trial comparing insulin detemir with NPH insulin as add-on therapy to oral glucose-lowering drugs in insulin-naive people with type 2 diabetes. Diabetes Care 2006;29(6):1269–74.

Intensive Insulin Therapy in Patients with Type 1 Diabetes Mellitus

Sean M. Switzer, BA[a], Emily G. Moser, BA[a,b],
Briana E. Rockler, BA[a], Satish K. Garg, MD[a,b,c],*

KEYWORDS

- Diabetes mellitus • Insulin therapy • Insulin analogs
- Glucose control • Glucose Monitoring

The Centers for Disease Control reported that as of 2011, 25.8 million Americans have diabetes,[1] with an estimated increase to 44.1 million people by the year 2033.[2] The associated cost for treating the current diabetic population is estimated at $218 billion annually with a projected increase to $336 billion annually by 2034 (**Fig. 1**).[2–4] Recent studies show the prevalence of diabetes to be 97 million in China and 62.4 million in India with a significant increase in patients with prediabetes in both countries.[5,6] The International Diabetes Federation predicts there will be 552 million people with diabetes by 2030.[7] Diabetes prevalence figures, however, are revised every 1 to 2 years; it may be prudent to consider predicting numbers for only the next 5 years rather than for decades at a time.[8]

Although the majority of increase in prevalence is in type 2 diabetes mellitus (T2D), the incidence of type 1 diabetes mellitus (T1D) is also increasing in many parts of the world and is trending toward earlier onset.[9] The incidence of T1D was estimated to be 40% higher in 2010 than in 1997.[10] These findings are supported by the Epidemiology and Prevention of Diabetes (EURODIAB) collaborative study consisting of 44 centers

Conflict of interest: Dr Satish Garg has received honoraria for giving lectures for sanofi-aventis, DexCom, and Merck. He has no stocks in any of the pharmaceutical or device companies. He has also received several grants from sanofi-aventis, DexCom, Merck, Cebix, Novo Nordisk, Medtronic MiniMed, Abbott, MannKind, the National Institutes of Health, JDRF, T1D Exchange through the Jaeb Center for Health Research, and Halozyme Therapeutics through the University of Colorado Denver. Sean Switzer, Emily Moser, and Briana Rockler do not report any conflict of interests.
[a] Barbara Davis Center for Childhood Diabetes, University of Colorado Denver, 1775 Aurora Court, A140, Aurora, CO 80045, USA
[b] School of Medicine, University of Colorado Denver, Aurora, CO, USA
[c] Diabetes Technology and Therapeutics, Aurora, CO, USA
* Corresponding author. Barbara Davis Center for Childhood Diabetes, University of Colorado Denver, 1775 Aurora Court, A140, Aurora, CO 80045.
E-mail address: Satish.Garg@ucdenver.edu

Endocrinol Metab Clin N Am 41 (2012) 89–104
doi:10.1016/j.ecl.2011.12.001
0889-8529/12/$ – see front matter © 2012 Elsevier Inc. All rights reserved.

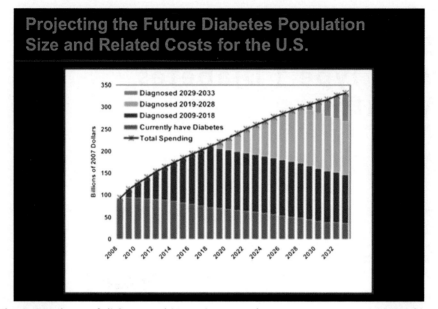

Fig. 1. Prevalence of diabetes and increasing costs. (*From* Huang ES, Basu A, O'Grady M, et al. Projecting the future diabetes population size and related costs for the US. Diabetes Care 2009;32:2225–9; with permission.)

across Europe and Israel, which reported an increase in incidence of T1D at a rate of 3% to 4% annually, with some regions reporting even higher growth rates.[9] Additionally, the incidence rates of increase—6.3%, 3.1%, and 2.4% in children ages 0 to 4 years, 5 to 9 years, and 10 to 14 years, respectively—further supports that T1D is trending toward earlier onset.

T1D is an autoimmune disease resulting from the immunologic destruction of insulin-producing pancreatic β-cells. A well-functioning pancreas monitors blood glucose levels and reacts appropriately by secreting either the insulin or glucagon necessary for maintaining euglycemia. This feedback loop is pivotal for glucose homeostasis. Over the course of a day, a healthy pancreas continuously releases a small amount of insulin (basal) and reacts to acute increases in blood glucose by releasing prandial/meal-time (bolus) insulin during meals (**Fig. 2**). When glucose levels are low, glucagon is secreted by α-cells to stimulate the release of liver glycogen stores and glucose through neoglucogenesis.

Autoimmunity may exist for years before β-cell destruction and the diagnosis of diabetes (**Fig. 3**). The disease can now be identified by testing for specific antibody markers (IAA, ICA512, GAD65, GADA, and ZnT8), especially in high-risk individuals.[11,12] After initial diagnosis of T1D and initiating insulin therapy, most patients go through a honeymoon phase, where β-cell function transiently improves.[13] This phase can last for a few weeks to a few years depending on the age of onset of the disease and other factors that remain unrecognized. Currently, there are several ongoing studies investigating ways to reduce ongoing β-cell destruction to extend the honeymoon phase.[14]

The destruction of the β cells responsible for insulin secretion requires T1D patients to administer exogenous insulin subcutaneously in an effort to control glycemia for the rest of their lives. The Diabetes Complications and Control Trial (DCCT), a 10-year,

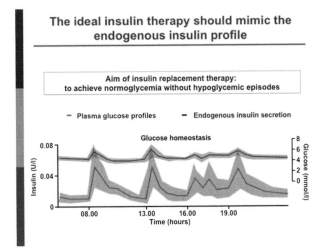

Fig. 2. Healthy pancreatic insulin secretion. (*From* Owens DR, Zinman B, Bolli GB. Insulins today and beyond. Lancet 2001;358:739–46; with permission.)

multicenter, randomized clinical trial designed to compare intensive insulin therapy (IIT) to conventional diabetes therapy with regard to their effects on early vascular and neurologic complications of T1D, concluded that there is an association between hyperglycemia and microvascular diabetic complications.[15] Subjects randomized to IIT, composed of multiple daily injections (MDI) or continuous subcutaneous insulin infusion (CSII) coupled with self-monitored blood glucose (SMBG), showed a 2% decline in glycoslyated hemoglobin (A1c) values, which were maintained for 5 years, as well as a reduction of microvascular complications of diabetes.[15] Follow-up of DCCT subjects for another decade by the Epidemiology of Diabetes Interventions

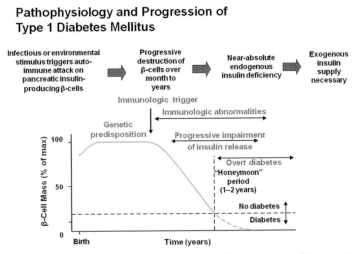

Fig. 3. Progression of T1D. (*Adapted from* Powers AC. Diabetes mellitus. In: Kasper DL, Harrison TR, editors. Harrison's principles of internal medicine, 16th edition. vol. 2. New York: McGraw-Hill; 2005. p. 2152–80; with permission.)

and Complications research group confirmed the legacy or memory effect on microvascular complications. These findings also demonstrated that despite similar A1c levels during the follow-up period, there was a significant reduction of macrovascular complications, such as cardiovascular disease and strokes.[16] These findings are the platform on which the need for IIT is built. Currently, the best therapeutic options for patients with T1D include a basal-bolus therapy, such as MDIs or CSII used in the DCCT. These therapy options must also be coupled with frequent SMBG and/or continuous glucose monitoring (CGM) (**Fig. 4**) to allow for proper insulin dosing and timing adjustments to avoid wide glucose excursions.[15]

INSULIN THERAPY OPTIONS
Multiple Daily Injections

In an effort to limit the debilitating long-term effects of hyperglycemia in T1D, treatment methodology continues to change as new products seek to exhibit normal physiologic glucose control.[15] Since the discovery of insulin in 1922, researchers and pharmaceutical companies have sought to develop new insulin analogs that emulate a healthy pancreas. Since the DCCT, attempts to achieve better glycemic control have often been in the form of IIT, which includes MDI or pump (ie, basal-bolus) therapy.[17] Because of a lack of insulin, both fasting and postprandial hyperglycemia present in T1D patients. Fasting hyperglycemia can be contained using long-acting basal insulin, which is administered once or twice a day, whereas postprandial hyperglycemia can be prevented by using premeal rapid-acting insulin. According to the DCCT, the biggest hurdle associated with IIT is a 3-fold increase in severe hypoglycemia and significant weight gain, making education and continued follow-up vital when instituting MDI therapy.[15]

Early insulins (porcine or bovine)[18] used for treatment in T1D patients varied significantly and contained many impurities that resulted in a rise of circulating insulin antibodies. The first long-acting (basal) insulin, protamine zinc, developed in the 1930s, was used twice a day without regular rapid-acting insulin.[18] Diabetes treatment was

Features	DexCom SEVEN PLUS[a] 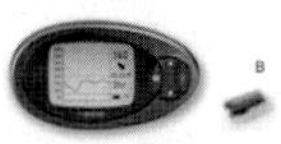	Medtronic Guardian 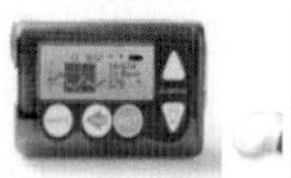	MiniMed Paradigm 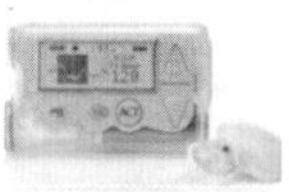
Approved Age Group	≥18 years	≥7 years	≥7 years
Integration with pump	[b]Yes	Yes	Yes
Integration with glucometer	No	Yes	Yes
Predictive alarm	Yes	Yes	Yes
Rate of change alarm	Yes	Yes	Yes
Sensor wear (days)	7 [c]10-14	3 [c]5-6	3 [c]5-6
Frequency of glucose measurements (minutes)	5	5	5

Fig. 4. Continuous glucose monitors. [a] GEN-4 was recently approved in Europe. [b] Not approved in the US but recently approved by the EMEA. [c] Off-label use.

transformed in the 1950s with the development of neutral protamine Hagedorn (NPH) and Lente insulin (Ultralente, Semilente, and Lente) as patients began a regiment of twice-daily NPH (basal) coupled with regular insulin (prandial) to provide better glycemic control. These treatment options are commonly referred to as conventional care. Insulin development continued to progress in the 1980s as purified pork insulin and recombinant human insulin were used to make therapeutic insulin, almost eliminating insulin allergies and antibody formation. In spite of this, these early products exhibited varied absorption rates contributing to unpredictable glycemic control.[19] The duration of action was inadequate and there was a significant peak after 4 to 6 hours leading to nocturnal hypoglycemic events.[19] These weaknesses made it clear that better long-acting insulin analogs (LAIAs) were necessary, which led to the development of the current insulins used in MDI treatment.

Currently, the LAIAs used in basal-bolus therapy are the insulins glargine (Lantus) and detemir (Levemir). These LAIAs were created by modifying the amino acid sequence on the β chain. They exhibit much improved pharmacokinetics and pharmocodynamics[20] (**Fig. 5**A) without a peak effect and maintain a longer duration of action.[19] The changes to the β-chain created a molecule that decreases the rate of absorption resulting in a longer duration of action of these insulin analogs without any peak effect. This development has allowed for a significant decrease in A1c values with reduced hypoglycemia compared with NPH.[21] Furthermore, these LAIAs have more predictable absorption rates and less intra-indivual and inter-individual variability,[19,20] significantly improving glycemic control in addition to limiting hypoglycemia, especially nocturnal.[22]

The action profiles of detemir and glargine show that LAIAs have a duration of up to 24 hours with minimum peak action (see **Fig. 5**B). Other LAIAs are the Eli Lilly insulin LY2605541, which is currently in clinical trial, and Novo Nordisk's degludec, which awaits Food and Drug Administration (FDA) and evaluation of the European Medicines Evaluation Agency (EMEA) approval to be released on the market.

Based on pharmacokinetic/pharmacodynamics data, degludec is reported to have a glucose-lowering effect (based on glucose infusion rates) for over 24 hours in addition to a smooth action profile (see **Fig. 5**B).[23] Degludec has a C-16 fatty acid chain attached to the end of the of the β-chain (see **Fig. 5**A). This change results in an increase in molecular size and an extended duration and allows the insulin to bind with either subcutaneous or vascular albumin. To date, various studies of T1D and T2D have documented similar decreased hypoglycemia by 20% to 30% with similar A1c values and the possibility of injecting basal insulin only 3 days a week due to its

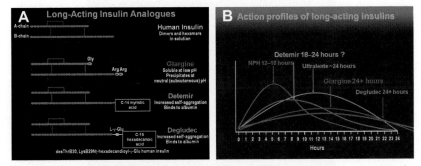

Fig. 5. (A) Amino acid structure of insulins glargine and detemir. (B) Action profile of insulins glargine, detemir, and degludec versus prior LAIAs.

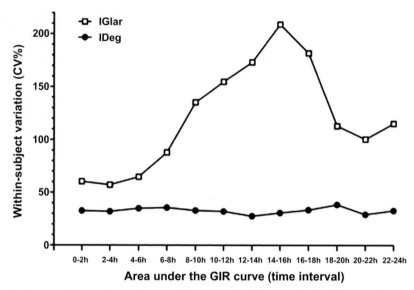

Fig. 6. Pharmacodynamic variability of insulin degludec versus insulin glargine. (*From* Heise T, Hermanski L, Nosek L, et al. The pharmacodynamic variability of insulin degludec is consistently lower than insulin glargine over 24 hours at steady state. Diabetes 2011; 60(Suppl 1):A263; with permission.)

longer duration of action.[23–25] In addition to a longer duration, degludec has also shown less variability in clinical trials compared with glargine (**Fig. 6**).

Although the pharmacokinetics/pharmacodynamics of today's LAIAs have shown vast improvements compared with their predecessors in meta-analysis studies,[23] new basal insulins are more costly. While some studies have shown these increased costs associated with LAIAs are warranted,[26] it is still a financial burden on T1D patients as well as health care systems around the world.

Just as LAIAs imitate the basal insulin delivery by the pancreas, rapid-acting insulin analogs (RAIAs) imitate the bolus insulin secretion necessary to avoid postprandial hyperglycemia (**Fig. 7**). Rapid-acting insulin injections are administered before meals based on premeal glucose levels as well as the carbohydrate, protein, and fat content of the meal. RAIAs exhibit a rapid onset of action with a shorter duration[20] and are

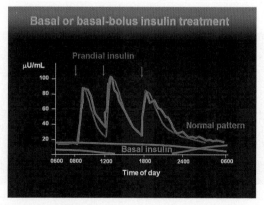

Fig. 7. Desired RAIA action profiles.

created by changing the amino acids at the end of the β-terminal of the insulin mole-cule (**Fig. 8**).[20] Insulin lispro (Humalog) was the first human analog introduced in 1996. Since lispro, 2 other RAIAs, insulin aspart (NovoLog) and glulisine (Apidra), have been introduced with similar benefits. Along with the ability to take insulin closer to meal-time, all 3 analogs have similar efficacy in A1c reduction, decreased postprandial hyperglycemia, and reduced late-onset postprandial hypoglycemia.[27]

Despite the established benefits of RAIAs for T1D management, there are draw-backs to these insulins. Just as with LAIAs, RAIAs represent an extra cost compared with conventional insulin therapy. Further analysis is necessary to determine if increased costs associated with IIT are offset by decreasing the cost associated with acute and long-term complications.[27] Although dystrophy (atrophy or hyper-trophy) is a side effect that has greatly decreased since the introduction of human recombinant insulin, there are still cases reported with the use of RAIAs and LAIAs[28] necessitating patient education of proper insulin use and rotating injection sites.

Another option for IIT therapy includes the use of premixed insulin analogs, composed of both LAIAs and RAIAs administered 2 to 4 times a day. Premixed insulin analogs seek to mimic physiologic endogenous insulin secretion.[29] These insulins come in a variety of ratios, including 80/20 (80% lispro/aspart and 20% neutral prot-amine lispro), 70/30, 60/40, 40/60, 30/70, 20/80, and so forth, which are available in Europe. Only 70/30 (70% insulin aspart protamine suspension and 30% insulin aspart), 75/25 (insulin lispro protamine suspension and 25% insulin lispro), and 50/50 (50% high lispro/protamine mix) mixtures are approved in the United States.[29] The idea behind premixed insulin is to provide T1D patients with basal and prandial insulin while limiting the number of daily injections, but studies have shown considerable vari-ability in onset and duration of action as well as inconsistent peak effects.[29] Due to

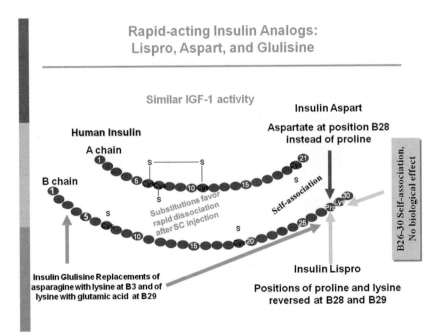

Fig. 8. Amino acid structure of lispro, aspart, and glulisine. (*From* Garg SK, Ellis SL, Ulrich H. Insulin glulisine: a new rapid-acting insulin analogue for the treatment of diabetes. Expert Opin Pharmacother 2005;6(4)1–9; with permission.)

these findings, premixed insulins are not typically suggested and other forms of IIT are generally used for more accurate glycemic control.

Delivery systems used in IIT for RAIAs, LAIAs, and premixed insulins include pens (prefilled disposable pens or pens with replaceable cartridges) or vials and syringes (**Fig. 9**). In Europe, pens are a more popular delivery system; however, due to higher costs in the United States, only approximately 20% of patients use pens.

Data collected by frequent SMBG and more recently from CGM use have brought to light the need to develop ultra-RAIAs, which can truly mimic pancreatic secretion of mealtime insulin. The ultra-RAIAs under development are VIAject made by Biodel, Halozyme, and Technosphere made by MannKind. VIAject uses EDTA, citric acid, and other reagents generally regarded as safe to dissociate insulin hexamers for rapid absorption.[30] Halozyme uses human recombinant hyaluronidase enzymes to promote rapid insulin absorption and dispersion.[27] Technosphere is inhaled insulin currently in a phase III study to establish noninferiority to insulin aspart.

Continuous Subcutaneous Insulin Infusion

CSII is another form of IIT that has been shown to have several advantages over MDI. Made possible by insulin pumps (see **Fig. 8**), CSII has been shown in studies to increase treatment satisfaction among patients and lower hypoglycemia with a reduced insulin dose.[31] The first insulin pumps were introduced in the late 1970s, using a single basal rate for insulin delivery along with incremental insulin secretions for mealtime bolus.[32] As pump technology has improved, pumps have become much smaller and compatible with commercial insulin without dilution. Pumps now have smaller, more durable batteries and built-in alarms. They are also easier to use than their predecessors with the same basic insulin delivery method, which uses a subcutaneously placed catheter.[32]

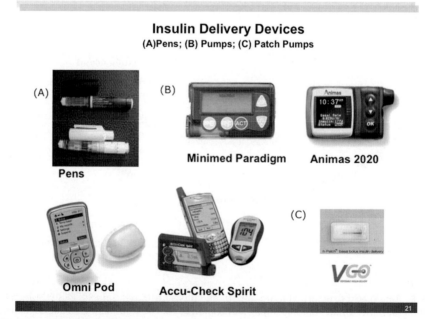

Insulin Delivery Devices
(A)Pens; (B) Pumps; (C) Patch Pumps

(A) Pens

(B) Minimed Paradigm   Animas 2020

Omni Pod   Accu-Check Spirit   (C) VGo

Fig. 9. Insulin delivery devices.

Current insulin pumps available are the MiniMed Paradigm by Medtronic, Animas by the Animas Corporation, Spirit by Accu-Chek, Omnipod, t:slim by Tandem, and V-Go patch pumps by Valeritas. The new patch pumps eliminate tubing because users interface with an infusion component that is directly on the skin instead of connected through a catheter.[32] This allows for ease of use and mobility by patch pump users. The OmniPod Insulin Management System (Insulet) delivers both basal and bolus insulin to the body through a pod that contains the pump, insulin, and cannula that interfaces with a separate controller.[33] Valeritas has introduced the V-Go, a transdermal hydraulic device without electronics, which received FDA approval in December 2010 and approval in Europe in July 2011. The Tandem t:slim, which is 25% smaller than other pumps and has a color touch screen interface, was approved by the FDA in November 2011. Roche is working on the Solo, a micropump and reservoir unit that attaches to a cradle with a cannula. Although this pump has received FDA approval, it is yet to be available for sale. The future may see smaller patch pumps with CGM incorporation that last longer than the current 2 to 3 days per insertion.

Advances in pump technology have resulted in pumps with fewer malfunctions and features that ensure greater control of insulin delivery.[34] Such features include the ability to program multiple basal rates for different times of day as well as the capacity to calculate recommended bolus doses based on both manually imputted blood glucoses and mealtime carbohydrate content. These pumps also include bolus profiling, temporary basal rate programming, and basal suspension for times of exercise or illness.[32] The ability to program and fine tune basal rates allows physicians to alter IIT for individual patients and their specific needs.[35] In addition, data management systems give a more accurate view of patient compliance, blood glucose levels, dosage, and timing to help aid in clinical care decisions and patient education.[31]

The primary advantage of CSII is improved glycemic control as measured by A1c, specifically for individuals with higher baseline A1c on MDI.[36] Studies have shown varying results regarding CSII and improved glycemic control in T1D patients. One study comparing CSII to MDI found little difference in therapies with an A1c values differing by only 0.5%,[37] whereas a subsequent study in hypoglycemic-prone subjects found an improvement in A1c of 1.5%.[38] Despite a confirmed benefit of CSII over MDI, advantages of CSII include a modest reduction in hypoglycemia while maintaining similar A1c values, a reduction in total insulin dose, and better patient compliance. Although improved glycemic control in CSII is not fully understood, it has been shown that individuals with higher baseline A1cs improve the most on CSII therapy.[39]

Despite recent innovations in pump technology, patients using a pump without proper education may miss or disregard additional boluses before meals, resulting in postprandial hyperglycemia. Increased A1cs can result in patients missing an average of 1 mealtime bolus per week.[40] Other disadvantages for pump users include higher costs, greater risk for diabetic ketoacidosis in the event of pump malfunction, skin irritation, and the inconvenience of being attached to the pump itself.[31,41] Continued education is pivotal during the transition from MDI to CSII.[31] Improved nonclogging catheters, insertion devices, and ultra–fast-acting insulin analogs may also facilitate better health outcomes for CSII.[32]

BLOOD GLUCOSE TESTING
Self-Monitored Blood Glucose

Frequent testing of blood glucose in T1D is an important aspect of diabetes management to ensure proper insulin doses are administered and to decrease glucose variability (GV). Studies have shown that frequent testing of blood glucose by self-monitoring blood glucose (SMBG) devices is associated with decreased A1c values.[42] Like other devices used in the treatment of T1D, SMBG monitors have undergone significant improvements to adhere to FDA accuracy guidelines.[43] A study conducted in 2010 found that 11 out of 27 meters currently on the market did not meet accuracy guidelines. Device companies have since improved these products to meet the FDA guidelines so that their products are within ±15 mg/dL of the reference method at blood glucose concentrations less than or equal to 75 mg/dL and within ±20 mg/dL at blood glucose concentrations greater than or equal to 75 mg/dL at least 95% of the time.[43] Improvements in SMBG devices have also included resistance to interference from molecules, such as maltose, to ensure accurate readings for hospitalized patients with diabetes.[44]

Continuous Glucose Monitors

Patients with T1D may also benefit greatly from the use of CGMs. These devices work by sampling a patient's interstitial fluid and presenting blood glucose values every 1 to 5 minutes.[45] Patients are informed of their blood glucose in real time, which allows them to appropriately adjust their insulin dosage based on their glucose trends. CGMs can provide abundant information regarding a patient's glucose control, variability, and significant highs/lows, whereas SMBGs only provide patients with a single blood glucose measurement.[45] Alarm functions on CGMs assist in reducing hypoglycemia and hyperglycemia, especially at night.[46] By tracking blood glucose continuously, CGMs allow both patients and their providers to better understand hypoglycemic and hyperglycemic trends and adjust their insulin doses and timing of insulin injections appropriately. This may result in better glucose control, minimized glycemic excursions, and reduce glucose variability (GV).[47]

There are 3 FDA approved CGMs currently available, including the SEVEN PLUS by DexCom and the Paradigm REAL-Time and Guardian REAL-Time by Medtronic. The FreeStyle Navigator by Abbott Diabetes Care has recently been discontinued by the FDA due to ongoing quality control issues. The DexCom SEVEN PLUS CGM System takes glucose measurements every 5 minutes and displays glucose values via a transmitter to the unit. Each sensor can be worn for 7 days and requires a 2-hour start-up period with necessary SMBG calibrations every 12 hours to ensure accuracy. This device features alarms that can be set to notify a patient of hypoglycemic and hyperglycemic glucose levels, allowing patients to spend more time in euglycemic ranges. The SEVEN PLUS can display blood glucose changes and trends over 1, 3, 6, 12, and 24 hours and has the ability to monitor meal times, insulin administration, and physical activity. This allows for a more complete picture of glucose excursions and their causes to patients and treating physicians to assist in clinical care decisions. The Medtronic MiniMed Paradigm REAL-Time Insulin Pump and Continuous Glucose Monitoring System is much like the SEVEN PLUS in that it requires a 2-hour start-up and SMBG calibrations every 12 hours but it is only approved for 3-day use. The MiniMed Paradigm REAL-Time requires 2 different insertion sites, 1 for the sensor and 1 for insulin delivery. The MiniMed Guardian REAL-Time CGM is a similar device designed for patients using MDIs. Both of these CGMs allow patients and physicians access to glucose trend graphs for 3 to 24 hours and feature alarms to warn of hypoglycemic and hyperglycemic glucose levels. Medtronic is also currently working on a new sensor, the Enlite that can communicate with the Medtronic pump. It is approved for 6-day use in Europe but is still being investigated for approval by the FDA in the United States.

As with any developing technology, there are drawbacks to CGMs. Due to the physiologic lag time between blood glucose values and those read in the interstitial fluid by the CGM, CGMs only supplement SMBGs, which should be measured to confirm glucose readings before treatment actions are taken.[18] The FDA and EMEA have only approved these products as adjunctive to SMBG. This lag time is accentuated with a high rate of change greater than 2 mg/dL/min.[48] Other disadvantages to CGMs include site erythema, edema, and skin irritation from the sensor/adhesive.[49,50] Patients may also be prone to overcorrecting hypoglyclemia and hyperglycemia, which may accentuate glucose excursions.[48]

CLOSED-LOOP THERAPY

Studies have found that CSII coupled with CGMs improves glycemic control when the CGM is being used regularly.[32] Therefore, it has been argued that a minimally invasive system using CGMs, insulin pumps, and algorithms is the most feasible step in closing the loop in T1D patients.[51] In an effort to create a system that functions as an artificial pancreas (bionic pancreas), algorithms and mathematical modeling must be used to link CGM with insulin delivery.[51] These algorithms will be evaluated on their ability to match β-cell physiology and recreate glucose and insulin profiles of healthy individuals.[52]

A closed-loop system using a validated algorithm would help eliminate the possibility of human errors, such as forgotten insulin doses and overcorrection. It is at the forefront of diabetes research and is currently limited by the lack of accurate glucose sensors that do not experience lag time associated with reading interstitial fluid rather than blood glucose levels.[52,53] In addition, all CGMs need to be calibrated at least 2 times per day using SMBG values; thus, errors in SMBG readings can further complicate accuracy of CGM glucose values.[54] Currently, two main approaches to closed-loop systems exist. The extracorporeal uses subcutaneous glucose monitoring coupled with subcutaneous insulin (sc–sc) delivery whereas the implantable uses intravenous glucose sampling and intraperitoneal insulin (iv–ip) delivery.[53] The sc–sc approach to a closed-loop system is the minimally invasive option and has the greatest potential for widespread application.[53] It is inhibited by substantial lag times, however, between rising glucose levels and the peak effect of the secreted insulin, increasing the likelihood of significant glycemic excursions.[53] Although lag times are decreased in the iv–ip system, they are still longer than a typical physiologic response time in a healthy individual. Furthermore, implantable pumps are expensive, need surgical implantation, and are associated with major complications, such as pump-pocket infections and device failures.[55]

Although some researchers have suggested that the iv–ip method is the only feasible way to truly close the loop, other research has shown promising results using external pump systems.[53] In a 2008 study, 17 T1D patients were randomized to a fully closed-loop (FCL) system or a hybrid closed-loop (HCL) system.[56] The FCL arm had no interaction with their insulin delivery system whereas those in the HCL arm administered a premeal priming bolus of insulin that accounted for 25% to 50% of the anticipated carbohydrates.[56] The conclusion of this study found that both the FCL and HCL systems were superior to traditional care despite the risk of nocturnal hypoglycemia associated with delayed insulin absorption.[56] Other ongoing studies include a proposed in-home study using the Medtronic Paradigm Veo closed-loop system. This system incorporates a low glucose suspend, which is designed to prevent hypoglycemia, especially when patients are sleeping. This pump is currently approved in Europe. Clinical trials in the United States are awaiting FDA approval and will be initiated at the start of 2012.[57]

Clinical trials are also in progress to assess closed-loop systems that incorporate bihormonal infusion of insulin and glucagon to mimic a well-functioning pancreas.[58,59]

In an effort to combat hypoglycemia associated with IIT and closed-loop systems, studies have shown that low glucose suspend may not be enough and that the use of glucagon in conjunction with insulin analogs may provide better glycemic control and decrease hypoglycemia.[58,59]

Ultimately, closed-loop systems and the creation of a functioning artificial pancreas are the future of IIT in T1D patients. Currently, hypoglycemia due to lag times from glucose sensors remains one of the largest barriers to an FCL system[53] as is hyperglycemia due to catheter occlusion. The future of closed-loop systems is dependent on substantially more research to test combinations of pumps and CGMs as well as bihormonal and implanted pumps.

GLUCOSE VARIABILITY

A healthy individual exhibits a narrow blood glucose range. Glucose homeostasis is maintained at appropriate levels by pancreatic β-cells, which are sensitive to glucose in a concentration-dependent manner.[60] Several studies, such as the DCCT and the UK Prospective Diabetes Study, have debated the role of GV and its relationship with microvascular complications.[61] There are other clinical trials that show GV as an independent risk factor for microvascular and macrovascular complications. Furthermore, wide fluctuations in GV can increase the risk for severe hypoglycemia.[62]

Other short-term (acute) studies have demonstrated that GV is associated with oxidative stress markers that may be associated with the endothelial damage seen in vascular complications.[63] Additional long-term studies are necessary to confirm that reducing GV causes a reduction in microvascular and macrovascular complications. This notion has inspired subsequent studies relating to GV in T1D patients in an effort to better understand GV and its effects. In one such study, the incidence of retinopathy in a group of adolescents with T1D fell substantially between 1990 and 2002 despite A1c levels remaining static,[64] further supporting the findings by the DCCT. One speculative explanation for this phenomenon is that conventionally treated patients received fewer insulin injections than those of the intensive therapy arm of the study and experienced a greater number of glycemic excursions.[65] These findings promote the theory that IIT can help reduce glycemic fluctuations. It has consequently been proposed that T1D treatment goals should not only be to avoid short-term complications, such as hypoglycemia and diabetic ketoacidosis, but also to minimize variability in blood glucose to limit excess risk of long-term complications.[61]

SUMMARY

Improving glucose control limits long-term micromascular and macrovascular diabetes complications.[16] Intensive insulin treatment using MDI or CSII is the best choice for subjects with T1D. Several advances in new insulin preparations (such as LAIAs and RAIAs) have facilitated implementation of IIT. Glucose monitoring with SMBG and/or CGM should be an integral part of IIT, especially to limit hypoglycemia and GV. Today, use of new insulin analogs, frequent SMBG, and use of real-time CGMs has significantly decreased severe hypoglycemia compared with DCCT. The future may lie in development of an artificial pancreas (bionic pancreas), which incorporates CGM with CSII.

ACKNOWLEDGMENTS

We sincerely thank the staff at the Barbara Davis Center for Childhood Diabetes helping us in preparing this article.

REFERENCES

1. National Diabetes Fact Sheet: national estimates and general information on diabetes and prediabetes in the United States 2011. Available at: http://www.cdc.gov/diabetes/pubs/pdf/ndfs_2011.pdf. Accessed August 26, 2011.
2. Huang ES, Basu A, O'Grady M, et al. Projecting the future diabetes population size and related costs for the US. Diabetes Care 2009;32:2225–9.
3. Diabetes and prediabetes cost in the U.S. $218 billion in 2007: en route to $336 billion by 2034. Diabetes Health; 2010. Available at: http://diabeteshealth.com/read/2010/02/03/6551/diabetes-and-pre-diabetes-cost-the-us-218-billion-in-2007-en-route-to-336-billion-by-2034/. Accessed August 26, 2011.
4. Diabetes and pre-diabetes accounted for $218 billion in costs in 2007, health affairs paper demonstrates 2008. Available at: http://press.novonordisk-us.com/index.php?s=43&item=230. Accessed August 26, 2011.
5. Yang W, Lu J, Weng J, et al. China National Diabetes and Metabolic Disorders Study Group: Prevalence of diabetes among men and women in China. N Engl J Med 2010;362:1090–101.
6. Anjana RM, Pradeepa R, Deepa M, et al. Prevalence of diabetes and prediabetes (impaired fasting glucose and/or impaired glucose tolerance) in urban and rural India: Phase I results of the Indian Council of Medical Research–INdia DIABetes (ICMR – INDIAB) study. Diabetologia 2011. DOI: 10.1007/s00125-011-2291-5.
7. International Diabetes Federation. IDF Diabetes Atlas. 5th edition. Brussels (Belgium): International diabetes federation; 2011. Available at: http://eatlas.idf.org. Accessed November 11, 2011.
8. Garg SK. Rising epidemic of diabetes and hypertension in Asia. Diabetes Technol Ther 2011;14(1): DOI: 10.1089/dia.2011.0257.
9. Atkinson MA, Eisenbarth GS. Type 1 diabetes: new perspectives on disease pathogenesis and treatment. Lancet 2001;358:221–9.
10. Onkamo P, Vonnen S, Karvonen M, et al. Worldwide increase in incidence of Type 1 diabetes—the analysis of the data on published incidence trends. Diabetologia 1999;42:1395–403.
11. Imagawa A, Toshiaki H, Jun-ichiro M, et al. A novel subtype of type 1 diabetes mellitus characterized by a rapid onset and absence of diabetes-related antibodies. N Engl J Med 2000;342:301–7.
12. Verge CF, Stenger D, Bonifacio E, et al. Combined use of autoantibodies (IA-2 autoantibody, GAD autoantibody, insulin autoantibody, cytoplasmic islet cell antibodies) in type 1 diabetes: combinatorial islet autoantibody workshop. Diabetes 1998;47(12):1857–66.
13. Greenbaum CJ. Insulin resistance in type 1 diabetes. Diabetes Metab Res Rev 2002;18(3):192–200.
14. Abdul-Rasoul M, Habib H, Al-Khouly M. 'The honeymoon phase' in children with type 1 diabetes mellitus: frequency, duration, and influential factors. Pediatr Diabetes 2006;7(2):101–7.
15. The Diabetes Control and Complications Trial Research Group. The effect of intensive treatment of diabetes on the development and progression of long-term complications in insulin-dependent diabetes mellitus. N Engl J Med 1993;329:977–86.
16. Writing Team for the Diabetes Control and Complications Trial/Epidemiology of Diabetes Interventions and Complications Research Group. Sustained effect of intensive treatment of type 1 diabetes mellitus on development and progression

of diabetic nephropathy: the Epidemiology of Diabetes Interventions and Complications (EDIC) study. JAMA 2003;290:2159–67.

17. Ratner RE, Diabetes Prevention Program Research. An update on the diabetes prevention program. Endorc Pract 2006;12(1):20–4.

18. Hirsch IB. Insulin delivery devices—pumps and pens. Diabetes Technol Ther 2010;12(Suppl 1):S115–6.

19. Pickup JC, Renard E. Long-acting insulin analogs versus insulin pump therapy for the treatment of type 1 and type 2 diabetes. Diabetes Care 2008;31(Suppl 2): S140–5.

20. Garg SK, Ellis SL, Ulrich H. Insulin glulisine: a new rapid-acting insulin analogue for the treatment of diabetes. Expert Opin Pharmacother 2005;6(4):1–9.

21. Rosenstock J, Dailey G, Massi-Benedetti M, et al. Reduced hypoglycemia risk with insulin glargine: A meta-analysis comparing insulin glargine with human NPH insulin in type 2 diabetes. Diabetes Care 2005;28(4):950–5.

22. Owens DR, Bolli GB. Beyond the era of NPH insulin—long-acting insulin analogs: chemistry comparative pharmacology, and clinical application. Diabetes Technol Ther 2008;10:333–49.

23. Zinman B, Fulcher G, Rao PV, et al. Insulin degludec, an ultra-long-acting basal insulin, once a day or three times a week versus insulin glargine once a day in patients with type 2 diabetes: a 16-week, randomized, open-label, phase 2 trial. Lancet 2011;377:924–31.

24. Kudra Y, Basu A. Ultra-long-acting insulins for lifestyle-related pandemic. Lancet 2011;377:880–9.

25. Birkeland K, Home P, Wendish U, et al. Insulin degludec in type 1 diabetes: a randomized controlled trial of new-generation ultra-long-acting insulin compared with insulin glargine. Diabetes Care 2011;34(3):661–5.

26. Radermecker RP, Scheen AJ. Continuous subcutaneous insulin infusion with short-acting insulin analogues or human regular insulin: efficacy, safety, quality of life, and cost-effectiveness. Diabetes Metab Res Rev 2004;20(3):178–88.

27. Vaughn DE, Yocum RC, Muchmore DB, et al. Accelerated pharmacokinetics and glucodynamics of prandial insulins injected with recombinant human hyaluronidase. Diabetes Technol Ther 2009;11:345–52.

28. del Olmo MI, Campos V, Abellan P, et al. A case of lipoatrophy with insulin detemir. Diabetes Res Clin Pract 2008;80(1):e20–1.

29. Garber AJ. Premixed insulin analogues for the treatment of diabetes mellitus. Drugs 2006;66(1):31–49.

30. Steiner S, Hompesch M, Pohl R, et al. A novel insulin formulation with a more rapid onset of action. Diabetologia 2008;51:1602–6.

31. Meneghini L, Sparrow-Bodenmiller J. Practical aspects and considerations when switching between continuous subcutaneous insulin infusion and multiple daily injections. Diabetes Technol Ther 2010;12(Suppl 1):109–14.

32. Skyler JS. Continous subcutaneous insulin infusion—a historical perspective. Diabetes Technol Ther 2010;12(Suppl 1):S5–9.

33. Anhalt H, Bohannon NJ. Insulin patch pumps: their development and future in closed-loop systems. Diabetes Technol Ther 2010;12(Suppl 1):S51–8.

34. Scaramuzza AE, Zuccotti GV. Commentary on 'Continuous subcutaneous insulin infusion (CSII) versus multiple insulin injections for type 1 diabetes mellitus' with a response from the review authors. Evid Base Child Health 2010;5: 1870–2.

35. Maahs DM, Horton LA, Chase HP. The use of insulin pumps in youth with type 1 diabetes. Diabetes Technol Ther 2010;12(Suppl 1):S51–8.

36. Pickup JC, Kidd J, Burmiston S, et al. Determinants of glycaemic control in type 1 diabetes during intensified therapy with multiple daily insulin injections or continuous subcutaneous insulin infusion: importance of blood glucose variability. Diabetes Metab Res Rev 2006;22:232–7.
37. Pickup JC, Mattock MB, Kerry S. Glycaemic control with continuous subcutaneous insulin infusion compared to intensive insulin injection therapy in type 1 diabetes: meta-analysis of randomized controlled trials. BMJ 2002;324:705–8.
38. Pickup JC, Kidd J, Burmistion S, et al. Effectiveness of continuous subcutaneous insulin infusion in hypoglycaemic-prone type 1 diabetes: implications for NICE guidelines. Pract Diabet Int 2005;22:10–4.
39. Retnakaran R, Hochman J, DeVries JH, et al. Continuous subcutaneous insulin infusion versus multiple daily injections: the impact of baselin A1c. Diabetes Care 2004;27:2590–6.
40. Burdick J, Chase HP, Slover RH, et al. Missed insulin meal boluses and elevated hemoglobin A1c levels in children receiving insulin pump therapy. Pediatrics 2004;113:221–4.
41. Linkeschova R, Raoul M, Bott U, et al. Less severe hypoglycaemia, better metabolic control, and improved quality of life in type 1 diabetes mellitus with continuous subcutaneous insulin infusion (CSII) therapy; an observational study of 100 consecutive patients followed for a mean of 2 years. Diabet Med 2002;19: 746–51.
42. Garg SK, Hirsch IB. Self-monitoring of blood glucose. Int J Clin Pract 2010; 64(Suppl):1–10. DOI: 10.1111/j.1742-1241.2009.02271.x.
43. Freckmann G, Baumstark A, Jendrike N, et al. System accuracy evaluation of 27 blood glucose monitorying systems according to DIN EN ISO 15197. Diabetes Technol Ther 2010;12:245–7.
44. Hirsch IB, Verderese CA. Interference of home blood glucose measurements and poor outcomes: a solvable problem requiring broader exposure. Diabetes Technol Ther 2010;12:245–7.
45. Garg SK. Role of continuous glucose monitoring in patients with diabetes using multiple daily insulin injections. Infusystems International 2009;8:17–21.
46. Garg SK, Hoff HK, Chase HP. The role of continuous sensors in diabetes care. Endocrinol Metab Clin North Am 2004;33:163–73.
47. Gilliam LK, Hirsch IB. Practical aspects of real-time continuous glucose monitoring. Diabetes Technol Ther 2009;11:93–103.
48. Ellis SL, Bookout T, Garg SK, et al. Use of continuous glucose monitoring to improve diabetes mellitus management. Endocrinol Metab Clin North Am 2007; 36(Suppl 2):46–8.
49. Garg SK, Zisser H, Schwartz S, et al. Improvement in glycemic excursions with a transcutaneous, real-time continuous glucose sensor: a randomized controlled trial. Diabetes Care 2006;29:44–50.
50. Garg SK, Potts RO, Ackerman NR, et al. Correlation of fingerstick blood glucose measurements with Gluco Watch biographer glucose results in young subjects with type 1 diabetes. Diabetes Care 1999;22:1708–14.
51. Kovatchev BP, Brenton M, Man CD, et al. In Silico preclinical trials: a proof of concept in closed-loop control of type 1 diabetes. J Diabetes Sci Technol 2009;3(1):44–55.
52. Steil GM, Panteleon AE, Rebrin K. Closed-loop insulin-delivery—the path to physiological glucose control. Adv Drug Deliv Rev 2004;56:125–44.
53. Hovorka R. Continuous glucose monitoring and closed-loop systems. Diabet Med 2005;23:1–12.

54. Mazze R, Strock E, Borgman S. Evaluating the accuracy, reliability, and clinical applicability of continuous glucose monitoring (CGM): Is CGM ready for real time? Diabetes Technol Ther 2009;11:11–8.
55. Selam JL. External and implantable insulin pumps: current place in the treatment of diabetes. Exp Clin Endocrinol Diabetes 2001;109:S333–40.
56. Weinzimer SA, Steil GM, Swan KL, et al. Fully automated closed-loop insulin delivery versus semiautomated hybrid control in pediatric patients with type 1 diabetes using an artificial pancreas. Diabetes Care 2010;33:121–7.
57. Danne T, Kordonouri O, Holder M, et al. Prevention of hypoglycemia by using low glucose suspend function in sensor-augmented pump therapy. Diabetes Technol Ther 2011;10:1129–34.
58. El-Khatib FH, Russel SJ, Nathan DM, et al. A bihormonal closed-loop artificial pancreas for type 1 diabetes. Sci Transl Med 2010;2:27ra.
59. Castle JR, Engle JM, El Youssef J, et al. Novel use of glucagon in a closed-loop system for prevention of hypoglycemia in type 1 diabetes. Diabetes Care 2010; 33:1282–7.
60. Henquin JC. Perspectives in diabetes: triggering and amplifying pathways of regulation of insulin secretion by glucose. Diabetes 2000;49:1751–60.
61. Kilpatrick ES, Rigby AS, Atkin SL. The effect of glucose variability on the risk of microvascular complications in type 1 diabetes. Diabetes Care 2006;29(7): 1486–90.
62. White NH, Chase HP, Arslanian S, et al. Comparison of glycemic variability associated with insulin glargine and intermediate-acting insulin when used as the basal component of multiple daily injections for adolescents with type 1 diabetes. Diabetes Care 2009;32(3):387–93.
63. Monnier L, Mas E, Ginet C, et al. Activation of oxidative stress by acute glucose fluctuations compared with sustained chronic hyperglycemia in patients with type 2 diabetes. JAMA 2006;295(14):1681–7.
64. Mohsin F, Craig ME, Cusumano J, et al. Discordant trends in microvascular complications in adolescents with type 1 diabetes from 1990 to 2002. Diabetes Care 2005;28:1974–80.
65. Hirsch IB, Brownlee M. Should minimal blood glucose variability become the gold standard of glycemic control? J Diabetes Complications 2005;19:178–81.

Closed-Loop Insulin Delivery in Type 1 Diabetes

Hood Thabit, MD[a,b], Roman Hovorka, PhD[a],*

KEYWORDS

- Closed loop • Continuous glucose sensor
- Insulin pump • Algorithm

Advances in diabetes technology have led to significant improvements in the quality of life and care received by individuals with diabetes. Despite this, achieving tight glycemic control through intensive insulin therapy and modern insulin regimens is challenging because of the barrier of hypoglycemia,[1] the most feared complication of insulin therapy as reported by patients, caregivers, and physicians.[2]

Recent research in therapeutic devices for type 1 diabetes focuses on improving glucose monitoring and insulin-delivery devices with the view of integrating these into an artificial pancreas, a closed-loop insulin delivery system.[3] Coupling subcutaneous continuous glucose monitoring[4] and subcutaneous insulin pump delivery,[5] closed-loop systems deliver insulin in a continued glucose-responsive manner **(Fig. 1)**. This novel approach differs from the conventional pump therapy by the use of a control algorithm, which directs insulin delivery based on real-time sensor glucose levels.[6] The artificial pancreas may transform the management of type 1 diabetes and improve the quality of life, acting as a bridge to cure until stem cell therapy or islet cell transplantation becomes available.

The first effort to develop components of the artificial pancreas started with the studies on semicontinuous glucose monitoring by Weller and colleagues[7] in 1960. The first portable insulin pump was designed by Kadish[8] in 1964. Prototypes of the

Funding support: Juvenile Diabetes Research Foundation, National Institute of Diabetes and Digestive and Kidney Diseases, NIHR Cambridge Biomedical Research Centre, Medical Research Council Centre for Obesity and Related Metabolic Diseases, Diabetes UK, European Commission Framework Program 7.

Conflicts of interest: R.H. reports having received speaker honoraria from Minimed Medtronic, Lifescan, and Novo Nordisk; serving on advisory panel for Animas and Minimed Medtronic; receiving license fees from BBraun and Becton Dickinson; and having served as a consultant to Becton Dickinson, BBraun, and Profil. H.T. has no competing interests.

[a] Institute of Metabolic Science, Addenbrookes Hospital, University of Cambridge, Box 289, Level 4, Cambridge CB2 0QQ, UK
[b] Faculty of Medicine, University of Malaya, Kuala Lumpur, Malaysia
* Corresponding author.
E-mail address: rh347@cam.ac.uk

Endocrinol Metab Clin N Am 41 (2012) 105–117
doi:10.1016/j.ecl.2011.12.003
0889-8529/12/$ – see front matter © 2012 Elsevier Inc. All rights reserved.

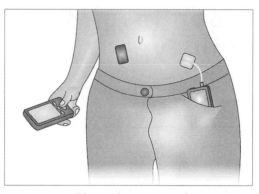

Fig. 1. A closed-loop system comprising a glucose sensor (*rectangle* on the left-hand side of the abdomen), an insulin pump (device in the pocket connected to patient via an infusion set), and a mobile-sized device containing the control algorithm (in patient's hand). Each component communicates with the other wirelessly. (*From* Hovorka R. Closed-loop insulin delivery: from bench to clinical practice. Nat Rev Endocrinol 2011;7:385–95; with permission.)

artificial pancreas adopting intravascular sensing and delivery, devised in the 1970s by Albisser and colleagues as well as Pfeiffer and colleagues,[9,10] then paved the way for the first commercial closed-loop bedside device in 1974, the Biostator (Miles Laboratories, Elkhart, IN, USA). Attempts to miniaturize the Biostator concept followed,[11] but given the infection risk and lack of commercially available devices supporting the intravascular route, focus turned in the late 1990s to alternative body-access ports.

Prototypes that are currently in use adopt the subcutaneous route for the measurement of interstitial glucose level and insulin delivery.[12] Other means of insulin delivery and glucose sensing have been studied. The delivery of insulin intraperitoneally has been demonstrated to be feasible by Renard and colleagues,[13] but the focus firmly remains on the subcutaneous route.

This article outlines the individual components of the closed-loop system together with the existing clinical evidence. The artificial pancreas prototypes currently used in clinical studies are reviewed as well as obstacles and limitations facing the technology. Additional information can be found elsewhere.[3,14,15]

COMPONENTS OF THE CLOSED-LOOP SYSTEMS
Continuous Glucose Monitoring

The advent of real-time glucose sensing has been a crucial step in glucose-monitoring technology.[4] In contrast to earlier devices that provided Holter-type retrospective data,[16] real-time glucose monitoring allows the patient to make immediate adjustments to their insulin doses, food intake, and physical activity by inspecting glucose values and trends and by responding to low and high glucose alarms.

The present generation of continuous glucose monitors (CGMs) provides a minimally invasive method to measure glycemic variations and report glucose trends.[17] Most widely used devices use a subcutaneously implanted needle-type amperometric enzyme electrode, which measures the interstitial glucose concentration by detecting changes in the electric current caused by the enzymatic catalyzation of glucose by glucose oxidase into hydrogen peroxide.[18] Examples of CGMs include Enlite (Medtronic MiniMed, Northridge, CA, USA), Dexcom SEVEN PLUS (DexCom Inc, San Diego, CA, USA), and Freestyle Navigator (Abbot Laboratories, Alameda, CA,

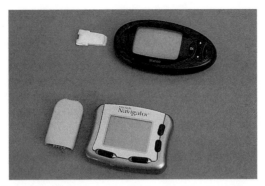

Fig. 2. Examples of continuous glucose monitoring devices: the Dexcom SEVEN PLUS (*top*) and the Freestyle Navigator (*bottom*).

USA) (**Fig. 2**). The devices display a new glucose reading every 1 to 5 minutes for up to 7 days of continuous wear per sensor insertion.

Reverse iontophoresis was used by GlucoWatch (Cygnus, Redwood City, CA, USA) to measure interstitial glucose ex vivo[19]; this device is no longer available. Microdialysis[20] with ex vivo sensing of glucose oxidase is used by the GlucoMen device (Menarini Diagnostics, Firenze, Italy) using a fine, hollow dialysis fiber implanted in the subcutaneous tissue and perfused with isotonic fluid, which then carries glucose to a glucose-oxidase sensor placed ex vivo.[21]

The advantage of continuous glucose monitoring in clinical practice is in identifying trends of glucose values and reducing the frequency and severity of hypoglycemia events. A meta-analysis[22] of randomized controlled trials evaluating continuous glucose monitoring in adults and youths documented a significant reduction in hemoglobin A_{1c} (HbA_{1c}) levels, particularly in those with the highest HbA_{1c} level at baseline, and in frequent users of continuous glucose monitoring. Exposure to hypoglycemia is also reduced during continuous glucose monitoring. Criticism has been leveled at the need to use the sensors 80% of the time to achieve benefits,[23] but continuous glucose monitoring in combination with intensive insulin therapy seems to be more cost-effective than self-monitoring of blood glucose.[24]

Insulin Pump

Insulin pump therapy uses a portable electromechanical pump to mimic nondiabetic insulin delivery. The pump infuses insulin at preselected rates, normally a slow basal rate with patient-activated boosts at mealtimes.[5] The use of insulin pump therapy is growing but is varied across developed countries; an estimated 20% to 25% of individuals with type 1 diabetes use an insulin pump in the United States, compared with 10% in Sweden and Germany, and fewer than 1% in Denmark.[25]

Most modern insulin pumps are approximately the size of a pager and comprise an insulin reservoir, a small battery-operated motor that is linked to a computerized control mechanism, and a subcutaneous infusion set (cannula and tubing system). Sensor-augmented insulin pumps, such as the MiniMed Paradigm Veo (Medtronic MiniMed, Northridge, CA, USA) (**Fig. 3**) or Vibe (Animas, West Chester, PA, USA) feature integration with a continuous glucose monitor, with documented benefits on HbA_{1c} reduction.[26] A recent innovation in pump design has been the introduction of the patch pump (Omnipod; Insulet, MA, USA), which has a reservoir unit that adheres

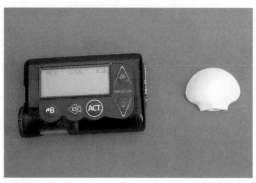

Fig. 3. A sensor-augmented insulin pump: the MiniMed Paradigm Veo integrated with the Enlite continuous glucose sensor.

directly to the patient's skin and houses an integrated infusion set and automated inserter, thus making it free of tubing.[27]

An insulin pump normally delivers rapid-acting insulin analogues.[28] Modern smart pumps have a built-in customizable bolus calculator and monitor insulin on board to reduce the risk of insulin stacking.[29]

Control Algorithm

Two main families of control algorithm have been used in closed-loop clinical studies[6]: the classic feedback proportional-integral-derivative (PID) controller[30–34] and the model predictive controller (MPC).[35–38] The PID controller adjusts insulin delivery by assessing glucose excursions from 3 viewpoints: the departure from target glucose level (the proportional component), the area under the curve between ambient and target glucose levels (the integral component), and the rate of change in ambient glucose level (the derivative component).[32] PID controllers have been used with intra-vascular and subcutaneous glucose sensing and insulin delivery,[11,39,40] as well as during intraperitoneal insulin delivery.[13]

Most recent research focuses on the MPC approach,[41] as it can more easily accommodate delays associated with insulin absorption and also account for meal intake and prandial insulin boluses. The vital ingredient of the MPC is a mathematical model that links insulin delivery and meal ingestion to glucose excursions.[36] The MPC approach works by comparing the model-predicted glucose levels with the actual glucose levels, updating the model, and calculating future insulin infusion rates to minimize the difference between the model-predicted glucose concentration and target glucose concentration. Other clinically evaluated control approaches include fuzzy logic,[42] which modulates insulin delivery on the basis of approximate rules and may be suitable to express empirical knowledge acquired by the diabetes practitioners. Algorithms may include a safety module to constrain insulin delivery,[43] limiting the amount of insulin on board[44] or the maximum rate of insulin delivery or suspending insulin delivery when glucose levels are low or decreasing.[45]

ARTIFICIAL PANCREAS PROTOTYPES

Research prototypes of the artificial pancreas adopting the subcutaneous route include the Artificial Pancreas Software, a modular system[46] supporting wireless connection to a range of glucose sensors and insulin pumps. The physiologic insulin delivery system comprises a Medtronic glucose sensor and pump, and uses the PID algorithm with recent modification for insulin feedback.[47] The Florence platform expands on the manual Cambridge system[48] and uses the Navigator continuous glucose monitor, the Aviator insulin pump, and an MPC controller (**Fig. 4**). The Boston prototype for dual-hormone delivery uses manual closed-loop control adopting venous blood glucose measurement (GlucoScout; International Biomedical, Austin, TX, USA), and an MPC algorithm for insulin delivery and a PID controller for glucagon delivery.[37] The Oregon prototype for dual-hormone delivery uses manual closed-loop control with a fading-memory proportional derivative controller.[33]

CLOSED-LOOP APPROACHES
Overview

It is anticipated that closed-loop systems will evolve with increasing technological sophistication and more comprehensive treatment objectives.[49] Early generations are likely to provide benefits in terms of reduced incidence of hypoglycemia. Follow-up closed-loop applications may address hyperglycemia, postprandial control, and lifestyle activities including exercise. Meals and exercise can be indicated to the control algorithm and prandial insulin boluses can be delivered by the patient, thus simplifying the closed-loop operation. In a more challenging fully closed-loop configuration, the control algorithm is not aware of meals and exercise, and delivers insulin solely based on sensor glucose levels. Glucagon coadministration can be used to counteract peripheral overinsulinization following insulin boluses or delayed insulin absorption. Closed-loop approaches and associated results are listed in **Table 1**.

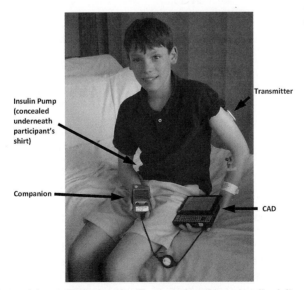

Fig. 4. A study participant displaying the Florence closed-loop insulin delivery system, consisting of a handheld device (Companion), which receives and displays glucose value data from the Freestyle Navigator Transmitter, communicating with the Control Algorithm Device (CAD) and controlling the subcutaneous insulin pump.

Table 1
Summary of achieved results with various closed-loop delivery approaches

Objective/Approach	Status	Results	References
Low glucose suspend	Postmarketing studies	Reduced nocturnal hypoglycemia in those with greatest risk; well accepted by patients	51,52
Suspend to prevent low glucose	Laboratory studies; home studies planned	Nocturnal hypoglycemia prevention of 80% events; effective as part of overnight closed loop	53,72
Treat to range	Laboratory testing underway	—	—
Overnight	Laboratory studies; home studies planned	Increased time spent in target glucose range by 20% in adolescents and adults; reduced risk of nocturnal hypoglycemia	38,48
Meal announcement	Laboratory studies	Feasibility documented in children, adults, pregnant women using various control algorithms; preferred option by most investigators	59,60,73
Fully closed loop	Laboratory studies	Feasibility documented in children and adults; addition of small prandial bolus improves control; delayed insulin absorption/action remains a challenge	13,32,34,42,47
Fully closed loop with glucagon coadministration	Laboratory studies	Feasibility documented in adults; glucagon helpful but cannot always overcome insulin overdelivery	33,37

Low Glucose Suspend Function

The low glucose suspend function is the first example of a commercial application of closed-loop insulin delivery. An insulin pump with an integrated continuous glucose monitoring (Paradigm Veo; Medtronic Diabetes, Northridge, CA, USA) automatically suspends insulin delivery for up to 2 hours when hypoglycemia is detected and the hypoglycemia alarm is not acknowledged by the patient. The low glucose suspend function aims to reduce the severity of hypoglycemia because prolonged low-sensor glucose levels may lead to seizures.[50]

Postmarketing studies on the low glucose suspend function in adults and children documented significant reductions in the frequency and duration of nocturnal hypoglycemia, particularly in those with greatest risk.[51,52] Despite the occasional suboptimal sensor accuracy, no adverse events such as severe hyperglycemia, ketosis, or other safety issues were noted. Patients found the low glucose suspend function useful and were in favor of its regular use.[51]

Hypoglycemia Prevention

The low glucose suspend function aims to reduce severity but does not prevent hypoglycemia, which is an objective of the work by Buckingham and colleagues,[53] who tested an algorithm to discontinue insulin delivery when pending hypoglycemia was predicted. The approach prevented hypoglycemia on 75% of nights (84% events) without hyperglycemia rebound. Up to 4 hours' and, rarely, longer suspension of insulin delivery is also present during overnight closed loop. Assessment of safety and efficacy has been made for PID[54] and MPC[45] controllers in children and adolescents, indicating that prolonged suspension is safe and useful.

Overnight Closed-Loop Studies

The most severe hypoglycemic events occur after midnight.[55] Young children are vulnerable to the adverse effects of neuroglycopenia such as seizures that are related to hypoglycemia when they sleep.[56] Thus, overnight closed-loop delivery to reduce the risk of hypoglycemia may provide a solution to an important clinical problem of concern to many parents and caregivers.[57]

Randomized crossover studies in young patients demonstrated that overnight closed-loop control significantly increased the time spent in the target glucose range and reduced the time spent in hypoglycemia.[38] No nocturnal hypoglycemic episodes were documented and rescue carbohydrates were not required during closed loop, which was an important step toward realizing the clinical potential of the closed-loop system. Randomized closed-loop studies in adults have shown similar promising results. Closed-loop delivery increased the overnight time spent within target glucose levels and reduced the overnight time in hypoglycemia.[48] Similar to studies in children, overnight hypoglycemia (blood glucose level<55 mg/dL [3.0 mmol/L]) was eliminated by closed-loop insulin delivery in adults.

Risk analysis using extensive in silico testing to assess the impact of calibration errors and sensor artifacts suggested that overnight closed loop may reduce substantially the incidence of nocturnal hypoglycemia.[58] These improvements encourage the progress to ambulatory testing.

Day and Night Closed-Loop Studies

Waking hours present a unique set of challenges, including variable dietary and exercise patterns. The postprandial period is particularly challenging because of delays associated with the absorption of subcutaneously delivered insulin and the variable appearance of glucose from the meal. This situation can lead to late postprandial hypoglycemia, as closed-loop systems may deliver too much insulin in an attempt to correct high postprandial glucose levels. During conventional pump therapy, the delayed action of insulin may lead to insulin stacking, thus increasing the risk of hypoglycemia, and similar concerns apply also to the closed loop.

A practical solution is to combine closed-loop operation with conventional manual delivery of prandial boluses. A PID algorithm with meal announcement (a hybrid closed-loop system) gave significantly better postprandial glucose levels than a fully-closed-loop system[34] using small prandial boluses given 10 to 15 minutes before meals. A multinational study evaluating an MPC controller documented the reduced frequency of nocturnal hypoglycemia events, and after breakfast the closed loop controlled glucose levels as effectively as patient-directed conventional insulin pump therapy. A sample glucose profile from a closed-loop study with an MPC controller during adolescence[59] is shown in **Fig. 5**.

The feasibility and efficacy of MPC-based closed-loop insulin delivery was demonstrated in women throughout different stages of pregnancy.[60] A randomized study of a well-controlled cohort of pregnant women suggested a reduced risk of very low glucose levels with closed-loop insulin delivery, but otherwise similar glucose outcomes.[61]

Dual-hormone or bihormonal delivery systems incorporate the delivery of insulin with counterregulatory hormones such as glucagon. The advantage of using glucagon is that it acts rapidly, mimicking the physiologic response to hypoglycemia without the need for fast-acting oral glucose. Glucagon coadministration has been

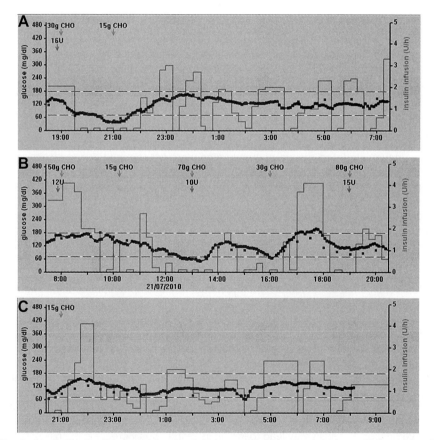

Fig. 5. (A–C) Glucose levels and insulin delivery profiles observed during a 36-hour closed-loop study in a young subject. The bold line shows the continuous subcutaneous glucose trace and the black squares indicate reference plasma glucose values (not used to determine the insulin delivery but shown to demonstrate deviation between sensor and plasma glucose levels). Insulin infusion rates during closed-loop delivery are denoted by the gray line. Vertical arrows indicate meals and snacks (*light gray arrow*) and insulin boluses (*dark gray arrow*). Carbohydrate contents of the meal/snack and insulin doses are also shown. Horizontal dashed lines illustrate the target range of 90 to 180 mg/dL (3.9–10 mmol/L).

investigated with the fully closed-loop approach.[33,37] Although effective, glucagon could not fully counteract insulin overdelivery, and on occasions hypoglycemia presented.[37]

LIMITATIONS AND OBSTACLES
Accuracy of CGMs

Suboptimal accuracy and reliability remain one of the biggest obstacles for closed-loop systems.[12,14] Commercially available CGMs can achieve a median relative absolute difference between sensor and reference glucose measurements of 15% or less, which should be commensurate with closed-loop glucose control. However, transient and persistent deviations of greater magnitude occur. Transient deviations relate to temporal loss or increase of sensor sensitivity, or mechanical perturbation including temporal sensor dislodgment.[62] Persistent deviations are caused by erroneous calibration, an inappropriate calibration algorithm, or slow drift of sensor sensitivity. When a sensor overreads blood glucose levels, the persistent deviations pose the greatest challenge to safe closed-loop insulin delivery, as insulin overdelivery may occur, thus increasing the risk of hypoglycemia.

A 5- to 15-minute time lag between glucose levels in the interstitial fluid and blood glucose values contributes to the sensor deviations and reflects the transport of glucose from blood to the interstitial fluid.[63–66]

Insulin Absorption

Even with modern rapid-acting insulin analogues, it takes approximately 90 to 120 minutes for a subcutaneously delivered insulin analogue to reach its maximum glucose-lowering capacity, and its action can continue well beyond this peak. The administration of several correction boluses in close sequence causes insulin stacking and a high risk of hypoglycemia, which, if not accounted for by the control algorithm, can pose a safety hazard for closed-loop systems.[44] High glucose levels may have to be normalized slowly even during closed-loop delivery, complicating postprandial glucose control. Control during and after exercise may require preemptive carbohydrate intake or dual-hormone treatment to eliminate the risk of hypoglycemia.[67]

Individual Variability

Insulin absorption and insulin action vary substantially between and within subjects.[68] Intersubject variability is attributable to factors influencing insulin sensitivity, such as body mass, age, gender, physical activity, and smoking. Intrasubject variability reflects the day-to-day and hour-to-hour variations related to circadian and diurnal cycles, dawn phenomenon,[69] acute illness, stress,[70] and the delayed effects of exercise and alcohol.[71] These variations in insulin requirements need to be compensated for by closed-loop operations, and adaptive systems may be required to compensate fully for these variations.

FUTURE DIRECTIONS

The next research priority is to test the artificial pancreas outside the confines of a controlled laboratory environment and ultimately in the patient's home. Artificial pancreas studies at home may involve short-term testing, possibly at a transitional hotel-like facility, followed by long-term testing to compare closed-loop control with conventional insulin therapy.

The introduction of the artificial pancreas into clinical practice will likely be a staged process focusing initially on hypoglycemia prevention followed by tightening of glucose control. It is important to set realistic goals, as clinically meaningful improvement of glycemic control expressed by HbA_{1c} may occur gradually. Wider use may depend on the establishment of appropriate infrastructures that can provide support, both technical and clinical, to patients and practitioners who will be using the artificial pancreas.

REFERENCES

1. Cryer PE. The barrier of hypoglycemia in diabetes. Diabetes 2008;57(12): 3169–76.
2. Unger J, Parkin C. Hypoglycemia in insulin-treated diabetes: a case for increased vigilance. Postgrad Med 2011;123(4):81–91.
3. Hovorka R. Closed-loop insulin delivery: from bench to clinical practice. Nat Rev Endocrinol 2011;7(7):385–95.
4. Klonoff DC. Continuous glucose monitoring: roadmap for 21st century diabetes therapy. Diabetes Care 2005;28(5):1231–9.
5. Pickup J, Keen H. Continuous subcutaneous insulin infusion at 25 years: evidence base for the expanding use of insulin pump therapy in type 1 diabetes. Diabetes Care 2002;25(3):593–8.
6. Bequette BW. A critical assessment of algorithms and challenges in the development of a closed-loop artificial pancreas. Diabetes Technol Ther 2005;7(1): 28–47.
7. Weller C, Linder M, Macaulay A, et al. Continuous in vivo determination of blood glucose in human subjects. Ann N Y Acad Sci 1960;87:658–68.
8. Kadish A. Automation control of blood sugar. I. A servomechanism for glucose monitoring and control. Am J Med Electron 1964;3:82–6.
9. Albisser AM, Leibel BS, Ewart TG, et al. An artificial endocrine pancreas. Diabetes 1974;23(5):389–96.
10. Pfeiffer EF, Thum C, Clemens AH. The artificial beta cell—a continuous control of blood sugar by external regulation of insulin infusion (glucose controlled insulin infusion system). Horm Metab Res 1974;6(5):339–42.
11. Renard E, Costalat G, Chevassus H, et al. Closed loop insulin delivery using implanted insulin pumps and sensors in type 1 diabetic patients. Diabetes Res Clin Pract 2006;74(Suppl 2):S173–7.
12. Hovorka R. Continuous glucose monitoring and closed-loop systems. Diabet Med 2006;23(1):1–12.
13. Renard E, Place J, Cantwell M, et al. Closed-loop insulin delivery using a subcutaneous glucose sensor and intraperitoneal insulin delivery: feasibility study testing a new model for the artificial pancreas. Diabetes Care 2010;33(1): 121–7.
14. Steil GM, Rebrin K. Closed-loop insulin delivery—what lies between where we are and where we are going? Expert Opin Drug Deliv 2005;2(2):353–62.
15. Renard E, Costalat G, Chevassus H, et al. Artificial beta-cell: clinical experience toward an implantable closed-loop insulin delivery system. Diabetes Metab 2006; 32(5 Pt 2):497–502.
16. Mastrototaro J. The MiniMed Continuous Glucose Monitoring System (CGMS). J Pediatr Endocrinol Metab 1999;12(Suppl 3):751–8.
17. Oliver NS, Toumazou C, Cass AE, et al. Glucose sensors: a review of current and emerging technology. Diabet Med 2009;26(3):197–210.
18. Feldman B, Brazg R, Schwartz S, et al. A continuous glucose sensor based on wired enzyme technology—results from a 3-day trial in patients with type 1 diabetes. Diabetes Technol Ther 2003;5(5):769–79.

19. Tamada JA, Garg S, Jovanovic L, et al. Noninvasive glucose monitoring: comprehensive clinical results. Cygnus Research Team. JAMA 1999;282(19):1839–44.
20. Bolinder J, Ungerstedt U, Arner P. Microdialysis measurement of the absolute glucose concentration in subcutaneous adipose tissue allowing glucose monitoring in diabetic patients. Diabetologia 1992;35(12):1177–80.
21. Valgimigli F, Lucarelli F, Scuffi C, et al. Evaluating the clinical accuracy of GlucoMen®Day: a novel microdialysis-based continuous glucose monitor. J Diabetes Sci Technol 2010;4(5):1182–92.
22. Pickup JC, Freeman SC, Sutton AJ. Glycaemic control in type 1 diabetes during real time continuous glucose monitoring compared with self monitoring of blood glucose: meta-analysis of randomised controlled trials using individual patient data. BMJ 2011;343:d3805.
23. Peters A. Do we really need continuous glucose monitoring? Diabetes Technol Ther 2009;11(Suppl 1):S128–30.
24. McQueen R, Ellis S, Campbell J, et al. Cost-effectiveness of continuous glucose monitoring and intensive insulin therapy for type 1 diabetes. Cost Eff Resour Alloc 2011;9:13.
25. Selam S. CSII in Europe: where are we, where are we going? An analysis of articles published in Infusystems International. Diabetes Res Clin Pract 2006; 74(Suppl 2):S23–126.
26. Bergenstal RM, Tamborlane WV, Ahmann A, et al. Effectiveness of sensor-augmented insulin-pump therapy in type 1 diabetes. N Engl J Med 2010;363(4):311–20.
27. Zisser H, Jovanovic L. OmniPod Insulin Management System: patient perceptions, preference, and glycemic control. Diabetes Care 2006;29(9):2175.
28. Bode BW. Comparison of pharmacokinetic properties, physicochemical stability, and pump compatibility of 3 rapid-acting insulin analogues—aspart, lispro, and glulisine. Endocr Pract 2011;17(2):271–80.
29. Zisser H, Wagner R, Pleus S, et al. Clinical performance of three bolus calculators in subjects with type 1 diabetes mellitus: a head-to-head-to-head comparison. Diabetes Technol Ther 2010;12(12):955–61.
30. Clemens AH. Feedback control dynamics for glucose controlled insulin infusion system. Med Prog Technol 1979;6(3):91–8.
31. Marchetti G, Barolo M, Jovanovic L, et al. An improved PID switching control strategy for type 1 diabetes. IEEE Trans Biomed Eng 2008;55(3):857–65.
32. Steil GM, Rebrin K, Darwin C, et al. Feasibility of automating insulin delivery for the treatment of type 1 diabetes. Diabetes 2006;55(12):3344–50.
33. Castle JR, Engle JM, El Youssef J, et al. Novel use of glucagon in a closed-loop system for prevention of hypoglycemia in type 1 diabetes. Diabetes Care 2010; 33(6):1282–7.
34. Weinzimer SA, Steil GM, Swan KL, et al. Fully automated closed-loop insulin delivery versus semiautomated hybrid control in pediatric patients with type 1 diabetes using an artificial pancreas. Diabetes Care 2008;31(5):934–9.
35. Magni L, Raimondo DM, Bossi L, et al. Model predictive control of type 1 diabetes: an in silico trial. J Diabetes Sci Technol 2007;1(6):804–12.
36. Hovorka R, Canonico V, Chassin LJ, et al. Nonlinear model predictive control of glucose concentration in subjects with type 1 diabetes. Physiol Meas 2004;25(4):905–20.
37. El-Khatib FH, Russell SJ, Nathan DM, et al. A bihormonal closed-loop artificial pancreas for type 1 diabetes. Sci Transl Med 2010;2(27):27ra27.
38. Hovorka R, Allen JM, Elleri D, et al. Manual closed-loop insulin delivery in children and adolescents with type 1 diabetes: a phase 2 randomised crossover trial. Lancet 2010;375(9716):743–51.

39. Steil GM, Panteleon AE, Rebrin K. Closed-loop insulin delivery-the path to physiological glucose control. Adv Drug Deliv Rev 2004;56(2):125–44.

40. Shimoda S, Nishida K, Sakakida M, et al. Closed-loop subcutaneous insulin infusion algorithm with a short-acting insulin analog for long-term clinical application of a wearable artificial endocrine pancreas. Front Med Biol Eng 1997;8(3):197–211.

41. Camacho EF, Bordons C. Model predictive control. London: Springer-Verlag; 1999.

42. Atlas E, Nimri R, Miller S, et al. MD-logic artificial pancreas system: a pilot study in adults with type 1 diabetes. Diabetes Care 2010;33(5):1072–6.

43. Kovatchev B, Patek S, Dassau E, et al. Control to range for diabetes: functionality and modular architecture. J Diabetes Sci Technol 2009;3(5):1058–65.

44. Ellingsen C, Dassau E, Zisser H, et al. Safety constraints in an artificial pancreatic beta cell: an implementation of model predictive control with insulin on board. J Diabetes Sci Technol 2009;3(3):536–44.

45. Elleri D, Allen JM, Nodale M, et al. Suspended insulin infusion during overnight closed-loop glucose control in children and adolescents with Type 1 diabetes. Diabet Med 2010;27(4):480–4.

46. Dassau E, Zisser H, Palerm C C, et al. Modular artificial beta-cell system: a prototype for clinical research. J Diabetes Sci Technol 2008;2(5):863–72.

47. Steil GM, Palerm CC, Kurtz N, et al. The effect of insulin feedback on closed loop glucose control. J Clin Endocrinol Metab 2011;96(5):1402–8.

48. Hovorka R, Kumareswaran K, Harris J, et al. Overnight closed loop insulin delivery (artificial pancreas) in adults with type 1 diabetes: crossover randomised controlled studies. BMJ 2011;342:d1855.

49. Kowalski AJ. Can we really close the loop and how soon? Accelerating the availability of an artificial pancreas: a roadmap to better diabetes outcomes. Diabetes Technol Ther 2009;11(Suppl 1):S113–9.

50. Buckingham B, Wilson DM, Lecher T, et al. Duration of nocturnal hypoglycemia before seizures. Diabetes Care 2008;31(11):2110–2.

51. Choudhary P, Shin J, Wang Y, et al. Insulin pump therapy with automated insulin suspension in response to hypoglycemia: reduction in nocturnal hypoglycemia in those at greatest risk. Diabetes Care 2011;34(9):2023–5.

52. Danne T, Kordonouri O, Holder M, et al. Prevention of hypoglycemia by using low glucose suspend function in sensor-augmented pump therapy. Diabetes Technol Ther 2011;13(11):1129–34.

53. Buckingham B, Chase HP, Dassau E, et al. Prevention of nocturnal hypoglycemia using predictive alarm algorithms and insulin pump suspension. Diabetes Care 2010;33(5):1013–7.

54. Cengiz E, Swan KL, Tamborlane WV, et al. Is an automatic pump suspension feature safe for children with type 1 diabetes? An exploratory analysis with a closed-loop system. Diabetes Technol Ther 2009;11(4):207–10.

55. Epidemiology of severe hypoglycemia in the diabetes control and complications trial. The DCCT Research Group. Am J Med 1991;90(4):450–9.

56. Davis EA, Keating B, Byrne GC, et al. Hypoglycemia: incidence and clinical predictors in a large population-based sample of children and adolescents with IDDM. Diabetes Care 1997;20(1):22–5.

57. Elleri D, Acerini CL, Allen JM, et al. Parental attitudes towards overnight closed-loop glucose control in children with type 1 diabetes. Diabetes Technol Ther 2010;12(1):35–9.

58. Wilinska ME, Budiman ES, Taub MB, et al. Overnight closed-loop insulin delivery with model predictive control: assessment of hypoglycemia and hyperglycemia risk using simulation studies. J Diabetes Sci Technol 2009;3(5):1109–20.

59. Elleri D, Allen JM, Kumareswaran K, et al. Day-and-night closed loop (CL) glucose control in adolescents with type 1 diabetes (T1D). Diabetes 2011;60(Suppl 1):A41.

60. Murphy HR, Elleri D, Allen JM, et al. Closed-loop insulin delivery during pregnancy complicated by type 1 diabetes. Diabetes Care 2011;34(2):406–11.

61. Murphy HR, Kumareswaran K, Elleri D, et al. Safety and efficacy of 24-h closed-loop insulin delivery in well-controlled pregnant women with type 1 diabetes: a randomized crossover case series. Diabetes Care 2011;34(12):2527–9.

62. McGarraugh G, Bergenstal R. Detection of hypoglycemia with continuous interstitial and traditional blood glucose monitoring using the FreeStyle Navigator Continuous Glucose Monitoring System. Diabetes Technol Ther 2009;11(3):145–50.

63. Garg SK, Voelmle M, Gottlieb PA. Time lag characterization of two continuous glucose monitoring systems. Diabetes Res Clin Pract 2010;87(3):348–53.

64. Weinstein RL, Schwartz SL, Brazg RL, et al. Accuracy of the 5-day FreeStyle Navigator Continuous Glucose Monitoring System: comparison with frequent laboratory reference measurements. Diabetes Care 2007;30(5):1125–30.

65. Keenan DB, Mastrototaro JJ, Voskanyan G, et al. Delays in minimally invasive continuous glucose monitoring devices: a review of current technology. J Diabetes Sci Technol 2009;3(5):1207–14.

66. Wei C, Lunn DJ, Acerini CL, et al. Measurement delay associated with the Guardian RT continuous glucose monitoring system. Diabet Med 2010;27(1):117–22.

67. Tsalikian E, Kollman C, Tamborlane WB, et al. Prevention of hypoglycemia during exercise in children with type 1 diabetes by suspending basal insulin. Diabetes Care 2006;29(10):2200–4.

68. Heinemann L. Variability of insulin absorption and insulin action. Diabetes Technol Ther 2002;4(5):673–82.

69. Carroll MF, Schade DS. The dawn phenomenon revisited: implications for diabetes therapy. Endocr Pract 2005;11(1):55–64.

70. Riazi A, Pickup J, Bradley C. Daily stress and glycaemic control in Type 1 diabetes: individual differences in magnitude, direction, and timing of stress-reactivity. Diabetes Res Clin Pract 2004;66(3):237–44.

71. Turner BC, Jenkins E, Kerr D, et al. The effect of evening alcohol consumption on next-morning glucose control in type 1 diabetes. Diabetes Care 2001;24(11):1888–93.

72. Buckingham B, Cobry E, Clinton P, et al. Preventing hypoglycemia using predictive alarm algorithms and insulin pump suspension. Diabetes Technol Ther 2009;11(2):93–7.

73. Kovatchev B, Cobelli C, Renard E, et al. Multinational study of subcutaneous model-predictive closed-loop control in type 1 diabetes mellitus: summary of the results. J Diabetes Sci Technol 2010;4(6):1374–81.

Insulin Therapy in Type 2 Diabetes Mellitus

Jack L. Leahy, MD

KEYWORDS

• Insulin therapy • Type 2 diabetes mellitus • Glucose control

INTRODUCTION

The worldwide burden of diabetes continues to increase at an alarming rate, with the latest statistics from the US Centers for Disease Control showing an 11.3% incidence of diabetes and 35% for prediabetes in adult Americans.[1] Also, the International Diabetes Federation predicts that the global incidence will increase from 366 million currently to 552 million in 2030, with developing nations particularly affected.[2] The increase is multifactorial: most obvious are the diet and lifestyle changes that accompany Westernization, but genetic variances, inadequate prenatal care or childhood malnutrition predisposing to obesity or diabetes later in life, gastrointestinal microflora-related immunologic and metabolic effects, food additives, and environmental toxins are all active research topics.[3] Furthermore, epidemiologic studies have shown that persons with type 2 diabetes have a higher incidence than the general population of numerous other serious health problems.[4,5] So it is not a surprise that the worldwide threat posed by type 2 diabetes and other noncommunicable diseases is viewed as potentially cataclysmic.[6]

The strategy to counter the threat is to optimize health care through early diagnosis and treatment algorithms and standards of care.[7–9] Although there has been considerable discussion of late about treatment guidelines because of recent disappointing highly publicized large clinical trials (see the review by Yuen and Riddle elsewhere in this issue), the consensus continues to be that there is compelling evidence for the benefits of intensive blood glucose control (usually defined by an A1c value of less than 7%) for prevention of diabetes complications in most patients with type 2 diabetes.[10–13] One can argue that the legacy effect against macrovascular and microvascular complications still present many years after completion of the Steno 2[14] and United Kingdom Prospective Diabetes Study (UKPDS)[15] trials in type 2 diabetes, and

Conflicts of Interest: Advisory boards for Merck, Sanofi, Bristol Myers Squibb, Novo-Nordisk, Takeda. Research grant support with salary from Takeda.
Division of Endocrinology, Diabetes and Metabolism, Department of Medicine, University of Vermont, Colchester Research Facility, Room 110, 208 South Park Drive, Colchester, VT 05446, USA
E-mail address: jleahy@uvm.edu

Endocrinol Metab Clin N Am 41 (2012) 119–144
doi:10.1016/j.ecl.2012.03.004
0889-8529/12/$ – see front matter © 2012 Elsevier Inc. All rights reserved.

endo.theclinics.com

the DCCT/EDIC in type 1 diabetes,[16,17] has unequivocally proved the importance of optimal blood glucose control as early as possible.

Another issue is the increase in the number of pharmaceuticals to treat type 2 diabetes, with a new class of agents having appeared almost yearly for the last decade. The positive effect is that health care providers and patients have lots of choice, with many issues besides blood glucose control now routinely considered: cost, hypoglycemia risk, side effects, impact on weight and cardiovascular risk factors. However, the negative effect is that the blood glucose improvement with all of these agents is limited. The one therapy with unlimited potential (at least theoretically) is insulin. Also, new insulins and delivery devices have come to market over the last decade with a high level of patient safety and acceptance.[18] Still, for many patients[19–21] and providers,[22] insulin remains a last resort, with enormous negative connotations. What often goes undiscussed with patients is the many studies that show glucose control is achievable with insulin safely in most patients with type 2 diabetes. A recent publication reported a high degree of patient acceptance when discussions had occurred with their health care providers related to disease progression and the patient's anxieties.[23] A personal conviction of the author is that effective diabetes management at the primary care or specialty level requires a belief in the importance of insulin therapy in uncontrolled patients with type 2 diabetes. This review details the theories, observed outcomes, and how-tos regarding insulin use in type 2 diabetes.

PROGRAMS FOR STARTING INSULIN IN TYPE 2 DIABETES
Basal Insulin Therapy

The usual transition from oral agents to insulin in type 2 diabetes is to add a long-acting insulin to bring the fasting glucose to a target level: less than 100 mg/dL (5.5 mmol/L) is a common goal in clinical trials, although few attain that level, but instead typically average 110 to 120 mg/dL (6.1–6.7 mmol/L), so-called basal insulin therapy (**Fig. 1**). The result is a decrease of the 24-hour glucose profile (ie, both premeal and postmeal in absolute terms). Semantically, this is a premeal or basal strategy because most studies show that the delta increase and decrease in glucose after a meal is unchanged, but starts at a lower baseline.[24–26] The important point is the belief of some that reversal of glucose toxicity, and consequently improved insulin release at meals, is a crucial part of how basal insulin acts. In part this situation is because the first reports of glucose toxicity were based on studies that showed recovery of endogenous insulin secretion after intensive insulin therapy in relatively short duration type 2 diabetes.[27,28] Instead, modern studies mostly show little to no improvement in prandial insulin secretion with basal insulin.[29] One reason may be that insulin is usually started after failure of oral agents, thus in patients with advanced disease and presumably little chance for recovery of β-cell function. Consistent with that idea are several studies of short-term insulin therapy in new-onset patients with type 2 diabetes that show large improvements in β-cell function and often reversal of the diabetes,[30–32] including a highly discussed study from China[33] in which the diabetes remission was still present 1 year off all therapy. Another issue is the defective incretin regulation of mealtime insulin and glucagon secretion in type 2 diabetes; little is known about how this system is affected by basal insulin therapy.[34,35]

Basal insulin therapy goes back many years to BIDS insulin therapy (bedtime insulin, daytime sulfonylurea), which added NPH (neutral protamine Hagedorn) insulin at bedtime to the only available oral therapy in the United States at the time.[36,37] Another variation added 70:30 NPH/regular insulin at suppertime.[38] However, the influx of new oral agents that began in the mid-1990s took interest away from insulin so its use

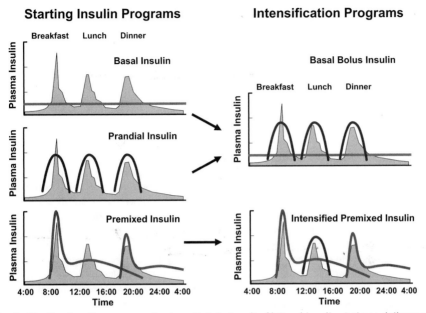

Fig. 1. Starting insulin programs for type 2 diabetes. (*Left*) Basal insulin, 3-times daily prandial insulin, and twice-daily analogue premix. (*Right*) Intensification programs: basal-bolus insulin, twice-daily premixed analogue with prandial insulin added at lunch. The background of each diagram depicts the normal pattern of insulin levels in nondiabetic individuals eating 3 daily meals. The arrows show the progression from starting to intensification insulin programs in the 4-T trial,[94] as described in the text.

markedly decreased in the United States.[39,40] It is mostly forgotten that the first thiazolidinedione (troglitazone) was initially approved by the US Food and Drug Administration only for uncontrolled insulin-taking type 2 diabetes patients, with the expectation that many could eventually be withdrawn from insulin. Interest in insulin started to return in the late 1990s and early 2000s because of several issues: awareness that many patients were uncontrolled with the new oral agents, evidence that progressive β-cell dysfunction was a characteristic feature of type 2 diabetes and accounted in large part for the oral agent failure in the UKPDS study[41] along with the UKPDS substudy that showed continued blood glucose control by starting insulin early (when fasting glucose exceeded 108 mg/dL or 6 mmol/L) in sulfonylurea-treated patients,[42] and the advent of new insulins (insulin analogues).

Interest intensified with the Treat to Target study, which compared bedtime glargine versus NPH insulin added to patients failing metformin and sulfonylurea therapy.[43] Several factors accounted for why this study was viewed as groundbreaking. The study population was large (756 patients), with the kind of patients seen commonly by both primary care providers and specialists: A1c level average of 8.6% on the most common combination of oral agents at the time. Also, the protocol detailed clear goals (fasting glucose less than 100 mg/dL or 5.5 mmol/L) and used a titration schema of weekly increases of 0 to 8 units that could be replicated in any clinical setting, as was later proved by a large study performed in primary care providers' offices.[44] Most important, both insulins worked: A1c level was decreased to 6.9%, thus taking the average patient to goal (A1c level <7%) as opposed to the many less successful studies that added another oral drug. The other important finding of the study was a decreased incidence of nonserious nocturnal hypoglycemia with glargine. Nearly identical results were seen in a similar Treat to Target study comparing detemir and NPH insulin.[45] Also numerous studies and meta-analyses subsequently reported comparable results, accounting for the well-known dogma that the advantage of analogue basal insulins over NPH is safety (nonserious hypoglycemia) not efficacy.[46–48]

An issue is whether there are meaningful clinical differences between glargine and detemir. A 1-year head-to-head comparison in 582 insulin-naive patients failing 1 or 2 oral agents with average A1c level 8.2% showed equivalent decrease of the A1c level to 7.1%, and the same safety in terms of hypoglycemia.[49] What differed was slightly less weight gain with detemir. Also, the protocol started everyone on once-daily dosing of the randomized insulin but allowed a move to twice-daily detemir if the fasting glucose level was controlled and the presupper blood glucose level exceeded that value (patients on glargine stayed on once-daily dosing no matter what) and 55% of the patients received detemir twice daily. However, the most discussed difference was the higher insulin doses with detemir: 0.44 units/kg glargine, 0.78 units/kg once-daily detemir, 1.0 units/kg twice-daily detemir. Higher dosing with detemir compared with the other basal insulins also was noted in a pooled analysis of several trials,[50] and agreed with pharmacodynamic studies, especially at higher body mass index (calculated as weight in kilograms divided by the square of height in meters).[51,52] In contrast, a single investigator study found no difference in dosing between glargine and detemir in crossover patients assessed with continuous glucose monitoring.[53] The general opinion today is that both insulins are highly effective in type 2 diabetes, and any variance in dosage or number of daily injections is a minor issue.

New basal insulins are under development. Farthest along is degludec, which forms multihexamer assemblies in the subcutaneous space, resulting in a duration of action that exceeds 24 hours (see the review by Borgaño and Zinman elsewhere in this issue). Published results have shown efficacy and safety in type 1 diabetes,[54] type 2 diabetes,[55] and as a premix with aspart insulin in type 2 diabetes.[56] However, this finding poses an interesting dilemma as to what new insulins will improve on, because today's basal analogues are generally viewed as effective and safe. A current focus is degludec having a lower rate of hypoglycemia than the existing basal insulins, and it is expected that there will soon be an active debate about what is an acceptable versus optimal risk of hypoglycemia in insulin-treated type 2 diabetes.[57]

Thus, basal insulin therapy is simple and safe and has a high degree of success in getting patients to an A1c level of 7% or less. A comprehensive review of published randomized trials of basal insulin therapy in type 2 diabetes found on average more than 40% of patients met that goal, with many starting with high A1c levels.[58] Also, a pooled data analysis found a correlation with the baseline level of A1c: glargine started before the A1c level exceeded 8% resulted in a 75% success rate at getting to 7% or less along with less weight gain and no more hypoglycemia than higher A1c levels.[59,60]

Premixed Insulin Therapy

An alternate approach to starting patients with type 2 diabetes on insulin is premixed insulin (human insulin or an analogue mix) at breakfast and supper (see **Fig. 1**), based on the rationale that uncontrolled diabetes represents both premeal and postmeal hyperglycemia.[61,62] Also often cited is the possibility that postprandial hyperglycemia is most atherogenic.[63] The counterargument is that a single injection is preferable to a multishot program, and there is concern about hypoglycemia because of the lack of titratability from the fixed ratio of prandial and basal insulin. Head-to-head trials have provided important insight.

Janka[64] compared twice-daily 70:30 (NPH/regular) versus glargine insulin for 24 weeks in 371 insulin-naive patients with average A1c level 8.8%. The major findings were a better decrease of A1c level with glargine (–1.6% vs –1.3%), and more of that group reaching a combined outcome of A1c level less than 7% without nocturnal hypoglycemia (46% of glargine-treated vs 29% with premix). Also, the rate of confirmed hypoglycemia with the premixed insulin was more than double that of glargine. Subsequent cost analyses from Germany[65] and Ontario, Canada[66] found glargine was more cost-effective than premixed human insulin, although the generalizability is unknown.

Analogous to basal insulins, interest in premixes has shifted to the analogues (aspart or lispro combinations) for better postmeal glucose control and less hypoglycemia.[67–69] The INITIATE trial[70] compared twice-daily aspart 70:30 and glargine for 28 weeks in 233 insulin-naive patients with average A1c level 9.8% on metformin with or without other oral agents. The major finding was a better decrease of A1c level with the premixed insulin (to 6.9% vs 7.4% with glargine), although significance was lost if the starting A1c level was less than 8.5%. However, the rate of minor hypoglycemia was 5 times higher with the premixed insulin, and there was greater weight gain (+5.4 kg with premix and +3.5 kg with glargine) as well as higher insulin doses. Similar findings have been reported by others.[71] The DURABLE (Durability of Basal Versus Lispro Mix 75/25 Insulin Efficacy) trial compared twice-daily lispro 75:25 and glargine in more than 2000 patients with average A1c level 9.1%. At 24 weeks, A1c level was slightly lower with the premix (to 7.2% with premix vs 7.3% with glargine), but with higher insulin doses and more weight gain.[72] As expected, overall nonserious hypoglycemia was increased with the premix, but paradoxically nocturnal hypoglycemia was less than with glargine. This trial was continued for another 2 years in the individuals whose A1c level at 24 weeks was less than 7% to study the durability of control, and a modestly longer treatment success was noted with the premix over glargine (average 17 months vs 14 months).[73]

Thus premixed insulins, particularly analogue mixes, are highly effective for glycemic control, especially with high A1c values, but on average have more weight gain and a higher risk of hypoglycemia than basal insulin alone; this same conclusion was made in the previously cited comprehensive analysis of insulin regimens in type 2 diabetes.[58] Using premixes 3 times daily likely maintains the high efficacy, but with fewer side effects.[74–77] Regardless, the simplicity and safety of basal insulin has led most experts to recommend it as the starting insulin program in type 2 diabetes. A related idea is studies that switched patients who are inadequately controlled on premixed insulin to basal insulin and oral antidiabetic agents, with modest success.[78,79]

Prandial Insulin Therapy

Another starting program is to add prandial insulin at each meal without basal insulin (see **Fig. 1**). The APOLLO trial compared once-daily glargine with mealtime lispro (3 times daily) for 44 weeks in 418 patients failing various oral agents with mean A1c level 8.7%.[26,80] The decrease in A1c level was the same (–1.7% with glargine and –1.9% with lispro) as was weight gain, but there was 5 times the rate of hypoglycemia with the lispro program. Also, patient satisfaction was better with glargine.

INTENSIFICATION OF INSULIN THERAPY IN TYPE 2 DIABETES
Basal-Bolus Insulin Therapy Versus Premixed Insulin

When blood glucose control is lacking with one of the starting programs, the usual next step is a full basal-bolus program, usually an analogue basal insulin once or twice daily and a rapid-acting analogue at each meal (see **Fig. 1**). Bergenstal and colleagues[81] studied carbohydrate counting versus set dosing of mealtime glulisine as part of a basal-bolus insulin program in patients with type 2 diabetes failing various insulin regimens. Although the main finding was no clear benefit of carbohydrate counting over the simpler approach to mealtime insulin, this study can be viewed as showing the effectiveness and safety of basal-bolus therapy in type 2 diabetes. From that viewpoint, the A1c level was decreased from 8.1% to 8.3% at the outset to 6.5% to 6.7% after 24 weeks on glargine and mealtime glulisine along with optimization of the insulin doses. The insulin doses were large (daily average of 207 units of combined basal and prandial insulin with the simple mealtime regimen and 176 units with carbohydrate counting). Even with these doses, severe hypoglycemia was modest (0.7–0.9 episodes per year) as was weight gain (2.4–3.6 kg). Thus, basal-bolus insulin therapy is highly effective in type 2 diabetes, and is safe, but takes the know-how to optimize the program and typically lots of insulin. There do not seem to be important differences between glargine and detemir as the basal insulin.[82,83] In contrast, a small single-center study found better results with glargine versus NPH insulin.[84]

Another approach to intensification is twice-daily or thrice-daily premixed insulin. In the PREFER study, patients failing various oral agents with average A1c level 8.6% received twice-daily aspart 70:30 or once-daily detemir and mealtime aspart for 26 weeks[85] The decrease of A1c level was modestly better with basal-bolus insulin (to 7.0% vs 7.2% with premix) along with slightly more major, but not minor hypoglycemia, in the basal-bolus–treated patients. The GINGER study randomized patients with type 2 diabetes on premixed insulin with or without metformin and average A1c level 8.6% to a basal-bolus regimen with glargine and glulisine versus intensification of their premixed insulin.[86] Again. there was better A1c level decrease with the basal-bolus program (47% basal-bolus–treated patients reached A1c level <7% vs 28% with the premixed insulin), but now with similar hypoglycemia. Rosenstock and colleagues[87] compared basal-bolus insulin with 3-times-a-day lispro mix 50:50, and found a modestly higher percentage of patients reached A1c level less than 7% with the basal-bolus regimen, with no difference in hypoglycemia. Collectively these results show that basal-bolus and premixed insulins are both effective in type 2 diabetes failing oral agents or less intensive insulin programs. However, on balance there seems to be the potential for a better decrease of A1c level with the basal-bolus therapy over premixes, with at least as good safety.

Stepwise Addition of Bolus Insulin to Basal Insulin

A simpler approach than advancing directly from basal insulin to a full basal-bolus program would be welcome. Given that modern eating habits are often to bunch many of the daytime calories into a single large meal, it has been proposed to cover that meal with 1 prandial injection, then add additional mealtime injections later if needed (**Fig. 2**). The concept started as theoretical,[88] but **Fig. 3** shows the 7-point glucose profile from the previously cited INITIATE trial, which compared glargine insulin with twice-daily aspart 70:30 in patients failing oral agents.[70] The results in the glargine-treated group showing acceptable control through the day followed by an increase in blood glucose level after supper support the plausibility of the concept.

The first testing was the OPAL study, which compared 2 treatment strategies (adding glulisine at breakfast or to the meal with the largest postprandial glucose excursion) for 24 weeks in patients optimized on glargine and oral agents with average A1c level 7.4%.[89] The main finding was similar efficacy and safety no matter which meal was chosen. Also, the final A1c level in both groups was 6.9% to 7.0%, with 30% of the patients 6.5% or less, confirming that 1 prandial injection is adequate in many patients failing basal insulin therapy.

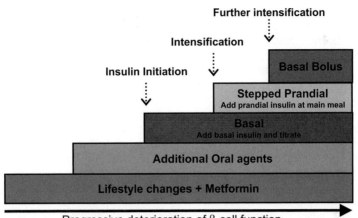

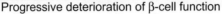

Fig. 2. Sequential stages for therapy for type 2 diabetes, including a step between basal insulin and basal-bolus insulin therapy: the sequential addition of 1, then 2 prandial injections if needed before moving to a full basal-bolus program. This therapy is usually referred to as stepped prandial therapy or basal plus therapy.

However, baseline blood glucose control in the OPAL study was better than the average patient failing basal insulin. Subsequent studies tested individuals with higher levels of A1c, often taking them through a program of first optimizing basal insulin, and then adding 1 meal insulin injection if needed. A proof-of concept study performed in patients with average A1c level 8.6% to 8.8% optimized glargine for 3 months followed by 3 months of glulisine added at the largest meal in those with A1c level

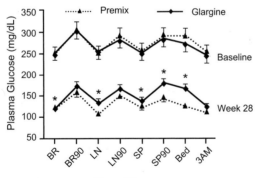

Time of Day

Fig. 3. Daylong glucose profiles at baseline and after 24 weeks in patients with type 2 diabetes failing oral agents treated with twice-daily aspart 70:30 mix (*stippled line*) or glargine insulin (*solid line*). Asterisks represent significant differences (*P*<.05) between the groups at that time point. Glucose monitoring samples were taken before breakfast (BR), 90 minutes later (BR90), before lunch (LN) and 90 minutes later (LN90), before supper (SP) and 90 minutes later (SP90), bedtime and 3 AM. Note that the highest glucose values in the glargine-treated group are from a supper-related step-up. (*Adapted from* Raskin P, Allen E, Hollander P, et al. Initiating insulin therapy in type 2 diabetes: a comparison of biphasic and basal insulin analogs. Diabetes Care 2005;28:263; with permission.)

greater than 7% on glargine alone.[90] At the first 3-month point, A1c level had fallen to 7.8% to 8.0%, with an additional 0.4% decrease with the 1 injection of glulisine. In the ELEONOR study,[91] patients with average A1c level of 8.8% on various oral agents had glargine added for 8 to 16 weeks to bring the fasting glucose level less than 126 mg/dL (7 mmol/L); more than 90% of the patients met that goal. In these patients, glulisine was added for 24 weeks at the meal with the highest postprandial glucose excursion. The tested issue was whether optimization of insulin dosing and blood glucose control differed using standard home glucose monitoring or telecare electronic communication of blood glucose results with the investigator; it did not. Relevant to this discussion, the A1c level decreased from 8.8% at baseline to 7.9% with glargine alone, and 7.1% with the 1 injection of glulisine, with 45% to 55% of those patients reaching A1c level 7.0% or less.

A different way of testing the stepped prandial concept is to compare a single injection versus multiple prandial injections after optimization of basal insulin. The All-to-Target study, which to date has been presented only in abstract form, is a 60-week study of 3 treatment strategies in 572 patients with average A1c level 9.4% on oral therapy: optimize glargine and then add once-daily glulisine (+1), optimize glargine followed by stepped addition of glulisine to a maximum of 3 injections (+0 to 3), or twice-daily aspart 70:30 throughout.[92] The same number of patients reached A1c level less than 7% with glargine + 1 (49%) as glargine + 0 to 3 (45%). Other results were that both of these approaches were superior to the premixed insulin (39% to A1c level <7%), and the glargine regimens had less hypoglycemia than the premixed insulin.[93]

In summary, adding prandial insulin in a stepwise fashion to patients with optimized basal insulin is still being validated. However, there is sufficient evidence to conclude that not all patients with type 2 diabetes failing basal insulin need a full basal-bolus program, and many can reach an A1c level less than 7% with just 1 prandial injection. Given that one-by-one addition of mealtime insulin is less intimidating for most patients and providers, as this approach becomes better known, one expects that it will be widely adopted for optimizing insulin treatment in type 2 diabetes.

The 4-T Trial: Head-to-Head Comparison of the Various Insulin Regimens

The 4-T trial studied the optimal starting insulin program in type 2 diabetes, and then how best to intensify insulin therapy. As such, this single study tested the conclusions of the many head-to-head comparisons of insulin regimens described earlier. Patients (708) failing sulfonylurea and metformin therapy with mean A1c level 8.4% to 8.6% were randomized to premeal aspart (prandial insulin), once-daily detemir (basal insulin), or twice-daily aspart 70:30 (premixed) for 1 year.[94] Those whose A1c level was more than 7% at the end of that year (which was most of the patients) were advanced to an intensified program for another 2 years by adding detemir to the prandial insulin (prandial/basal), mealtime aspart to the basal insulin (basal/prandial), or lunchtime aspart to the premixed insulin.[95] At the 1-year point, A1c level decrease was better with the prandial insulin (to 7.2%) and biphasic aspart (to 7.3%) than with detemir (to 7.6%), but with more weight gain (+5.7 kg prandial, +4.7 kg premix, +1.9 kg basal) and grade 2 or higher hypoglycemia (12, 5.7, 2.3 yearly events, respectively).[94] The 2-year intensification resulted in good glycemic control in all of the regimens: A1c level was 7.1% with premix, 6.8% with prandial/basal, and 6.9% with basal/prandial. What differed was a higher rate of hypoglycemia and more weight gain with the premix and prandial/basal insulin versus starting with detemir and progressing if needed to a full basal-bolus program.[95] Thus, these results closely mirror the theme of the many studies detailed earlier; on balance, starting with basal insulin followed by adding prandial insulin as needed seems to provide a modestly better balance of efficacy and safety over starting with premixed or prandial insulin.

Insulin Pump Therapy in Type 2 Diabetes

Insulin pumps are being increasingly used in type 2 diabetes,[96] sometimes with U-500 insulin.[97] Open-label, nonrandomized studies have shown them to be effective and safe.[98–100] The more controversial issue is whether they are superior to subcutaneous insulin, and thus justify the cost. Raskin and colleagues[101] randomized 132 uncontrolled insulin-taking patients with type 2 diabetes for 24 weeks to an insulin pump versus an intensified multiple daily injection (MDI) regimen of NPH and aspart insulin. The decrease in A1c level was the same (baseline 8.0% to 8.2% to 7.6% for the pump and 7.5% for the MDI program) and there was no difference in hypoglycemia. What did differ is that 93% of those using the pump preferred it over their previous injections. The investigators concluded that the pump "provided efficacy and safety comparable to MDI therapy for type 2 diabetes...indicating pump therapy should be considered when initiating intensive insulin therapy for type 2 diabetes." In contrast, Monami and colleagues[102] performed a meta-analysis of the few randomized studies that had compared pump and basal-bolus therapy in type 2 diabetes. They also found no difference. However, the lack of superiority led them to conclude "available data do not justify the use of CSII...in type 2 diabetes." Ergo the controversy. What may eventually help is patch-pump technology and the potential for comparable efficacy to traditional pumps, but with less complexity and expense.[103] Ref.[104] is a comprehensive review of patch pumps, although it is focused more on their applicability to closed-loop systems for type 1 diabetes.

INCRETIN-BASED THERAPY: IN PLACE OF OR TOGETHER WITH INSULIN IN TYPE 2 DIABETES?

As new pharmaceuticals have appeared for type 2 diabetes, a hope of many has been to obviate insulin. A few years ago, the focus was whether adding a thiazolidinedione in patients failing combination sulfonylurea and metformin (triple therapy) could replace basal insulin.[105] Head-to-head comparisons showed similar decrease of A1c level from a baseline up to 9% to 9.5%, with the expected higher incidence of hypoglycemia with insulin, and weight gain with the thiazolidinedione.[106,107] Because of this positive result, switching patients off insulin to a thiazolidinedione was studied,[108] and a polypill with all 3 oral medications was developed[109] along with discussions about starting all 3 orals at diagnosis.[110] Enthusiasm has now disappeared because of the myriad of problems with thiazolidinediones.

The current discussion relates to incretin therapies: glucagonlike peptide 1 (GLP-1) receptor agonists or dipeptidyl peptidase-4 (DPP-4) inhibitors. The GLP-1 receptor agonists are of particular interest because they come not only with reasonable glycemic control, but a more desirable clinical profile than insulin: weight loss, minimal hypoglycemia, improved blood pressure and lipid levels, and the wow factor of new medications.[111,112] The question of relative effectiveness of basal insulin or a GLP-1 receptor agonist in patients failing orals has been addressed in several head-to-head trials. Heine and colleagues[24] compared exenatide or glargine added for 26 weeks in patients on metformin and sulfonylurea therapy with average A1c level 8.2%. A1c level improved equally to 7.1%, with weight gain (+1.8 kg) and more nocturnal hypoglycemia with the insulin, and weight loss (–2.3 kg) and gastrointestinal side effects with exenatide. What made the study highly discussed was the observation that this same A1c level improvement resulted from different mechanisms: a decrease of fasting and premeal glycemia with the insulin as opposed to flattening of the postbreakfast and postsupper glucose excursions with exenatide (**Fig. 4**). Generally comparable results were seen in a comparison of liraglutide and glargine insulin at the same baseline A1c level (8.2%), although the A1c level decrease was modestly better with liraglutide (−1.3% with liraglutide vs −1.1% with glargine).[113] Also, 24-week comparisons of exenatide with once-daily or twice-daily aspart 70:30 showed equal to better decrease of A1c level with the insulin, but with weight gain and more hypoglycemia.[114,115] Together these results show that GLP-1 receptor agonists and insulin are both good choices in persons failing oral agents, but with different clinical profiles. Still, one expects the efficacy will deviate in favor of insulin at high A1c levels; the cutoff point is not known, but a common guess is more than 8.5%. This situation raises concern that the concept of equivalency could be misinterpreted and foster avoidance of insulin, as was observed in an audit of persons with professional drivers licenses in the United Kingdom.[116] A related question is whether insulin can be replaced with a GLP-1 receptor agonist. That issue was tested in a 16-week pilot study of patients with average A1c level 8.1% who were switched from insulin to exenatide; glycemia was unchanged in 60%, but deteriorated in the rest, so half of them went back on insulin before the end of the trial.[117] The mostly negative view of these results is seen in the title of the accompanying editorial[118] "Missing the point: substituting exenatide for nonoptimized insulin: going from bad to worse!"

Currently the greatest enthusiasm is for insulin and incretin therapy used together based on their complimentary effects on basal and postprandial glucose (see **Fig. 4**), and hope that the weight loss and minimal risk of hypoglycemia with GLP-1 receptor agonists would lessen those issues with insulin. A pharmacokinetic and pharmacodynamic study of combination liraglutide and detemir showed no change in the PK profile

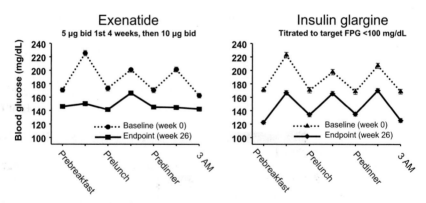

Fig. 4. Daylong glucose profiles at baseline (*stippled line*) and after 26 weeks of therapy in patients with type 2 diabetes failing oral agents treated with exenatide twice daily (*left panel*) or glargine insulin (*right panel*). Both treatments decreased the A1c level from 8.2% to 7.1%. Also, the characteristic clinical profile of these agents was observed: weight gain (+1.8 kg) and more nocturnal hypoglycemia with the insulin, and weight loss (−2.3 kg) and gastrointestinal side effects with exenatide. However, what makes this figure notable is the evidence that the improvement in A1c level stemmed from different effects on blood glucose: breakfast and suppertime postprandial control with exenatide, and decrease of the overall glucose profile with glargine. (*Data from* Heine RJ, Van Gaal LF, Johns D, et al. Exenatide versus insulin glargine in patients with suboptimally controlled type 2 diabetes: a randomized trial. Ann Intern Med 2005;143:559–69.)

of either agent, and confirmed there was the expected additive effect for a decrease in blood glucose levels.[119] Also, several observational studies of exenatide with insulin in clinical practice have enthusiastically supported the combination,[120–123] and a small study of poorly controlled patients on U-500 insulin reported the A1c level was decreased from 8.5% to 7.1% along with an 11-kg weight loss and 28% reduction in insulin doses with just 12 weeks of liraglutide additive therapy.[124] The first randomized trial was a 4-week proof-of-concept study that added exenatide or sitagliptin versus current therapy in patients on metformin and glargine insulin with average A1c level 7.9% to 8.4%.[125] Glargine optimization was also performed so the A1c level decreased in all groups, but more with exenatide (–1.9%) than sitagliptin (–1.5%) or the metformin and glargine (–1.2%). In addition, postmeal glucose excursions were markedly decreased with exenatide (less so with sitagliptin), the hypoglycemia rates were minimal with both incretin therapies, and there was modest weight loss with exenatide. Ergo, proof of concept.

Interest in the topic of combination insulin/GLP-1 receptor agonist therapy has skyrocketed because of a multicenter study that added exenatide or placebo in 259 patients with A1c level 8.3% to 8.5% on glargine and various oral agents.[126] The protocol optimized the glargine dose in both groups. After 30 weeks, the A1c level was decreased 1.7% in the exenatide-treated group versus 1.0% with placebo. Also, there was a 2.8-kg weight difference (–1.8 kg with exenatide and +1.0 kg with placebo), no difference in hypoglycemia, and the exenatide group needed less of an increase in glargine dose for optimization (**Fig. 5**). The intense discussion of this study has in part been critical because exenatide was not compared with mealtime insulin, which is the usual next step in patients failing basal insulin therapy. The investigators have countered that the next insulin-related step in a patient like this should be to properly adjust their basal insulin dosage, which is supported by the A1c level improvement they saw in the placebo group. Regardless, this study has mostly been praised as groundbreaking, because it shows with dramatic results what many believe is the future of how type 2 diabetes treatment is likely to evolve.

Several questions related to this topic are under discussion. Is it best to start with basal insulin followed by a GLP-1 receptor agonist, or the other way around? An abstract[127] from 2011 took the opposite approach to the study by Buse and

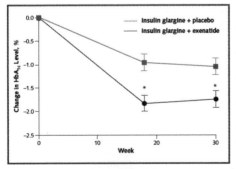

Fig. 5. A1c values over 30 weeks (*left panel*) and a listing of the major clinical results (*right panel*) in patients with type 2 diabetes who were failing metformin and glargine insulin with baseline A1c values of 8.3% to 8.5% treated with intensification of the glargine (placebo) or that along with addition of exenatide twice-daily. (*Data from* Buse JB, Bergenstal RM, Glass LC, et al. Use of twice-daily exenatide in basal insulin-treated patients with type 2 diabetes: a randomized, controlled trial. Ann Intern Med 2011;154:103–12.)

colleagues[126] by starting patients failing orals on liraglutide for 12 weeks followed by detemir insulin if needed; 60% of the patients reached A1c level 7% or less with liraglutide alone, and 43% of the rest after adding detemir. Thus either way works; whether 1 sequence is superior to the other is the subject of several trials under development. A related question is whether the GLP-1 receptor agonist works by improving β-cell function, and if so, would the benefit not be less in patients with a long duration of diabetes and poor β-cell reserve (ie, patients already on insulin)? GLP-1 receptor agonists in type 2 diabetes act not only to improve β-cell function but also by decreasing postmeal glucagon levels and slowing gastric motility; many believe that these effects account for most of the improvement in glycemia.[111,112] Contrary to the tenet of the question about the necessity for preserved β-cell functional capacity for a good clinical response to GLP-1 receptor agonists, small studies have shown impressive benefits of adding (not substituting) these agents in type 1 diabetes.[128,129] Is 1 GLP-1 receptor agonist preferable to another, and where will the weekly or bimonthly preparations fit? Current speculation is that the preferred agents will be those with the greatest decrease of postmeal glucose excursions, but the final answer awaits head-to-head trials.

Less information is available about usage of DPP-4 inhibitors with insulin in patients with type 2 diabetes. As might be expected from the clinical profile of these agents, glycemia improves only modestly, and they lack the weight-loss and insulin-sparing effects of GLP-1 receptor agonists. Vildagliptin added for 24 weeks in patients on a multishot insulin program with average A1c level 8.4% decreased the A1c level 0.2% versus a 0.5% increase in placebo-treated patients.[130] Sitagliptin for 24 weeks in insulin-taking patients with average A1c level 8.6% to 8.7% decreased the A1c level 0.6% versus 0.0% with placebo.[131]

WHICH ORAL AGENTS TO USE WHEN INSULIN IS STARTED IN TYPE 2 DIABETES?

An issue that is little discussed is which oral agents should be continued or stopped with insulin treatment in type 2 diabetes. Not controversial is metformin; several years ago we reviewed the available studies[132] and found better glucose control and less weight gain in type 2 diabetes patients using insulin and metformin versus insulin alone. Continuing incretin therapy (GLP-1 receptor agonists and probably DPP-4 inhibitors) with basal insulin also is well accepted, as detailed earlier, but what to do with basal-bolus insulin is untested. Thiazolidinedione use with insulin was controversial a few years ago because of the potential for additive effects on weight gain, edema, or congestive heart failure, although in clinical practice they were mostly continued for their insulin-sparing effect. It is less of an issue today because of the many side effects and safety issues with thiazolidinediones.

The question which has not been fully settled is whether to continue sulfonylureas with basal insulin; there has been a running debate of this issue for many years.[133–135] The argument for keeping them is that their discontinuation often leads to a deterioration of glycemic control.[136] Also, when basal insulin is added to the common combination of metformin and a sulfonylurea with or without a thiazolidinedione, the only medication that is directly acting on postmeal glycemia is the sulfonylurea. Opponents argue that the sulfonylurea raises the risk of hypoglycemia and weight gain. Also, some believe that being able to optimize the basal insulin (ie, fasting glucose) is sometimes prevented by a normal to low daytime glucose level from the sulfonylurea. And the fear of cardiovascular risks with sulfonylureas periodically flares.

Surprisingly few studies have critically assessed sulfonylurea use with insulin in type 2 diabetes. Yki-Järvinen and colleagues[137] tested bedtime NPH insulin with various other therapies for 1 year in patients with a starting A1c level of 9.9%: metformin, glyburide, metformin and glyburide, or increasing from once to twice-daily NPH. The best decrease of A1c level (–2.5%) and the least weight gain both occurred with metformin alone. More recently, a pooled analysis and meta-analysis of studies initiating glargine basal insulin therapy in patients with type 2 diabetes found the highest proportion of patients achieving A1c level 7% or less, the least weight gain, and the least hypoglycemia all occurred in those using metformin alone compared with a sulfonylurea alone or combination metformin and sulfonylurea.[138] Similarly, a post hoc analysis of a large clinical trial comparing glargine and detemir as basal insulin therapy, in which all patients were kept on metformin but whether to stop secretagogues was left to the discretion of the investigator, reported that the patients who continued secretagogues had equivalent levels of A1c but more weight gain and hypoglycemia than those taking only metformin.[139] Thus whether sulfonylureas have a positive or negative effect with basal insulin in type 2 diabetes remains an open question. Given the continued common use of these agents around the world, a well-designed trial to settle this issue would be helpful.

SUMMARY

Insulin remains a core therapy for type 2 diabetes even with the many new pharmaceuticals that have become available over the last 15 years. Despite claims that 1 or more would replace insulin in this disease, insulin is still the therapy with the greatest potential to work when all else fails. The downsides are convenience (it has to be injected), weight gain, and hypoglycemia. The inconvenience of injection has improved greatly with pen delivery systems and tiny (for the most part, painless) needles, and a major advantage of the insulin analogues is reducing the others. Still, the practice of many health care providers and patients is to hold off insulin as long as possible despite data showing that waiting to start basal insulin until the A1c level is more than 8% can worsen weight gain and decrease the chance of successful blood glucose control.[59,60] Also, unlike many of the newer therapies, except for hypoglycemia, there are few safety concerns with insulin. There are reports of cancer and cardiovascular risks with insulin therapy,[140,141] but the general belief (at least currently) is they are unproved. We will soon learn more about these issues from several studies including the ORIGIN (Outcome Reduction with an Initial Glargine Intervention) trial, an 8-year study of cardiovascular outcomes in more than 12,000 subjects with prediabetes or very early type 2 diabetes (average A1c level 6.4%) given glargine insulin versus traditional therapy.[142] Stepping back and looking at the extensive literature on insulin use along with clinical experience leads to the inescapable conclusion that in type 2 diabetes insulin is effective, safe, and well accepted by patients, especially when enthusiastically recommended by their health care provider. The controversy today is not whether to use insulin, but when and how best to start it and optimize it, and which benefits new insulins may bring. As detailed in the head-to-head trials described in this review, differences between the various insulin programs are generally minor. Still, on balance, the author agrees with most experts that starting with basal insulin followed by a stepwise addition of prandial insulin seems to be optimal in terms of simplicity and safety.

A major discussion is how treatment practices might evolve. Particularly influential are the recent studies that investigated the relative positioning of incretin therapies (in particular GLP-1 receptor agonists) versus insulin. Head-to-head trials of twice daily or once-weekly exenatide[24,143,144] or liraglutide[113] versus basal insulin in patients failing oral agents show reasonable equivalency or maybe even modestly superior glucose control up to an A1c level of 8.5%. However, what has the field buzzing is the potential of using them together, maybe in the same syringe, for better efficacy, weight control, minimal hypoglycemia, and improvement in cardiovascular risk factors. Assuming that current safety concerns regarding insulin and the incretin agents prove to be insignificant, there is a growing belief that this combination will be at the core of future diabetes therapy until something better comes along.

HOW-TOS OF INSULIN THERAPY IN TYPE 2 DIABETES

I end this review with a summary of how I start and optimize insulin in the average patient with type 2 diabetes (**Box 1**). Although generally in agreement with the studies described in this review, I want to emphasize that the specific details and nuances are my own.

Core elements of successful diabetes therapy are access to diabetes education and dieticians.[145,146] Also, recent studies have confirmed the benefits, albeit mild, of home blood glucose monitoring with insulin treatment in type 2 diabetes.[147,148] I typically do the following:

1. At the first visit in which insulin is discussed, the patient and I talk about why insulin and why not something else, and I emphasize the benefits and ease of use, and also identity and discuss the patient's fears. Not surprisingly it is nurturing, friendly, and positive; patients are usually afraid whether they admit it or not. Lots of questions are good; the patient is engaged. No questions are usually not good. The patient is then seen by a diabetes educator, who has them self-inject, shows them insulin pens, discusses the risks and treatment of hypoglycemia, and sets up a phone contact in the first few days after insulin is started. Also, gaps in diabetes education are discussed, with plans for future visits as needed. Typically, the time with me and the educator is 40 to 50 minutes and results in almost all patients being willing or enthusiastic to start then and there.
2. I mostly start with basal insulin, and almost always a basal analogue once daily unless it is unaffordable, when bedtime NPH insulin by syringe and vial instead are used. If glargine insulin is chosen, the patient can choose the time that is easiest for them to take it (most studies have not found a best time), whereas detemir is started at suppertime or bedtime. Also, I tend to continue the patient's other diabetes agents, including sulfonylureas, at least initially.
3. We negotiate a frequency of self-blood glucose monitoring; I know of no way to start and then adjust a dosage of basal insulin without daily fasting blood glucose values. I have found that simply explaining why we need home blood glucose values converts many who had repeatedly refused to perform home testing for their referring providers into reliable patients who come back knowing, and wanting to discuss, their glucose results. I also prefer a second daily test, either prelunch alternating with presupper alternating with bedtime on a rotating sequence, or presupper alternating with prebed (assuming at least 2 hours after supper). Obviously, I take more testing if offered, but twice a day is enough for successful therapy. Again, that strategy must be discussed with the patient; it is usually easily explained why that second glucose result is needed to know how to make future decisions about adjustments in basal insulin or addition of prandial insulin.
4. In agreement with the recommendations of the American Diabetes Association (ADA)/European Association for the Study of Diabetes (EASD) algorithm[7] and many others, I typically start 0.2 units/kg of the chosen insulin, although it is less if I am worried about a high risk of hypoglycemia such as in elderly or frail patients,

Box 1
Sequence of steps for initiating basal insulin therapy followed by stepped prandial insulin in type 2 diabetes. The specific details are gleamed from literature as cited in the text along with the author's personal experience

- Starting insulin therapy:
  - Discuss reason for insulin therapy, available insulins and programs, and how insulin is started and optimized. Identify the patient's fears
  - Diabetes educator: self-injection, hypoglycemia education, set up post-visit contact
- Insulin start:
  - Basal insulin: start 0.2 units/kg chosen insulin at appropriate injection time
  - Establish maximal dose: usually 0.4–0.5 units/kg
  - Home titration algorithm: favorite is increase 1 unit daily until fasting glucose is less than 120–130 mg/dL or maximal insulin dose is reached
  - Home blood glucose monitoring: 2 daily tests (fasting and alternating presupper and postsupper) or all 3 tests
  - Typically continue the patient's other diabetes medications
- Optimization of basal insulin:
  - Review blood glucose log and pattern
  - Adjust basal insulin dose as needed to attain target fasting glucose; if high daytime glucose values, discuss lifestyle efforts versus potential need for additional therapy such as prandial insulin or incretin therapy
- Insulin intensification: adding prandial insulin:
  - Blood glucose log shows fasting glucose at or close to target, but A1c level not at target along with increased daytime glucose values
  - Lifestyle efforts have been optimized as much as possible
  - Review prandial insulin versus adding incretin therapy
- Prandial insulin: stepped insulin therapy:
  - Add chosen insulin at largest meal or to the meal with greatest level of postprandial hyperglycemia (usually the same)
  - Start 4 units at the start of that meal
  - Home titration: twice-weekly increase 1 unit until 2-hour postmeal glucose is less than 160 mg/dL or 3 or more hour value less than 130 mg/dL
- Follow-up visits:
  - Review blood glucose log and A1c value
  - Review lifestyle efforts and other relevant factors
  - Adjust current insulins, or if needed add additional meal injection followed by titration

impaired renal, hepatic, or cardiac function. Also I sometimes start less in patients taking a thiazolidinedione as rarely they end up on surprisingly small doses of basal insulin. However, it is important to keep in perspective that this starting dose is small; clinical studies have shown on average that type 2 diabetes patients on glargine or NPH insulin end up on 0.47 units/kg,[58] and on detemir probably more.

5. I discuss with the patient the target fasting glucose and A1c values, and give most patients an algorithm for home insulin adjustment. Regarding the target, less than

100 mg/dL or 5.5 mmol/L is a common target in studies, but one that I find often hard to attain. I tend to start with a goal of "always less than 130 and 120 if doable. Then we'll see if we can do even better." For dose adjustments, many algorithms are available and tested in numerous clinical trials. The most recommended is that of the ADA/EASD of 2 unit increases every 3 days until the target fasting glucose is reached.[7] I prefer a 1-unit daily increase[149]; my belief (based on no data) is that there is less forgetting and slowness to advance when changes are made every day.

6. Unlike most investigators, I give patients a maximal dose of usually 0.4 to 0.5 units/kg. This strategy is in part because I have seen many patients who get lost to follow-up and reappear many months later on 1.5 or 2 units/kg of the basal insulin, often with inadequate fasting glucose values but nighttime hypoglycemia. What they need is suppertime prandial insulin (maybe more meals as well) and less basal insulin. Ergo I now give a maximal dose (where to stop before the next visit) plus I discuss all of this carefully with the patient so they understand what I am doing and why. For example, in a 100 kg patient, I would start 20 units of the chosen basal insulin with instructions to increase 1 unit daily until the fasting glucose is routinely below 120 mg/dL. If that does not happen by 45 units, then they stay at that dose until the next visit when we will review the home blood glucose results and decide whether to continue to increase the basal insulin versus adding prandial insulin or a GLP-1 receptor agonist.

7. I see patients back typically 1 month later, plus they have had phone contact with the Certified Diabetes Educator at least weekly over that month. The patient and I review together their blood glucose log and identify any pattern, and what that may mean in terms of future plans for their insulin therapy. Additional discussions are to reemphasize their blood glucose and A1c goals, how they are doing lifestyle-wise and with hypoglycemia, and whether we are going to continue or change their oral diabetes medications.

8. An important part of the studies of basal insulin therapy that are cited in this review is the understanding that some patients do not reach their target A1c level despite optimized dosing of the basal insulin. Further increases in basal insulin dosage are not the answer. That situation is identified by a blood glucose pattern with a fasting glucose that is at or close to goal, and higher glucose values during the day. If all premeal values are substantially higher, a full basal-bolus insulin program is needed, although adding a GLP-1 receptor agonist is another option for some patients. On the other hand, a pattern in which the blood glucose increases only after supper as seen in **Fig. 3** is common. In that case, I use the stepped approach of adding 1 mealtime injection. Either way, I tend to start a rapid-acting analogue at the identified meal(s) at about 0.05 to 0.1 unit/kg and then adjust 1 unit every few days to a 2-hour postprandial target of less than 140–160 mg/dL or 7.8–8.8 mmol/L individualized to the planned intensity of therapy for that patient, or to less than 130 mg/dL or 7.2 mmol/L if the testing is at least 3 hours after food. Many investigators recommend starting with less prandial insulin; 4 units is common,[7] but it does not matter. Success is based on successful titration, not what dosage was started. A controversy is what to do with sulfonylureas or DPP-4 inhibitors when mealtime insulin is started. Definitive data are not available. I tend to continue these agents with a single mealtime insulin injection, but stop them with a full basal-bolus program.

EPILOGUE

I often finish presentations on insulin therapy for type 2 diabetes with the slide shown in **Fig. 6**, so it seemed fitting to add it to this review. It is a tribute to Robert Turner, the

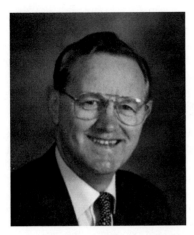

Robert Turner MA, MD, FRCP
Professor of Medicine
University of Oxford

1938-1999

*"We don't start insulin early enough, or use
it aggressively enough"*

Fig. 6. Tribute to Robert Turner showing his comment about the UK Prospective Diabetes Study in response to a question as to what was the major thing he had learned from the UKPDS trial. His answer shown on the figure is unfortunately still apt today.

famous UK diabetologist who led the UKPDS.[150] I made it after watching Dr Turner present the findings from the UKPDS at the Canadian Diabetes Association annual meeting in 1998. After his presentation, he was asked from a member of the audience "What is the major thing you learned from the UKPDS trial." His answer shown on the figure is unfortunately still true today.

REFERENCES

1. 2011 National Diabetes Fact Sheet. Available at: http://www.cdc.gov/diabetes/pubs/factsheet11/htm. Accessed January 28, 2012.
2. IDF Diabetes Atlas 5th edition. Available at: www.idf.org/diabetesatlas/5e/the-global-burden. Accessed January 28, 2012.
3. Leahy JL, Pratley RE. What is type 2 diabetes mellitus? Crucial role of maladaptive changes in beta cell and adipocyte biology. Translational Endocrinology and Metabolism 2011;2:9–42.
4. Emerging Risk Factors Collaboration, Sarwar N, Gao P, Seshasai SR, et al. Diabetes mellitus: fasting blood glucose concentration and risk of vascular disease: a collaborative meta-analysis of 102 prospective studies. Lancet 2010;375:2215–22.
5. Emerging Risk Factors Collaboration, Seshasai SR, Kaptoge S, Thompson A, et al. Diabetes mellitus: fasting glucose and risk of cause-specific death. N Engl J Med 2011;364:829–41.
6. Rosenbaum L, Lamas D. Facing a "slow-motion disaster"–the UN meeting on noncommunicable diseases. N Engl J Med 2011;365:2345–8.
7. Nathan DM, Buse JB, Davidson MB, et al. Medical management of hyperglycemia in type 2 diabetes: a consensus algorithm for the initiation and adjustment of therapy. A consensus statement of the American Diabetes Association and the European Association for the Study of Diabetes. Diabetes Care 2009;32: 193–203.

8. Rodbard HW, Jellinger PS, Davidson JA, et al. Statement by an American Association of Clinical Endocrinologists/American College of Endocrinology consensus panel on type 2 diabetes: an algorithm for glycemic control. Endocr Pract 2009;15:540–59. Available at: https://www.aace.com/sites/default/files/GlycemicControl/Algorithm.pdf. Accessed January 28, 2012.

9. American Diabetes Association. Standards of medical care in diabetes–2012. Diabetes Care 2012;35(Suppl 1):S11–63.

10. Skyler JS, Bergenstal R, Bonow RO, et al. Intensive glycemic control and the prevention of cardiovascular events: implications of the ACCORD, ADVANCE, and VA Diabetes Trials: a position statement of the American Diabetes Association and a scientific statement of the American College of Cardiology Foundation and the American Heart Association. Diabetes Care 2009;32:187–92.

11. Ray KK, Seshasai SR, Wijesuriya S, et al. Effect of intensive control on cardiovascular outcomes and death in patients with diabetes mellitus: a meta-analysis of randomized controlled trials. Lancet 2009;373:1765–72.

12. Turnbull FM, Abraira C, Anderson RJ, et al. Intensive glucose control and macrovascular outcomes in type 2 diabetes. Diabetologia 2009;52:2288–98.

13. Zhang CY, Sun AJ, Zhang SN, et al. Effects of intensive glucose control on incidence of cardiovascular events in patients with type 2 diabetes: a meta-analysis. Ann Med 2010;42:305–15.

14. Gæde P, Lund-Andersen H, Parving HH, et al. Effect of a multifactorial intervention on mortality in type 2 diabetes. N Engl J Med 2008;358:580–91.

15. Holman RR, Paul SK, Bethel MA, et al. 10-year follow-up of intensive glucose control in type 2 diabetes. N Engl J Med 2008;359:1577–89.

16. Nathan DM, Cleary PA, Backlund JY, et al. Intensive diabetes treatment and cardiovascular disease in patients with type 1 diabetes. N Engl J Med 2005;353:2643–53.

17. deBoer IH, Sun W, Cleary PA, et al. Intensive diabetes therapy and glomerular filtration rate in type 1 diabetes. N Engl J Med 2011;365:2366–76.

18. Hartman I. Insulin analogs: impact on treatment success, satisfaction, quality of life, and adherence. Clin Med Res 2008;6:54–67.

19. Polonsky WH, Fisher L, Guzman S, et al. Psychological insulin resistance in patients with type 2 diabetes: the scope of the problem. Diabetes Care 2005;28:2543–5.

20. Cefalu WT, Mathieu C, Davidson J, et al. Patients' perceptions of subcutaneous insulin in the OPTIMIZE study: a multicenter follow-up study. Diabetes Technol Ther 2008;10:25–38.

21. Polonsky WH, Hajos TR, Dain MP, et al. Are patients with type 2 diabetes reluctant to start insulin? An explanation of the scope and underpinnings of psychological insulin resistance in a large, international population. Curr Med Res Opin 2011;27:1169–74.

22. Nakar S, Yitzhaki G, Rosenberg R, et al. Transition to insulin in type 2 diabetes: family physicians' misconception of patients' fears contributes to existing barriers. J Diabetes Complications 2007;4:220–6.

23. Jenkins N, Hallowell N, Farmer AJ, et al. Initiating insulin as part of the Treating to Target in Type 2 Diabetes (4-T) trial: an interview study of patients' and health professionals' experiences. Diabetes Care 2010;33:2178–80.

24. Heine RJ, Van Gaal LF, Johns D, et al. Exenatide versus insulin glargine in patients with suboptimally controlled type 2 diabetes: a randomized trial. Ann Intern Med 2005;143:559–69.

25. Yki-Järvinen H, Kauppinen-Mäkelin R, Tiikkainen M, et al. Insulin glargine or NPH combined with metformin in type 2 diabetes: the LANMET study. Diabetologia 2006;49:442–51.
26. Bretzel RG, Nuber U, Landgraf W, et al. Once-daily basal insulin glargine versus thrice-daily prandial insulin lispro in people with type 2 diabetes on oral hypoglycaemic agents (APOLLO): an open randomized controlled trial. Lancet 2008; 371:1073–84.
27. Turner RC, McCarthy ST, Holman RR, et al. Beta-cell function improved by supplementing basal insulin secretion in mild diabetes. Br Med J 1976;1:1252–4.
28. Garvey WT, Olefsky JM, Griffin J, et al. The effect of insulin treatment on insulin secretion and insulin action in type II diabetes mellitus. Diabetes 1985;34: 222–34.
29. Bunck MC, Diamant M, Corner A, et al. One-year treatment with exenatide improves ß-cell function, compared with insulin glargine, in metformin-treated type 2 diabetic patients. Diabetes Care 2009;32:762–8.
30. Ilkova H, Glaser B, Tunckle A, et al. Induction of long-term glycemic control in newly diagnosed type 2 diabetic patients by transient intensive insulin therapy. Diabetes Care 1997;20:1351–6.
31. Ryan EA, Imes S, Wallace C. Short-term intensive insulin therapy in newly diagnosed type 2 diabetes. Diabetes Care 2004;27:1028–32.
32. Li Y, Xu W, Liao ZH, et al. Induction of long-term glycemic control in newly diagnosed type 2 diabetic patients is associated with improvement of beta-cell function. Diabetes Care 2004;27:2597–602.
33. Weng J, Li Y, Xu W, et al. Effect of intensive insulin therapy on beta-cell function and glycaemic control in patients with newly diagnosed type 2 diabetes: a multicentre randomized parallel-group trial. Lancet 2008;371:1753–60.
34. Hølberg PV, Zander M, Visbøll T, et al. Near normalization of blood glucose improves the potentiating effect of GLP-1 on glucose-induced insulin secretion in patients with type 2 diabetes. Diabetologia 2008;51:632–40.
35. Hølberg PV, Visbøll T, Robøl R, et al. Four-weeks of near-normalization of blood glucose improves the insulin response to glucagon-like peptide-1 and glucose-dependent insulinotropic polypeptide in patients with type 2 diabetes. Diabetologia 2009;52:199–207.
36. Riddle MC. New tactics for type 2 diabetes: regimens based on intermediate-acting insulin taken at bedtime. Lancet 1985;1:192–5.
37. Yki-Järvinen H, Kauppila M, Kajansuu E, et al. Comparison of insulin regimens in patients with non-insulin-dependent diabetes mellitus. N Engl J Med 1992;327: 1426–33.
38. Riddle M, Hart J, Bingham P, et al. Combined therapy for obese type 2 diabetes: suppertime mixed insulin with daytime sulfonylurea. Am J Med Sci 1992;303: 151–6.
39. Alexander GC, Sehgal NL, Moloney RM, et al. National trends in treatment of type 2 diabetes mellitus, 1994-2007. Arch Intern Med 2008;169(19):2088–94.
40. Li C, Ford ES, Zhao G, et al. Trends of insulin use among US adults with type 2 diabetes: the Behavioral Risk Factor Surveillance System, 1995-2007. J Diabetes Complications 2012;26(1):17–22.
41. UK Prospective Diabetes Study Group 16. Overview of 6 years' therapy of type II diabetes: a progressive disease. Diabetes 1995;44:1249–58.
42. Wright A, Burden AC, Paisey RC, et al. Sulfonylurea inadequacy: efficacy of addition of insulin over 6 years in patients with type 2 diabetes in the UK Prospective Diabetes Study (UKPDS 57). Diabetes Care 2002;25:330–6.

43. Riddle MC, Rosenstock J, Gerich J, et al. The Treat-to-Target Trial: randomized addition of glargine or human NPH insulin to oral therapy of type 2 diabetic patients. Diabetes Care 2003;26:3080–6.

44. Kennedy L, Herman WH, Strange P, et al. Impact of active versus usual algorithmic titration of basal insulin and point-of-care versus laboratory measurement of HbA1c on glycemic control in patients with type 2 diabetes: the Glycemic Optimization with Algorithms and Labs at Point of Care (GOAL A1C) trial. Diabetes Care 2008;29:1–8.

45. Hermansen K, Davies M, Derezinski T, et al. A 26-week, randomized, parallel, treat-to-target trial comparing insulin detemir with NPH insulin as add-on therapy to oral glucose-lowering drugs in insulin-naive people with type 2 diabetes. Diabetes Care 2006;29:1269–74.

46. Rosenstock J, Dailey G, Massi-Benedetti M, et al. Reduced hypoglycemia risk with insulin glargine: a meta-analysis comparing insulin glargine with human NPH insulin in type 2 diabetes. Diabetes Care 2005;28:950–5.

47. Monami M, Marchiommi N, Mannucci E. Long-acting insulin analogues versus NPH human insulin in type 2 diabetes: a meta-analysis. Diabetes Res Clin Pract 2008;81:184–9.

48. Home PD, Fritsche A, Schinzel S, et al. Meta-analysis of individual patient data to assess the risk of hypoglycaemia in people with type 2 diabetes using NPH insulin or insulin glargine. Diabetes Obes Metab 2010;12:772–9.

49. Rosenstock J, Davies M, Home PD, et al. A randomised, 52-week, treat-to-target trial comparing insulin detemir with insulin glargine when administered as add-on to glucose-lowering drugs in insulin-naive people with type 2 diabetes. Diabetologia 2008;51:408–16.

50. Dailey G, Admane K, Mercier F, et al. Relationship of insulin dose, A1c lowering, and weight in type 2 diabetes: comparing insulin glargine and insulin detemir. Diabetes Technol Ther 2010;12:1019–27.

51. Lucidi P, Porcellati F, Rossetti P, et al. Pharmacokinetics and pharmacodynamics of therapeutic doses of basal insulins NPH, glargine, and detemir after 1 week of daily administration at bedtime in type 2 diabetic subjects: a randomized crossover study. Diabetes Care 2011;34:1312–4.

52. Porcellati F, Lucidi P, Rossetti P, et al. Differential effects of adiposity on pharmacodynamics of basal insulins NPH, glargine, and detemir in type 2 diabetes mellitus. Diabetes Care 2011;34:2521–3.

53. King AB. No higher dose requirements with insulin detemir than glargine in type 2 diabetes: a crossover, double-blind, and randomized study using continuous glucose monitoring. J Diabetes Sci Technol 2010;4:151–4.

54. Birkeland KI, Home PD, Wendisch U, et al. Insulin degludec in type 1 diabetes: a randomized controlled trial of a new-generation ultra-long-acting insulin compared with insulin glargine. Diabetes Care 2011;34:661–5.

55. Zinman B, Fulcher G, Rao PV, et al. Insulin degludec, an ultra-long-acting basal insulin, once a day or three times a week versus insulin glargine once a day in patients with type 2 diabetes: a 16-week, randomized, open label, phase 2 trial. Lancet 2011;377:924–31.

56. Heise T, Tack CJ, Cuddihy R, et al. A new-generation ultra-long-acting basal insulin with a bolus boost compared with insulin glargine in insulin-naïve people with type 2 diabetes: a randomized, controlled trial. Diabetes Care 2011;34:699–774.

57. Little S, Shaw J, Home P. Hypoglycemia rates with basal insulin analogs. Diabetes Technol Ther 2011;13(Suppl 1):S53–64.

58. Giugliano D, Maiorino MI, Bellastella G, et al. Treatment regimens with insulin analogues and haemoglobin A1c target of <7% in type 2 diabetes: a systematic review. Diabetes Res Clin Pract 2011;92:1–10.
59. Riddle MC, Vlajnic A, Zhou R, et al. Baseline A1c predicts the likelihood of reaching the 7.0% A1c target with structured titration of add-on insulin glargine: patient-level analysis of 12 studies in type 2 diabetes. Diabetes 2009;58(Suppl 1):A125.
60. Leahy J, Vlajnic A, Rimler M, et al. Lower weight gain and better outcomes in patients with type 2 diabetes starting insulin treatment when baseline A1c <8%. Diabetologia 2011;54(Suppl 10):S273.
61. Riddle M, Umpierrez G, Digenio A, et al. Contributions of basal and postprandial hyperglycemia over a wide range of A1c levels before and after treatment intensification in type 2 diabetes. Diabetes Care 2011;34:2508–14.
62. Monnier L, Colette C, Owens D. Postprandial and basal glucose in type 2 diabetes: assessment and respective impacts. Diabetes Technol Ther 2011;12(Suppl 1):S25–32.
63. O'Keefe JH, Bell DS. Postprandial hyperglycemia/hyperlipidemia (postprandial dysmetabolism) is a cardiovascular risk factor. Am J Cardiol 2007;100:899–904.
64. Janka HU, Plewe G, Riddle MC, et al. Comparison of basal insulin added to oral agents versus twice-daily premixed insulin as initial insulin therapy for type 2 diabetes. Diabetes Care 2005;28:254–9.
65. Janka HU, Högy B. Economic evaluation of the treatment of type 2 diabetes with insulin glargine based on the LAPTOP trial. Eur J Health Econ 2008;9:165–70.
66. Tunis SL, Sauriol L, Minshall ME. Cost effectiveness of insulin glargine plus oral antidiabetes drugs compared with premixed insulin alone in patients with type 2 diabetes mellitus in Canada. Appl Health Econ Health Policy 2010;8(4):267–80.
67. McNally PG, Dean JD, Morris AD, et al. Using continuous glucose monitoring to measure the frequency of low glucose values when using biphasic insulin aspart 30 compared to biphasic human insulin 30: a double-blind crossover study in individuals with type 2 diabetes. Diabetes Care 2007;30:1044–8.
68. Qayyum R, Bolen S, Maruther N, et al. Systematic review: comparative effectiveness and safety of premixed insulin analogues in type 2 diabetes. Ann Intern Med 2008;149:549–59.
69. Heise T, Heinemann L, Hövelmann U, et al. Biphasic insulin aspart 30/70: pharmacokinetics and pharmacodynamics compared with once-daily biphasic human insulin and basal-bolus therapy. Diabetes Care 2009;32:1431–3.
70. Raskin P, Allen E, Hollander P, et al. Initiating insulin therapy in type 2 diabetes: a comparison of biphasic and basal insulin analogs. Diabetes Care 2005;28:260–5.
71. Kann PH, Wascher T, Zackova V, et al. Starting insulin therapy in type 2 diabetes: twice-daily biphasic insulin aspart 30 plus metformin versus once-daily insulin glargine plus glimepiride. Exp Clin Endocrinol Diabetes 2006;114:527–32.
72. Buse JB, Wolffenbuttel BH, Herman WH, et al. DURAbility of basal versus lispro mix 75/25 insulin efficacy (DURABLE) trial 24-week results: safety and efficacy of insulin lispro mix 75/25 versus insulin glargine added to oral antihyperglycemic drugs in patients with type 2 diabetes. Diabetes Care 2009;32:1007–13.
73. Buse JB, Wolffenbuttel BH, Herman WH, et al. The DURAbility of basal versus lispro mix 75/25 insulin efficacy (DURABLE) trial: comparing the durability of lispro mix 75/25 and glargine. Diabetes Care 2011;34:249–55.
74. Garber AJ, Wahlen T, Wahl T, et al. Attainment of glycaemic goals with once-, twice-, or thrice-daily dosing with biphasic insulin aspart 70/30 (The 1-2-3 study). Diabetes Obes Metab 2006;8:58–66.

75. Robbins DC, Beisswenger PJ, Ceriello A, et al. Mealtime 50/50 basal + prandial insulin analogue with a basal insulin analogue, both plus metformin, in the achievement of target HbA1c and pre- and postprandial blood glucose levels in patients with type 2 diabetes: a multinational, 24-week, randomized, open-label, parallel-group comparison. Clin Ther 2007;29:2349–64.

76. Clements MR, Tits J, Kinsley BT, et al. Improved glycaemic control of thrice-daily biphasic insulin aspart compared to twice-daily biphasic human insulin; a randomized, open-label trial in patients with type 1 or type 2 diabetes. Diabetes Obes Metab 2008;10:229–37.

77. Farcasiu E, Ivanyi T, Mozejko-Pastewka B, et al. Efficacy and safety of prandial premixed therapy using insulin lispro mix 50/50 3 times daily compared with progressive titration of insulin lispro mix 75/25 or biphasic insulin aspart 70/30 twice daily in patients with type 2 diabetes mellitus: a randomized, 16-week, open-label study. Clin Ther 2011;33:1682–93.

78. Davies M, Sinnassamy P, Storms F, et al. Insulin glargine-based therapy improves glycemic control in patients with type 2 diabetes sub-optimally controlled on pre-mixed insulin therapies. Diabetes Res Clin Pract 2008;79(2):368–75.

79. Schiel R, Müller UA. Efficacy and treatment satisfaction of once-daily insulin glargine plus one or two oral antidiabetic agents versus continuing premixed human insulin in patients with type 2 diabetes previously on long-term conventional insulin therapy: the SWITCH Pilot Study. Exp Clin Endocrinol Diabetes 2008;116:58–64.

80. Bretzel RG, Eckhard M, Landgraf W, et al. Initiating insulin therapy in type 2 diabetic patients failing on oral hypoglycemic agents. Basal or prandial insulin? The APOLLO trial and beyond. Diabetes Care 2009;32(Suppl 2): S260–5.

81. Bergenstal RM, Johnson M, Powers MA, et al. Adjust to target in type 2 diabetes: comparison of a simple regimen with carbohydrate counting for adjustment of mealtime insulin glulisine. Diabetes Care 2008;31:1305–10.

82. Hollander P, Cooper J, Bregnhøj J, et al. A 52-week, multinational, open-label, parallel-group, noninferiority, treat-to-target trial comparing insulin detemir with insulin glargine in a basal-bolus regimen with mealtime insulin aspart in patients with type 2 diabetes. Clin Ther 2008;30:1976–87.

83. Raskin P, Gylvin T, Weng W, et al. Comparison of insulin detemir and insulin glargine using a basal-bolus regimen in a randomized, controlled clinical study in patients with type 2 diabetes. Diabetes Metab Res Rev 2009;25:542–8.

84. Siegmund T, Weber S, Blankenfeld H, et al. Comparison of insulin glargine versus NPH insulin in people with type 2 diabetes mellitus under outpatient-clinic conditions for 18 months using a basal-bolus regimen with a rapid-acting insulin analogue as mealtime insulin. Exp Clin Endocrinol Diabetes 2007;115:349–53.

85. Liebl A, Prager R, Binz K, et al. Comparison of insulin analogue regimens in people with type 2 diabetes mellitus in the PREFER study: a randomized controlled trial. Diabetes Obes Metab 2009;11:45–52.

86. Fritsche A, Larbig M, Owens D, et al. Comparison between a basal-bolus and a premixed insulin regimen in individuals with type 2 diabetes–results of the GINGER study. Diabetes Obes Metab 2010;12:115–23.

87. Rosenstock J, Ahmann AJ, Colon G, et al. Advancing insulin therapy in type 2 diabetes previously treated with glargine plus oral agents: prandial premixed (insulin lispro protamine suspension/lispro) versus basal/bolus (glargine/lispro) therapy. Diabetes Care 2008;31:20–5.

88. Raccah D. Options for the intensification of insulin therapy when basal insulin is not enough in type 2 diabetes mellitus. Diabetes Obes Metab 2008;10(Suppl 2):76–82.

89. Lankisch MR, Ferlinz KC, Leahy JL, et al. Introducing a simplified approach to insulin therapy in type 2 diabetes: a comparison of two single-dose regimens of insulin glulisine plus insulin glargine and oral antidiabetic drugs. Diabetes Obes Metab 2008;10:1178–85.

90. Owens DR, Luzio SD, Sert-Langeron C, et al. Effects of initiation of a single pre-prandial dose of insulin glulisine while continuing titrated insulin glargine in type 2 diabetes: a 6-month "proof-of-concept". Diabetes Obes Metab 2011; 13:1020–7.

91. Del Prato S, Nicolucci A, Lovagnini-Scher AC, et al. Telecare provides comparable efficacy to conventional self-monitored blood glucose in patients with type 2 diabetes titrating one injection of insulin glulisine-the ELEONOR study. Diabetes Technol Ther 2012;14(2):175–82.

92. Riddle MC, Vlajnic A, Jones BA, et al. Comparison of 3 intensified insulin regimens added to oral therapy for type 2 diabetes: twice-daily aspart premixed vs glargine plus 1 prandial glulisine or stepwise addition of glulisine to glargine. Diabetes 2011;60(Suppl 1):A113.

93. Rosenstock J, Vlajnic A, Jones BA, et al. Time course of fasting glucose, hypoglycemia and body weight during systematic insulin dose titration: BID aspart premixed vs glargine +1 prandial glulisine or stepwise addition of glulisine to glargine in type 2 diabetes uncontrolled with oral agents. Diabetes 2011; 60(Suppl 1):A20.

94. Holman RR, Thorne KI, Farmer AJ, et al. Addition of biphasic, prandial, or basal insulin to oral therapy in type 2 diabetes. N Engl J Med 2007;357:1716–30.

95. Holman RR, Farmer AJ, Davies MJ, et al. Three-year efficacy of complex insulin regimens in type 2 diabetes. N Engl J Med 2009;361:1736–47.

96. Bode BW. Insulin pump use in type 2 diabetes. Diabetes Technol Ther 2010; 12(Suppl 1):S17–21.

97. Bulchandani DG, Konrady T, Hamburg MS. Clinical efficacy and patient satisfaction with U-500 insulin pump therapy in patients with type 2 diabetes. Endocr Pract 2007;13:721–5.

98. Edelman SV, Bode BW, Bailey TS, et al. Insulin pump therapy in patients with type 2 diabetes safely improved glycemic control using a simple insulin dosing regimen. Diabetes Technol Ther 2010;12:627–33.

99. Reznik Y, Morera J, Rod A, et al. Efficacy of continuous subcutaneous insulin infusion in type 2 diabetes mellitus: a survey on a cohort of 102 patients with prolonged follow-up. Diabetes Technol Ther 2010;12:931–6.

100. Frias JP, Bode BW, Bailey TS, et al. A 16-week open-label, multicenter pilot study assessing insulin pump therapy in patients with type 2 diabetes suboptimally controlled with multiple daily injections. J Diabetes Sci Technol 2011;5: 887–93.

101. Raskin P, Bode BW, Marks JB, et al. Continuous subcutaneous insulin infusion and multiple daily injection therapy are equally effective in type 2 diabetes: a randomized, parallel-group, 24-week study. Diabetes Care 2003;26:2598–603.

102. Monami M, Lamanna C, Marchionni N, et al. Continuous subcutaneous insulin infusion versus multiple daily insulin injections in type 2 diabetes: a meta-analysis. Exp Clin Endocrinol Diabetes 2009;117:220–2.

103. Skladany MJ, Miller M, Guthermann JS, et al. Patch-pump technology to manage type 2 diabetes mellitus: hurdles to market acceptance. J Diabetes Sci Technol 2008;2:1147–50.

104. Anhalt H, Bohannon NJ. Insulin patch pumps: their development and future in closed-loop systems. Diabetes Technol Ther 2010;12(Suppl 1):S51–8.
105. Dorkhan M, Frid A, Groop L. Differences in effects of insulin glargine or pioglitazone added to oral anti-diabetic therapy in patients with type 2 diabetes: what to add–insulin glargine or pioglitazone? Diabetes Res Clin Pract 2008;82:340–5.
106. Rosenstock J, Sugimoto D, Strange P, et al. Triple therapy in type 2 diabetes: insulin glargine or rosiglitazone added to combination therapy of sulfonylurea plus metformin in insulin-naïve patients. Diabetes Care 2006;29:554–9.
107. Triplitt C, Glass L, Miyazaki Y, et al. Comparison of glargine insulin versus rosiglitazone addition in poorly controlled type 2 diabetic patients on metformin plus sulfonylurea. Diabetes Care 2006;29:2371–7.
108. Hohberg C, Pfützner A, Forst T, et al. Successful switch from insulin therapy to treatment with pioglitazone in type 2 diabetes patients with residual beta-cell function: results from the PioSwitch study. Diabetes Obes Metab 2009;11:464–71.
109. Bell DS, Dharmalingam M, Kumar S, et al. Triple oral fixed-dose diabetes polypill versus insulin plus metformin efficacy demonstration study in the treatment of advanced type 2 diabetes (TrIED study-II). Diabetes Obes Metab 2011;13:800–5.
110. Lingvay I, Legendre JL, Kaloyanova PF, et al. Insulin-based versus triple oral therapy for newly diagnosed type 2 diabetes: which is better? Diabetes Care 2009;32:1789–95.
111. Lovshin JA, Drucker DJ. Incretin-based therapies for type 2 diabetes mellitus. Nat Rev Endocrinol 2009;5:262–9.
112. Garber AJ. Long-acting glucagon-like peptide 1 receptor agonists. A review of the efficacy and tolerability. Diabetes Care 2011;34(Suppl 2):S279–84.
113. Russell-Jones D, Vaag A, Schmitz O, et al. Liraglutide vs insulin glargine and placebo in combination with metformin and sulfonylurea therapy in type 2 diabetes mellitus (LEAD-5 met+SU): a randomised controlled trial. Diabetologia 2009;52:2046–55.
114. Bergenstal R, Leewin A, Bailey T, et al. Efficacy and safety of biphasic insulin aspart 70/30 versus exenatide in subjects with type 2 diabetes failing to achieve glycemic control with metformin and a sulfonylurea. Curr Med Res Opin 2009;25:65–75.
115. Gallwitz B, Böhmer M, Segiet T, et al. Exenatide twice daily versus premixed insulin aspart 70/30 in metformin-treated patients with type 2 diabetes: a randomized 26-week study on glycemic control and hypoglycemia. Diabetes Care 2011;34:604–6.
116. Thong KY, Ryder RE, Cull ML, et al. Insulin avoidance and treatment outcomes among patients with a professional driving license starting glucagon-like peptide 1 (GLP-1) agonists in the Association of British Clinical Diabetologists (ABCD) nationwide exenatide and liraglutide audits. Diabet Med 2012;29:690–2.
117. Davis SN, Johns D, Maggs D, et al. Exploring the substitution of exenatide for insulin with type 2 diabetes treated with insulin in combination with oral antidiabetes agents. Diabetes Care 2007;30:2767–72.
118. Rosenstock J, Fonseca V. Missing the point: substituting exenatide for nonoptimized insulin: going from bad to worse! Diabetes Care 2007;30:2972–3.
119. Morrow L, Hompesch M, Guthrie H, et al. Co-administration of liraglutide with insulin detemir demonstrates additive pharmacodynamic effects with no pharmacokinetic interaction. Diabetes Obes Metab 2011;13:75–80.
120. Viswanathan P, Chaudhuri A, Bhatia R, et al. Exenatide therapy in obese patients with type 2 diabetes mellitus treated with insulin. Endocr Pract 2007;13:444–50.

121. John LE, Kane MP, Busch RS, et al. Expanded use of exenatide in the management of type 2 diabetes. Diabetes Spectrum 2007;20:59–63.
122. Sheffield CA, Kane MP, Busch RS, et al. Safety and efficacy of exenatide in combination with insulin in patients with type 2 diabetes. Endocr Pract 2008; 14:285–92.
123. Yoon NM, Cavaghan MK, Brunelle RL, et al. Exenatide added to insulin therapy: a retrospective review of clinical practice over two years in an academic endocrinology outpatient setting. Clin Ther 2009;31:1511–23.
124. Lane W, Weinrib S, Rappaport J. The effect of liraglutide added to U-500 insulin in patients with type 2 diabetes and high insulin requirements. Diabetes Technol Ther 2011;13:592–5.
125. Arnolds S, Dellweg S, Clair J, et al. Further improvement in postprandial glucose control with addition of exenatide or sitagliptin to combination therapy with insulin glargine and metformin: a proof-of-concept study. Diabetes Care 2010; 33:1509–15.
126. Buse JB, Bergenstal RM, Glass LC, et al. Use of twice-daily exenatide in basal insulin-treated patients with type 2 diabetes: a randomized, controlled trial. Ann Intern Med 2011;154:103–12.
127. Rosenstock J, Devries JH, Seufert J, et al. A new type 2 diabetes treatment paradigm: sequential addition of liraglutide to metformin and then basal insulin detemir. Diabetes 2011;60(Suppl 1):A76.
128. Kielgast U, Krarup T, Holst JJ, et al. Four weeks of treatment with liraglutide reduces insulin dose without loss of glycemic control in type 1 diabetic patients with and without residual beta-cell function. Diabetes Care 2011;334:1463–8.
129. Varanasi A, Bellini N, Rawal D, et al. Liraglutide as additional treatment for type 1 diabetes. Eur J Endocrinol 2011;165:77–84.
130. Fonseca V, Schweizer A, Albrecht D, et al. Addition of vildagliptin to insulin improves glycaemic control in type 2 diabetes. Diabetologia 2007;50:1148–55.
131. Visbøll T, Rosenstock J, Yki-Järvinen H, et al. Efficacy and safety of sitagliptin when added to insulin therapy in patients with type 2 diabetes. Diabetes Obes Metab 2010;12:167–77.
132. Sasali A, Leahy JL. Insulin therapy for type 2 diabetes. Curr Diab Rep 2003;3: 378–85.
133. Yki-Järvinen Y. Combination therapies with insulin in type 2 diabetes. Diabetes Care 2001;24:758–67.
134. Riddle MC. Combined therapy with insulin plus oral agents: is there any advantage? Diabetes Care 2008;31(Suppl 2):S125–30.
135. Raskin P. Why insulin sensitizers but not secretagogues should be retained when initiating insulin in type 2 diabetes. Diabetes Metab Res Rev 2008;24:3–13.
136. Riddle M, Schneider J. Beginning insulin treatment of obese patients with evening 70/30 insulin plus glimepiride versus insulin alone. Glimepiride Combination Group. Diabetes Care 1998;21:1052–7.
137. Yki-Järvinen Y, Ryysy L, Nikkila K, et al. Comparison of bedtime insulin regimens in patients with type 2 diabetes mellitus: a randomized, controlled trial. Ann Intern Med 1999;130:389–96.
138. Fonseca V, Gill J, Zhou R, et al. An analysis of early insulin glarine added to metformin with or without sulfonylurea: impact on glycaemic control and hypoglycaemia. Diabetes Obes Metab 2011;13:814–22.
139. Swinnen SG, Dain MP, Mauricio D, et al. Continuation versus discontinuation of insulin secretagogues when initiating insulin in type 2 diabetes. Diabetes Obes Metab 2010;12:923–5.

140. Smith U, Gale AM. Does diabetes therapy influence the risk of cancer? Diabetologia 2009;52:1699–708.
141. Currie CJ, Johnson JA. The safety profile of exogenous insulin in people with type 2 diabetes: justification for concern. Diabetes Obes Metab 2012;14:1–4.
142. Origin Trial Investigators, Gerstein H, Yusuf S, et al. Rationale, design, and baseline characteristics for a large international trial of cardiovascular disease prevention in people with dysglycemia: the ORIGIN trial (Outcome reduction with an Initial Glargine Intervention). Am Heart J 2008;155:26–32.
143. Diamant M, Van Gaal L, Stranks S, et al. Once weekly exenatide compared with insulin glargine titrated to target in patients with type 2 diabetes (DURATION-3): an open-label randomised trial. Lancet 2010;375:2234–43.
144. Diamant M, Van Gaal L, Stranks S, et al. Safety and efficacy of once-weekly exenatide compared with insulin glargine titrated to target in patients with type 2 diabetes over 84 weeks. Diabetes Care 2012;35:683–9.
145. Funnell MM, Brown TL, Childs BP, et al. National standards for diabetes self-management education. Diabetes Care 2011;34(Suppl 1):S89–96.
146. Cochran J, Conn VS. Meta-analysis of quality of life outcomes following diabetes self-management training. Diabetes Educ 2008;34:815–23.
147. Poolsup N, Suksomboon N, Rattanasookchit S. Meta-analysis of the benefits of self-monitoring of blood glucose on glycemic control in type 2 diabetes patients: an update. Diabetes Technol Ther 2009;11:775–84.
148. Clar C, Barnard K, Cummins E, et al. Self-monitoring of blood glucose in type 2 diabetes: systematic review. Health Technol Assess 2010;14:1–140.
149. Gerstein HC, Yale JF, Harris SB, et al. A randomized trial of adding insulin glargine vs. avoidance of insulin in people with Type 2 diabetes on either no oral glucose-lowering agents or submaximal doses of metformin and/or sulphonylureas. The Canadian INSIGHT (Implementing New Strategies with Insulin Glargine for Hyperglycaemia Treatment) Study. Diabet Med 2006;23:736–42.
150. O'Rahilly S, Weir GC, Matthews DR. An appreciation of Robert Turner. Diabetes 2008;57:2819–21.

Insulin Therapy in Children and Adolescents

William V. Tamborlane, MD[a],*, Kristin A. Sikes, MSN, APRN, CDE[b]

KEYWORDS

• Insulin therapy • Pediatrics • MDI • Pump therapy

Insulin therapy is the mainstay of treatment in children and adolescents with type 1 diabetes (T1D) and is a key component in the treatment of type 2 diabetes (T2D) in this population as well. The Diabetes Control and Complications Trial (DCCT) established that intensive glycemic management leading to near normal glucose and A1c levels significantly reduced the risk of developing long-term complications and the benefits of this reduced risk outweighed the 3-fold increase in the risk of severe hypoglycemia.[1] Slowing the development of early retinopathy was observed in the DCCT subgroup of adolescents, as well as in adults in the study.[2] In the Epidemiology of Diabetes Interventions and Complications (EDIC) study, the observational follow-up to the DCCT, a continued increase in risk of complications was seen in the former conventional treatment group years after the end of the randomized control trial despite improved metabolic control, indicating that near normal glucose and A1c levels should be achieved and maintained in patients with T1D as early in the course of the disease as possible.[3]

There is no single standard for glycemic targets for children and adolescents with T1D. In 2005, the American Diabetes Association published a consensus statement indicating that A1c and glucose targets should be adjusted based on the age of the child and range from 7.5% to less than 8.5% in very young children, less than 8.0% in children aged 7 to 12 years, and less than 7.5% in teenagers.[4] Higher A1c levels were suggested for very young children apparently because of the potential risk of recurrent hypoglycemia on the developing brain. We believe that there are many problems with the approach taken by the American Diabetes Association, including the emerging evidence that chronic hyperglycemia is also detrimental to the developing brain. Consequently, our service follows the International Society for Pediatric and Adolescent Diabetes (ISPAD) guidelines that were published in 2009 and we recommend a target A1c of less than 7.5% for all pediatric patients, with strong emphasis placed on individualizing glucose targets to promote normoglycemia and preventing severe or frequent hypoglycemia.[5]

[a] Department of Pediatrics, Yale University School of Medicine, PO Box 208064, New Haven, CT 06520-8064, USA
[b] Yale Children's Diabetes Program, 2 Church Street South, Suite 404, New Haven, CT 02066, USA
* Corresponding author.
E-mail address: ks397@email.med.yale.edu

Endocrinol Metab Clin N Am 41 (2012) 145–160
doi:10.1016/j.ecl.2012.01.002
0889-8529/12/$ – see front matter © 2012 Published by Elsevier Inc.

endo.theclinics.com

AVAILABLE INSULIN FORMULATIONS

A major aim of current insulin replacement therapy is to simulate the normal pattern of insulin secretion as closely as possible. This aim can best be achieved with basal-bolus therapy using multiple daily injections (MDI) or continuous subcutaneous insulin infusion (CSII) pump therapy. Only a few years ago, options for insulin formulations were limited. There are now more than 10 varieties of biosynthetic human and analogue insulin, including regular insulin, neutral protamine Hagedorn (NPH) insulin, long-acting/basal insulin analogues, rapid-acting insulin analogues, and several different kinds of premixed insulin. The range of available insulin products is described in detail elsewhere in this issue.

Human Regular Insulin

Human regular insulin was a mainstay of insulin management in youth with T1D until about 15 years ago, but the advent of rapid-acting insulin analogues has virtually eliminated its use in children and adolescents. The delayed absorption and prolonged duration of action of the large premeal doses of regular insulin that are required by adolescents with T1D to overcome the insulin resistance of puberty undoubtedly contributed to problems with hyperglycemia and hypoglycemia in this age group. Regular insulin remains the insulin of choice in insulin drips in the treatment of diabetic ketoacidosis (DKA). A special formulation of regular insulin as U-500 (500 units/mL) is also available for use in patients with severe insulin resistance who require large daily doses of insulin.

Rapid-acting Analogues

Compared with regular insulin, the faster absorption of rapid-acting analogues (aspart [Novolog], lispro [Humalog], and glulisine [Apidra]) results in higher and sharper peaks and shorter duration of action, which, in turn, reduce late postprandial hypoglycemia and temper early postmeal glucose surges.[6]

Puberty does not seem to cause major alterations in the pharmacokinetics of premeal boluses of rapid analogues, but the insulin resistance of puberty reduces the ability of these insulins to stimulate glucose metabolism.[7] Rapid-acting insulin may be safely mixed with intermediate-acting insulin but mixing with long-acting insulin is not recommended. All 3 may be used in an insulin pump and studies have shown them to be safe and effective.[8,9] Lispro and aspart insulin may be diluted to concentrations less than U-100 such as U-50 or U-25 using diluents obtained from the manufacturer. Diluted insulin is used in very young children and others who are very sensitive to insulin and could benefit from more accurate dosing. Rapid-acting insulin analogues can be given intravenously, but they have not been shown to be superior to regular insulin.[10]

Intermediate-acting Insulin

Since the discontinuation of Lente insulin in 2005, NPH has been the only available intermediate-acting insulin. Although the delay in peak action of NPH provides a means to cover lunchtime glucose excursions in twice-a-day injection regimens, it makes NPH less than satisfactory for overnight basal insulin replacement.[11] As with regular insulin, the advent of the long-acting insulin analogues has largely replaced NPH in basal-bolus MDI treatment in pediatrics. However, NPH still plays a role in our approach to the treatment of patients newly diagnosed with T1D and it is still used in the treatment of T2D.

Long-acting Insulin Analogues

There are currently 2 commercially available long-acting insulin analogues that were developed to meet the body's basal insulin requirements for regulating hepatic glucose production: glargine (Lantus) and detemir (Levemir). Although glargine is the most frequently used basal insulin in MDI therapy in youth with T1D, the evidence supporting the enhanced safety of this insulin over NPH in adolescents has not been established. In a company-sponsored, randomized clinical trial in adolescents with T1D in the United States, changes in A1c levels did not differ between 2 treatment groups, but biochemical and clinical hypoglycemic episodes tended to occur more frequently in the glargine group than the twice-daily intermediate-acting insulin group.[12]

Compared with glargine, detemir has been shown to have a more consistent pharmacokinetic profile in children and a more consistent pharmacodynamic profile in adults with T1D.[13,14] On the other hand, the duration of detemir is shorter than that of glargine and thus may need to be given twice per day.[13]

Premixed Insulin

A variety of premixed insulin formulations, combining either rapid-acting or regular insulin with NPH or intermediate-acting insulin analogues, are available. The percentage of rapid-acting/regular to intermediate-acting varies with the formulation. The practical advantage of premixed insulin to cover both short-term and intermediate-term insulin needs in a single shot is also its greatest limitation. There is less flexibility when using premixed insulin for adjusting the individual insulin components, and this can be particularly problematic in young children or those with variable food intake. In our T1D practice, use of premixed insulin is restricted to those patients who have difficulty taking even 2 injections per day.

INSULIN DELIVERY OPTIONS FOR INJECTION THERAPY

Insulin syringes now come in a variety of sizes that are particularly useful in young children. In addition to the traditional 100-unit (1-mL) syringe marked in 2-unit increments, the 50-unit (0.5-mL) and 30-unit (0.3-mL) syringes are marked in single-unit increments, and 30-unit syringes with half-unit markings can also be ordered. These syringes are available with needle lengths from 8 to 13 mm.

Insulin pens are also available, both as disposable pens and as reusable pens with disposable cartridges. The disposable pens allow for only 1-unit doses, which may be problematic for very young children who might need half-unit dosing. On the other hand, there are reusable cartridge pens that allow for half-unit dosing.

INITIATING INSULIN THERAPY

Most newly diagnosed patients who present with symptoms of diabetes or are in DKA require upwards of 1 unit/kg/d at the start of insulin treatment. For asymptomatic patients who are incidentally diagnosed with diabetes during a routine sports physical or a well-child examination, starting doses may need to be only 0.5 unit/kg/d. The goal of initial insulin therapy in children with T1D should be the rapid achievement of normoglycemia to give the child the opportunity to enter the honeymoon, or partial remission, phase. The honeymoon period results from a combination of improved function of residual β-cells and reversal of the insulin resistance that accompanies uncontrolled diabetes. The ability to achieve target A1c levels with little or no severe hypoglycemia is greatly enhanced in patients with T1D with residual β-cell function.

All of our newly diagnosed patients are admitted to the hospital for initial diabetes education and insulin dose titration. Whereas most clinicians at other centers start patients on intensive insulin therapy with a basal-bolus MDI therapy at diagnosis, we use a variation on the twice-a-day insulin regimen. In this regimen, NPH and a rapid-acting analogue (usually aspart insulin) are freely mixed and given as a single injection with breakfast followed by separate injections of detemir and a rapid-acting analogue with dinner. The morning dose is divided into two-thirds NPH and one-third rapid and the evening dose is half rapid and half detemir. The rationale for this approach is that the predinner detemir provides the advantages of long-acting insulin analogues with respect to lowering the risk of nocturnal hypoglycemia compared with predinner NPH. Moreover, the NPH insulin in the prebreakfast mixture obviates lunch and afternoon snack doses of rapid-acting analogue, as well as a possible second dose of long-acting insulin in the morning.

During the 2 to 3 weeks after discharge, insulin doses are titrated toward target premeal glucose values of 70 to 130 mg/dL during daily telephone contact while the patients are maintained on an age-appropriate and weight-appropriate, fixed carbohydrate intake with each meal; patients are seen in follow-up clinic visits, approximately 2, 6, 13, 26, 39, and 52 weeks after diagnosis. The concepts of correction doses and insulin/carbohydrate ratios (ICRs) (based on the predinner dose of rapid-acting insulin analogue) are introduced during the first 2 follow-up visits. This more traditional approach to initial treatment provides time for families to acquire experience in basic management skills, including carbohydrate counting, as well as to learn advanced management concepts. Mean A1c levels that have been achieved and maintained in our patient population throughout the first year of treatment (ie, 6.9%–7.1%) compare favorably with HbA1c values reported in pediatric studies of newly diagnosed patients.[15]

A key reason that the twice-daily insulin regimen is effective during the honeymoon period is that insulin secretion from remaining β-cells smoothes out blood glucose (BG) variation during the day. As β-cell function declines, glucose levels become more variable and the limitations of this regimen become apparent. Increased variability of fasting BG levels is one of the first signs of waning β-cell function. When glycemic control becomes more difficult, our patients are switched to basal-bolus regimens, almost always via CSII pump therapy (see later discussion).

BASAL-BOLUS TREATMENT REGIMENS

The DCCT and EDIC studies established basal-bolus therapy using either MDI or CSII as the gold standard of treatment of T1D. However, insulin works only if it is taken, and other factors must be addressed when determining the best insulin regimen for an individual patient. These factors include the availability of an adult parent/guardian to supervise insulin administration, ability to count carbohydrates and monitor BG levels, and the willingness to take 4 or more injections of insulin daily. Moreover, periods of both hyperglycemia and hypoglycemia occur on a daily basis regardless of the regimen because no current insulin regimen can precisely simulate the function of the human β-cell. Thus, the goal of any insulin regimen is to minimize the frequency and severity of excursions into the hyperglycemic and hypoglycemic range.

MDI

For people without diabetes, β-cells provide continuous background insulin secretion in the fasting state to regulate hepatic glucose production. This background, or basal, insulin is then overlaid by spikes in insulin secretion in response to meals and snacks.

Basal-bolus insulin regimens attempt to replicate normal insulin secretion through the use of a long-acting insulin analogue to cover basal insulin needs along with bolus injections of rapid-acting insulin analogue with food intake and to correct increases in BG levels.

Either once-daily or twice-daily glargine or detemir may be used for basal insulin coverage. Typically, basal insulin accounts for approximately 40% to 50% of the insulin total daily dose (TDD).[10,16] However, children younger than 5 years often require basal insulin doses that are 30% to 40% of TDD. Once-daily glargine or detemir may be given either in the morning or in the evening, but it is important that it is given at the same time each day. As noted earlier, detemir may need to be given twice daily in many pediatric patients with T1D.[13] Some pediatric practitioners mix long-acting and rapid-acting insulin to reduce the number of injections, but studies from our laboratory indicate that such mixing is a bad idea because it markedly blunts the action of the rapid-acting insulin component of the mixture.[17]

Any of the rapid-acting insulin analogues may be used to cover bolus insulin needs. Ideally, the rapid-acting insulin bolus is given 10 to 15 minutes before eating, but this is a difficult goal to achieve in many youth with T1D. For the most precise dosing of bolus insulin, it is necessary to use both an insulin to carbohydrate ratio (ICR) and an insulin sensitivity or correction factor.

The ICR is defined as the grams of carbohydrate that 1 unit of insulin covers. This ratio may be determined using the 500 rule. Dividing 500 by the TDD gives a starting point for the carbohydrate ratio. For example, a teenager with a TDD of 50 units has a ratio as follows: 500/50 = 10. Thus, for this teen, 1 unit of insulin covers 10 g of carbohydrate. An alternative to using the 500 rule is to use an established ICR based on the child's age. **Table 1** lists the ICRs based on age that are used in our clinic. The ICR frequently differs by time of day, because more insulin is often needed per gram of carbohydrate before breakfast and less may be given to cover bedtime snacks.

Accuracy in determining the carbohydrate content of meals is of utmost importance but is often a problem in adolescents. We find that teens tend to underestimate the number of carbohydrates in their meal; refresher meetings with a dietitian can help reinforce the importance of maintaining mastery of this skill.

In addition to meal coverage, a correction dose of rapid-acting insulin is often given at mealtime to fix an increased BG level. It may also be given at other points in the day for the same reason. Traditional sliding-scale insulin doses based on BG levels have given way to a more sophisticated dosing algorithm based on an insulin sensitivity factor (ISF); namely, how much is BG lowered by 1 unit of insulin. The correction dose, based on the ISF, is calculated in relation to the target BG level, which can vary based on time of day and age/developmental level of the patient. Most patients in our clinic use a target value between 100 and 120 mg/dL.

Table 1 ISF and ICR by age		
Age of Child (y)	ISF (1 unit: ___ mg/dL)	ICR (1 unit per ___ g)
≤2	300–350	45–50 (breakfast often requires a more aggressive ICR, up to half of usual ICR)
3–5	200–250	45
6–8	180	30
9–11	100–150	20–22
12–13	75–100	12–15
14+	25–75	10

The ISF may be determined using the 1800 rule: divide 1800 by the TDD. For example, a teenager with a TDD of 50 units has an ISF as follows: 1800/50 = 36. Thus, for this teen, 1 unit of insulin decreases the BG 36 mg/dL. With this ratio and the target BG, a dose of insulin to correct an increased BG level may be calculated. The calculation to determine the insulin dose is (actual BG–target BG)/ISF = number of units of insulin. In the earlier example, if the teen has a BG level of 244 and the target BG is 100 mg/dL, the calculation would be (244–100)/36 = 4 units of insulin.

An alternative to using the 1800 rule is to use an established ISF based on the child's age. See **Table 1** for a list of the ISFs based on age that are used in our clinic. No matter how they are initially calculated, ICRs and ISFs are subsequently adjusted based on glucose monitoring results.

Particular advantages of basal-bolus MDI regimens are that they try to mirror the physiologic model of insulin secretion, increase flexibility in the timing and size of meals, and provide more opportunities to "course correct" throughout the day in response to abnormal glucose excursions. A particular disadvantage of these regimens is that they increase the number of daily injections needed to cover meals and large snacks compared with twice-a-day NPH-based regimens. In view of the flat time-action profile of the long-acting basal insulin analogues, basal-bolus MDI treatment puts a premium on compliance with premeal bolus dosing. Without bolus doses of rapid-acting insulin, long-acting basal insulin alone cannot prevent marked postprandial hyperglycemia. For some patients, especially adolescents, this situation means that they may have to inject insulin up to 8 times per day; 1 to 2 basal insulin injections, 3 meals and 3 snacks with bolus injections. As we have learned from our experience with CSII treatment, strict adherence to premeal bolusing is difficult for teenagers with T1D even when it is made as easy as possible to accomplish with an insulin pump.

Insulin Pump Therapy

The theoretic underpinnings and first forays into the use of CSII occurred more than 30 years ago, but it is only in the last 10 years that the use of CSII in children has taken off. Since then, CSII has been shown to be effective in lowering A1c compared with injection therapy in randomized and nonrandomized pediatric studies and to be associated with improved patient satisfaction and reduced frequency of hypoglycemia.[18] Some of the practical benefits of CSII compared with MDI are listed in **Box 1**. From the pediatric

---

Box 1
Practical benefits of CSII

- Basal infusion rates adjustable up to every 30 minutes
- Programmable temporary basal rates
- Ability to program multiple alternate basal rate profiles
- One site insertion every 2 to 3 days (vs many injections each day)
- Dose calculator
- Pump history functions and ability to upload to data management systems
- Customizable square-wave and dual-wave boluses
- Ability to deliver very small (0.025–0.05 units) doses of insulin

practitioner perspective, the memory features that record all pump-related activities are especially important. There are no secrets from the insulin pump and a bolus was delivered only if the pump says it was.

Although the pump has definite strengths, it is just another tool to manage a complex condition and should not be viewed as a cure for diabetes. Successful pump users work hard at managing their diabetes, often testing BG levels 8 to 10 times per day and using those data to make corrections throughout the day. We frequently remind patients that prolonged accidental or purposeful interruption of insulin delivery over several hours can lead to the development of ketones and DKA because they are receiving only rapid-acting insulin.[19] This risk can be reduced or eliminated when patients and their caregivers keep a close watch on BG values and follow recommendations for managing hyperglycemia.

Indications for CSII Treatment in Pediatrics

In our clinic, CSII is considered the best tool for achieving optimal glycemic control coupled with enhanced quality of life both for our patients and their families. We look at patients and ask "Why shouldn't they be on a pump?," rather than the more traditional model of proving that the patient deserves to be on a pump. To that end, the age of the patient and duration of diabetes play only a minor role in determining when patients transfer to CSII. It is increasingly clear that young infants, toddlers, and preschoolers are probably the ideal pediatric patients for CSII, because it lowers A1c, reduces the frequency of severe hypoglycemic episodes, and improves the quality of life of parents, who often describe the switch to pump therapy as "getting their child back."[20,21]

Patient selection should be referred to as family selection, because families play a key role in day-to-day diabetes management. Ideal candidates for CSII include motivated families who are committed to monitoring the BG at least 4 times per day and who have a working understanding of basic diabetes management, especially carbohydrate counting and using ICR and ISF to calculate insulin doses. A1c level also plays a role in determining readiness for CSII, although in our clinic it is less important than the factors listed earlier. We generally prefer to have A1c levels less than 8.5% before transition to pump treatment.

In 2006, a consensus conference of leading pediatric diabetes specialists was convened in Berlin to develop treatment guidelines for the use of CSII in children and adolescents. These experts agreed that CSII was indicated for pediatric patients:

- who have increased A1c levels on injection therapy
- who have frequent severe hypoglycemia
- who have widely fluctuating glucose levels (regardless of A1c)
- whose current regimen compromises lifestyle
- who show presence of microvascular complications or risk factors for macrovascular complications.

These experts also agreed that CSII may be beneficial in athletes, very young children, adolescents with eating disorders, those patients with a pronounced dawn effect, ketosis-prone patients, pregnant teens (ideally before conception), and children with pronounced needle phobia.[22]

Insulin Pump Basics

Insulin pump therapy uses only a rapid-acting insulin analogue to deliver constant insulin coverage. Conventional pump models are about the size of a pager and operate on a standard AAA or AA battery (**Table 2**). A reservoir for the pump is filled with several days' worth of insulin. Reservoir capacities range from 180 to 315 units of insulin. This reservoir attaches to a variable length (eg, 45–108 cm) of tubing, which in turn attaches to a small (eg, 6–17 mm) catheter or steel needle that is inserted into the subcutaneous tissue. Most common sites for insertion include the buttocks, abdomen, and upper leg/hip, and some children use their arms. The infusion set is inserted by either the child or caregiver and should be performed every 2 to 3 days or whenever persistently high BG values indicate a potential site failure. A "patch" pump, in which both the mechanics to drive the pump and the insulin are contained in a disposable pod is also commercially available. This pod is attached to the surface of the skin and includes an integrated catheter, which allows for subcutaneous delivery of the insulin. Insulin doses programmed by the patient/caregiver throughout the day are delivered by a handheld device that communicates wirelessly with the patch.

Most models of insulin pumps can be classified as smart pumps into which both ICRs and ISFs are programmed to create a bolus calculator. Patients or their caregivers must enter the carbohydrates to be consumed and the current BG value into the pump, and the calculator recommends an insulin dose based on the programmed ICR and ISF at that time of day. This dose of insulin is not delivered until it is confirmed by the patient or caregiver. Some pumps have the ability to transmit the BG value into the bolus calculator through a wireless link with a specific glucometer. Bolus doses can be administered over a few minutes or as square-wave and dual-wave boluses, which can be helpful for high-fat and prolonged meals. Ideally, bolus doses are delivered 10 to 15 minutes before the meal to minimize postmeal excursions.[23] However, delivery of the bolus after the meal can still minimize postprandial hyperglycemia and may be used in picky eaters, very young children, or in a setting, such as school, where there is less supervision to confirm that the carbohydrates that were entered into the pump are consumed.[24]

Basal insulin needs are covered by the rapid-acting insulin, which is delivered through a preprogrammed basal pattern. This pattern can be made up of multiple different rates; up to 48 different rates per day may be programmed, which allow for a waxing/waning pattern of basal insulin delivery. Furthermore, most pumps allow for multiple basal patterns to be stored in the memory. These multiple patterns are particularly handy when the variability of daily activities can affect BG levels. For example, many of our adolescents have a basal pattern for school days and another for weekends to account for their tendency to sleep the day away on a weekend or holiday from school. Because insulin pumps use only rapid-acting insulin, temporary changes can be made to the basal insulin pattern, and their effects can be seen within a matter of hours. This temporary adjustment of the basal rates is an effective tool for dealing with exercise or sick day management.

GETTING STARTED WITH CSII

Initiation of insulin pump therapy should be a multistep process that begins with determining which pump is best for the patient. When choosing an insulin pump, it is important to find the pump that offers the best fit for the patient. Some questions to think about include:

- Reservoir size: does the patient require a large TDD?
- Insulin sensitivity: would the patient benefit from small basal increments?

Table 2
Pump options and features

Pump	Minimal Basal Rate Increments (U/h)	Minimal Bolus Dose Increments (U)	Maximum Bolus Dose (U)	Insulin Reservoir Capacity (U)	Additional Features
Accu-Chek Spirit	0.1	0.1	25	315	Reversible display Includes personal digital assistant (PDA) device to calculate boluses and with database of foods Comes with backup pump AA battery Accu-Chek 360° (not Windows 7/Mac)
Animas One Touch Ping	0.025	0.05	35	200	Meter-remote can wirelessly beam BG and deliver insulin within 3 m CalorieKing database on meter Waterproof up to 3.6 m AA battery (meter-remote AAA battery) ezManager Max software (not Windows 7)
Insulet Omnipod	0.05	0.05	30	200	1000 common foods in PDA Freestyle meter in PDA component Pod is waterproof up to 2.4 m PDM requires AAA battery Abbott's CoPilot software (not Windows 7/Mac)
Medtronic Paradigm Revel 523/723	0.025	0.025 (to 0.975) then 0.05	25	180 (523) or 300 (723)	Available with real-time CGM AAA battery CareLink personal software (not Mac) Link with glucose meter can wirelessly beam BG level to insulin pump

Adapted from Sherr J, Tamborlane WV. Past, present, and future of insulin pump therapy: better shot at diabetes control. Mt Sinai J Med 2008;75(4):352–61.

- Carbohydrate counting savvy: would the patient/family benefit from having a food look-up program integrated into their pump?
- Continuous glucose monitor (CGM) use: would the patient/family benefit from a CGM receiver integrated in their pump?
- Remote control: would being able to bolus from a handheld device (vs directly on the pump itself) be beneficial?

It is less important which pump is chosen and more important that the patient, family, and caregiver develop a level of comfort and expertise with the particular model. **Box 2** summarizes the pump start process that is used at Yale Children's Diabetes Program.

Initial Starting Doses

Starting doses for insulin pump therapy depend on the type of regimen that the patient was previously receiving. For patients who are already on basal-bolus therapy, we typically transfer those doses directly to the pump. The initial total daily basal insulin dose equals:

- The daily dose of long-acting insulin analogue (-20% if A1c is $<7\%$) or
- 40% to 50% of the TDD of all insulin.

Box 2
The initiation of pump therapy at the Yale Children's Diabetes Program

2–6 weeks before start

- Review pros/cons of pump therapy
- Determine which model is best
- Initiate insurance process to secure coverage of pump
- Refer patient to online training resources or give them manual to review

1–2 weeks before start

- Have patient (depending on age) or caregivers complete online or written training
- Invite school nurse, baby sitters, other caregivers to pump training
- Family is contacted by official trainer from pump company to arrange the first of 2 visits
- Family receives insulin pump and should take pump out of box and start practicing button-pushing techniques
- First visit with official trainer to review ins/outs of pump model, practice button pushing, site insertion, and review diabetes mellitus management principles for pump users (may be done at family home or nearby site for convenience)

Day of start

- Typically scheduled for a Monday or Tuesday morning
- Usually done at clinic building
- Hold morning dose of long-acting insulin
- Initiate pump with insulin; family performs first site change
- Families instructed to test BG: before meals, 2 hours after meal, at bedtime, 12 AM, and 3 AM

Week after start

- Daily phone contact with nurse practitioner to titrate doses

The average hourly basal rate is determined as follows:

Total basal dose of insulin/24 = average hourly basal rate. From there, the hourly basal rates are adjusted based on the assumption that pediatric patients require more insulin during early-morning and early-evening hours and less insulin in the late-morning and overnight hours. This adjustment is typically made in increments of 0.1 units/h for those patients whose basal rates are more than 1 units/h, 0.05 units/h for those whose basal rates are 0.5 to 1 units/h, and 0.025 units/h for those whose basal rates are less than 0.5 units/h.

Initial bolus doses are straightforward for patients already using an ISF and ICR, because these ratios are transferred to the pump. Typically, a correction target of 100 mg/dL is used during the day and a target of 110 to 120 mg/dL is used for the overnight period. ISF and ICR can also be calculated using the 1800 and 500 rules or based on age (see **Table 1**). These are only starting rates and adjustments need to be made. Frequent BG monitoring is essential. BG levels should be checked before meals, 2 hours after meals, at bedtime, and at 12 AM and 3 AM for the first 1 to 2 weeks after starting pump therapy. In our clinic, advanced practice nurses speak with our new pump patients on a daily basis for the first 1 to 2 weeks to fine-tune the starting doses.

Pump-related problems: DKA prevention protocol

Special attention should be paid to acute hyperglycemia when using pump therapy, because use of this modality is a risk factor for DKA.[25] Because only rapid-acting insulin is administered, an interruption of insulin delivery results in increases in blood and urine ketone levels in 4 to 6 hours.[19] Such interruptions are most commonly caused by a problem with the infusion set; a partial disconnection or a kinking of the subcutaneous catheter. Thus, assessment of acute hyperglycemia should include an evaluation of the integrity of the infusion set and infusion site. If 2 consecutive BG levels are greater than 250 mg/dL (at least 2 hours apart) or fasting BG is greater than 275 mg/dL, the patient/parent is instructed to

- Check for ketones
- Change infusion set immediately
- Consider administering correction dose of insulin via syringe or insulin pen
  - May be calculated with insulin pump but delivered by injection
- Consider a temporary increase in basal rate (if ketones are present)
  - 125% to 150% for 2 hours for moderate ketones (>1.0–1.6 mmol/L)
  - 150% to 200% for 2 hours for large ketones (1.6–≥3.0 mmol/L)
- Repeat BG in 2 hours
  - Continued increase in BG levels or ketone levels or the presence of vomiting warrants call to the diabetes team.

Pump-related problems: stacking

All pump users should have a solid understanding of insulin action for the rapid-acting insulin used in their pumps. In glucose clamp studies in children and adolescents, our group has shown that blood levels of rapid-acting insulin peak 60 to 90 minutes after a bolus injection but that peak insulin action is delayed until ~40 minutes later. Moreover, the duration of action extends to 4 to 6 hours after bolus dosing.[7] Without this understanding, many patients and their families follow the more-is-better theory for diabetes management and take too many bolus doses of insulin too close together. This practice results in a phenomenon called stacking. Therefore, patients who check the BG 60 minutes after administration of a correction dose of insulin will not have seen the full effect of the insulin on glucose levels and may be tempted to take an additional correction dose, ending up overcorrecting, leading to hypoglycemia. Another advantage of pump therapy is that the pumps can be set to recommend against a correction dose of insulin within a certain period after a dose is given. For most pump models, this insulin action time can be individually adjusted. In our clinic, this time is typically set to 2 hours, or 3 hours for a few patients.

In general, insulin boluses that cover the carbohydrate content of a meal can be given sequentially over a short time span. However, in some of our teenagers who eat 8 snacks in a 2- to 3-hour period, these meal doses also stack up and cause late-onset hypoglycemia.

GLUCOSE MONITORING

A key component of intensive insulin management is regular adjustment of insulin doses based on changes in glucose control and on daily activity. Frequent BG monitoring, with a minimum of 4 tests per day, before meals and at bedtime, should be the goal. In addition to the traditional 4 BG tests, many patients benefit from strategically adding additional tests, such as 2 hours after meals, overnight, and before/after exercise, to develop a more robust picture of daily glucose trends. Testing should also be done whenever the symptoms of hypoglycemia occur. Regular glucose monitoring allows clinicians and families to make adjustments in the overall insulin regimen over a longer time span as well as to make dose-to-dose adjustments on a daily basis.

Even when families regularly test BG levels at least 4 times per day, they see only the tip of the iceberg when it comes to daily fluctuations in glucose levels.[26] Thus, the recent commercial introduction of continuous glucose monitoring (CGM) systems has the potential to revolutionize insulin management. Currently available CGM devices are inserted subcutaneously and provide glucose levels every few minutes as well as information on trends over 1 to 24 hours and on immediate glucose trends. This wealth of information allows for adjustments in insulin doses based on retrospective analysis as well as real-time in-the-moment adjustments. It is important to note that currently available CGM systems are not meant to replace fingerstick blood glucose monitoring but rather to complement it.

The Juvenile Diabetes Research Foundation CGM randomized controlled trial reported that adults who wear the devices on a near-daily basis can achieve improved A1c levels without an increase in hypoglycemia and those who have already achieved A1c targets can better maintain this level of control with the use of CGM.[27] This finding held true for youth who were willing to wear the sensor almost every day as well. However, many fewer children and adolescents were able to achieve the goal of almost daily wear. Thus, patients and families must be properly educated about the strengths and limitations of CGM to ensure success with this developing technology.

Insulin Dose Adjustment

Because the motto of pediatric diabetes management is that just when you think that you get things right, something changes, frequent review of glucose trends and regular adjustment of the insulin regimen can make the difference between achieving and maintaining target goals and not. It is important to regularly reinforce with patients and families that even those who meet the criteria for ideal glucose control still have glucose levels that are more than and less than the target range. The goal of insulin management should be to minimize the frequency and severity of these excursions. In general, premeal targets for BG are 80 to 120 mg/dL with 2-hour postprandial targets of less than 180 mg/dL. These targets should be adjusted based on individual need.

Adjusting Injection Regimens

Successful adjustment of injection regimens requires a working knowledge of the onset, peak, and duration of the insulin used. It is important to allow for sufficient time, often several days, so that trends and patterns can be identified and separated from the background noise of inherent day-to-day variability in BG levels. Regardless of when out-of-target glucose levels occur, clinicians should first try to determine a cause for the hyperglycemia or hypoglycemia. Typically, hypoglycemia is caused by excessive insulin, insufficient carbohydrate intake (or incorrect accounting of carbohydrate) and unplanned exercise. Hyperglycemia can occur with insufficient insulin, too much carbohydrate, missing premeal bolus doses, sedentary lifestyle, illness, and stress. Often there is no single cause, but a confluence of several. General principles for adjusting insulin doses are summarized in the following list. However, this list is not meant to be comprehensive.

- Doses are typically adjusted by 10% at any one time
- ICR: adjust based on 2-hour postprandial BG level
- ISF: adjust based on BG value 2 to 3 hours after correction (ideally carbohydrates are not eaten at the same time)
- Long-acting insulin: adjust based on fasting BG and abnormal levels outside meal/correction times
- NPH/split-mixed insulin: adjust based on fasting and predinner BG level
- Overnight: adjust long-acting or intermediate-acting insulin; may also need to adjust ICR/ISF if bedtime snack is eaten.

Adjusting Pump Settings

Most of the principles of bolus dose (ISF and ICR) adjustment in pump therapy are similar to those used for MDI treatment, except that the pump and dose calculator give the clinician more flexibility and precision in making small adjustments. Basal rates are designed to keep the BG levels steady between meals. Therefore, hyperglycemia or hypoglycemia that occurs beyond 2 to 3 hours after a meal or snack typically indicates a need for a basal rate adjustment. Testing at 12 AM and 3 AM for a few nights to determine when BG levels increase or decrease during the overnight period may also be useful.

INSULIN USE IN T2D

With the incidence of T2D in adolescents estimated at between 8% and 12% and even approaching 50% in some high-risk populations,[28] insulin is no longer reserved for use only in T1D. Although there are numerous medications for glucose control in adults, most have not been approved for pediatric use, and thus insulin remains a cornerstone for the management of BG levels in this population. Insulin is used at time of diagnosis for patients with significant hyperglycemia and in those for whom oral medications and lifestyle interventions are not sufficient to achieve optimal glycemic control.

In our clinic, patients with T2D who require insulin at diagnosis are started on the same regimen as those who are diagnosed with T1D. Our initial goals are to limit the effects of prolonged and pronounced hyperglycemia on β-cell function and to correct metabolic abnormalities. In many cases, after several weeks on insulin and initiation of metformin, insulin can be weaned and even eliminated.[29]

For those who are failing oral therapy alone, insulin is added as hyperglycemia increases. For those patients whose A1c remains near target, we typically add once-daily glargine. Small additions of insulin can make a big difference in overall glycemic control.[29] For those in whom the A1c has risen out of target, split-mixed insulin is started twice daily. The makeup of the split-mixed insulin depends on the eating patterns of the patient and on insurance coverage.

BG targets and strategies for adjusting insulin doses remain the same for T2D as for T1D. Thus, the information contained in the previous sections may be applied to insulin management of children with T2D. However, lifestyle changes and oral medications should remain a key part of the treatment regimen.

THE FUTURE: CLOSED-LOOP SYSTEMS AND THE ARTIFICIAL PANCREAS

Several investigator groups and pump and sensor manufacturers are working on the development of closed-loop systems that combine external insulin pumps with current CGM devices. These systems use controller algorithms that automatically regulate insulin infusion rates delivered by the pump based on sensor glucose readings every 1 to 5 minutes. These automated insulin infusion systems will have to be easily managed by the patient, protected against system problems that could lead to overdelivery of insulin, and able to respond to challenges of human physiology during normal daily activities, such as exercise and psychological stress. Although it has already been shown that closed-loop systems can control glucose levels effectively in short-term, inpatient, clinical research center studies,[30] much work needs to be done to ensure the safety of these systems before they are ready for outpatient use.

REFERENCES

1. DCCT Research Group. The effects of intensive diabetes treatment on the development and progression of long-term complication in insulin-dependent diabetes mellitus. The Diabetes Control and Complications Trial. N Engl J Med 1993;329: 977–86.
2. The DCCT Research Group. The effect of intensive diabetes treatment on the development and progression of long-term complications in adolescents with insulin-dependent diabetes mellitus: the Diabetes Control and Complications Trial. J Pediatr 1994;125:177–88.
3. DCCT Research Group, EDIC Research Group. Beneficial effects of intensive therapy of diabetes during adolescence: outcomes after the conclusion of the diabetes control and complications trial (DCCT). J Pediatr 2001;139(6):804–12.
4. Silverstein J, Klingensmith G, Copeland K, et al. Care of children and adolescents with type 1 diabetes. A statement of the American Diabetes Association. Diabetes Care 2005;28(1):186–212.
5. Rewers M, Pihoker C, Donaghue K, et al. Assessment and monitoring of glycemic control in children and adolescents with diabetes. Pediatr Diabetes 2009; 10(Suppl 12):71–81.
6. Vajo Z, Fawcett J, Duckworth WC. Recombinant DNA technology in the treatment of diabetes: insulin analogs. Endocr Rev 2001;22:706–17.
7. Swan KL, Weinzimer SA, Steil G, et al. Effect of puberty on the pharmacodynamic and pharmacokinetic properties of insulin pump therapy in youth with T1DM. Diabetes Care 2001;31:41–6.
8. Weinzimer SA, Ternand C, Campbell H, et al. A randomized trial comparing continuous subcutaneous insulin infusion of insulin aspart versus insulin lispro in children and adolescents with type 1 diabetes. Diabetes Care 2008;31(2):210–5.
9. Van Bon AC, Bode BW, Sert-Langeron C, et al. Insulin glulisine compared to insulin aspart and insulin lispro administered by continuous subcutaneous insulin

infusion in patients with type 1 diabetes: a randomized control trial. Diabetes Technol Ther 2011;13(6):607–14.

10. Bangstad HJ, Danne T, Deeb LC, et al. Insulin treatment in children and adolescents with diabetes. Pediatr Diabetes 2009;10(Suppl 12):82–99.

11. Lepore M, Panpanelli S, Fanelli C, et al. Pharmacokinetics and pharmacodynamics of subcutaneous injection of long-acting human insulin analog glargine, NPH insulin and ultralente human insulin and continuous subcutaneous infusion of insulin lispro. Diabetes 2000;49:2142–8.

12. Chase P, Arslanian S, White NH, et al. Insulin glargine vs. intermediate-acting insulin as the basal component of multiple daily injection regimens for adolescents with type 1 diabetes. J Pediatr 2008;153:547–53.

13. Danne T, Datz N, Endahl L, et al. Insulin detemir is characterized by a more reproducible pharmacokinetic profile than insulin glargine in children and adolescents with type 1 diabetes: results from a randomized, double-blind controlled trial. Pediatr Diabetes 2008;9:554–60.

14. Heise T, Nosek L, Ronn BB, et al. Lower within-subject variability of insulin detemir in comparison to NPH insulin and insulin glargine in people with type 1 diabetes. Diabetes 2004;53(6):1614–20.

15. Cengiz E, Sherr JL, Erkin-Cakmak A, et al. A bridge to insulin pump therapy: bid regimen with NPH and detemir insulin during initial treatment of youth with type 1 diabetes (T1D). Endocr Pract 2011;6:1–17.

16. Mooradian A, Bernbaum M, Albert SG. Narrative review: a rational approach to starting insulin therapy. Ann Intern Med 2006;145(2):125–34.

17. Cengiz E, Tamborlane W, Martin-Fredericksen M, et al. Early pharmacokinetic and pharmacodynamic effects of mixing lispro with glargine insulin. Diabetes Care 2010;33(5):1009–12.

18. Sherr J, Tamborlane WV. Past, present, and future of insulin pump therapy: better shot at diabetes control. Mt Sinai J Med 2008;75(4):352–61.

19. Attia N, Jones TW, Holcombe J, et al. Comparison of human regular and lispro insulins after interruption of continuous subcutaneous insulin infusion and in the treatment of acutely decompensated IDDM. Diabetes Care 1998;21:817–21.

20. Weinzimer SA, Ahern JH, Boland EA, et al. Continuous subcutaneous insulin infusion is safe and effective in infants and toddlers. Diabetes 2003;52(Suppl 2): A402.

21. Sullivan-Bolyai S, Knafl K, Tamborlane W, et al. Parents' reflections on the use of the insulin pump with their young children. J Nurs Scholarsh 2004;6:316–23.

22. Moshe P, Battelino T, Rodriguez H, et al. Use of insulin pump therapy in the pediatric age-group: consensus statement from the European Society for Paediatric Endocrinology, the Lawson Wilkins Pediatric Endocrine Society and the International Society for Pediatric and Adolescent Diabetes, endorsed by the American Diabetes Association and the European Association for the Study of Diabetes. Diabetes Care 2007;30(6):1653–62.

23. Luijf YM, Van Bon AC, Hoekstra JB, et al. Premeal injection of rapid acting insulin reduces postprandial glycemic excursions in type 1 diabetes. Diabetes Care 2010;30(10):2152–5.

24. Danne T. Flexibility of rapid-acting insulin analogues in children and adolescents with diabetes mellitus. Clin Ther 2007;29(Suppl D):S145–52.

25. Wolfsdorf J, Crag ME, Daneman D, et al. Diabetic ketoacidosis in children and adolescents with diabetes. Pediatr Diabetes 2009;10(Suppl 12):118–33.

26. Boland EA, DeLucia M, Brandt C, et al. Limitations of conventional methods of self blood glucose monitoring: lessons learned from three days of continuous

glucose monitoring in pediatric patients with type I diabetes. Diabetes Care 2001; 24:1858–62.

27. Juvenile Diabetes Research Foundation Continuous Glucose Monitoring Study Group. Effectiveness of continuous glucose monitoring in a clinical care environment: evidence from the Juvenile Diabetes Research Foundation continuous glucose monitoring (JDRF-CGM) trial. Diabetes Care 2010;33(1):17–20.

28. Writing group for the SEARCH for Diabetes in Youth Study Group. Incidence of diabetes in youth in the United States. JAMA 2007;297(24):2716–24.

29. Rosenbloom RL, Silverstein JH, Amemiya S, et al. Type 2 diabetes in children and adolescents. Pediatr Diabetes 2009;10(Suppl 12):17–32.

30. Weinzimer SA, Steil GM, Swan KL, et al. Fully automated closed-loop insulin delivery vs. semi-automated hybrid control in pediatric patients with type 1 diabetes using an artificial pancreas. Diabetes Care 2008;31:934–9390.

Insulin Therapy in Pregnancy

Aidan McElduff, FRACP[a,b],*, Robert G. Moses, MD[c]

KEYWORDS

• Pregnancy • Diabetes • Gestational diabetes • Insulin

Before the discovery and commercial availability of insulin after 1922, the life of any person with type 1 diabetes was extraordinarily restrictive, with a rapidly progressive disability and an inevitable premature death. Young girls diagnosed with type 1 diabetes rarely reached childbearing age, and, for women who developed type 1 diabetes while potentially fertile, pregnancy was positively discouraged. The number of successful pregnancies for women with type 1 diabetes was extremely small and, in truth, probably either represented a very early stage of diagnosis before insulin deficiency was fully established or was an example of type 2 diabetes. There was almost universal perinatal mortality and a very high maternal mortality.[1]

The advent of insulin greatly improved the fetal and maternal outcomes for pregnancy, but it remained unacceptably high for at least a generation. In 1947, the perinatal mortality rate in pregnancies complicated by preexisting diabetes was reported at about 40% in studies from Europe and the United States.[2] In the early 1950s, the concept of specialty clinics for pregnancies complicated by diabetes was introduced.[3] These clinics resulted in an almost 50% reduction in the perinatal mortality rate and were widely adopted. The clinics involved both centralized expertise and an interactive team approach for the management of diabetes and pregnancy. There was a subsequent gradual decline in the perinatal mortality rate over the next 20 to 25 years. A population study from Norway,[4] during the years 1967 to 1976, documented a decrease in perinatal mortality from 17.7% to 6.1%, whereas the total population figures were 2.4% and 1.8%, respectively. Thus in 1976 in Norway, the perinatal mortality associated with preexisting diabetes, predominantly type 1, was still 3 to 4 times that of the total population.

Two major advances have led to a further improvement in management, and these were not related to refinements of insulin therapy. The first was the increasingly

The authors declare no conflicts of interest.
[a] Discipline of Medicine, Sydney University, Sydney, NSW, Australia
[b] Northern Sydney Endocrine Centre, 1/38-40, Pacific Highway, St Leonards, NSW 2065, Australia
[c] Illawarra Diabetes Service, PO Box W58, Wollongong West, NSW 2500, Australia
* Corresponding author. Northern Sydney Endocrine Centre, 1/38-40, Pacific Highway, St Leonards, NSW 2065, Australia.
E-mail address: aidanm@med.usyd.edu.au

Endocrinol Metab Clin N Am 41 (2012) 161–173
doi:10.1016/j.ecl.2011.12.002
0889-8529/12/$ – see front matter © 2012 Elsevier Inc. All rights reserved.

widespread use of effective means of maternal glucose monitoring using portable home glucose meters. The other related to the measurement of glycosylated hemoglobin as an integrated measure of maternal glucose control. The first of these allowed for outpatient management of pregnancy rather than prolonged hospitalization. The second allowed for an objective assessment of glycemic control and of the relationship between glycemic control and outcomes. However, although the absolute risk of perinatal mortality has declined in both the general population and in women with diabetes, the relative risk remains approximately 3 times higher in the subgroup with diabetes.[5] The difficult continuing challenge is to eliminate this difference, a large part of which relates to preconception care and the need to reduce major congenital abnormalities.[6]

INSULIN THERAPY IN PREGNANCY: WHAT PHYSICIANS ARE TRYING TO MIMIC

In the fasting state, glucose levels are maintained by endogenous hepatic glucose production and release. This is highly regulated by pancreatic insulin secretion into the portal vein (basal insulin). After a meal, insulin is released into the portal vein, largely determined by the quantity and quality of the ingested carbohydrate (bolus insulin). The amount and proportion of insulin required for each phase will vary from individual to individual and from time to time. We try to mimic these 2 phases of insulin secretion with basal and bolus subcutaneous injections. In pregnancy, the fasting glucose level is lower and the relative postprandial rise is higher than that in the nonpregnant state.[7] Furthermore, the postprandial excursion returns to baseline more rapidly, particularly as pregnancy progresses. These changes need to be considered in adjusting and monitoring insulin therapy during pregnancy.

A further complication is the variation in hepatic glucose output known as the dawn phenomenon. More basal insulin is required during the early hours of morning to control the increased hepatic glucose output attributed to increasing levels of cortisol and growth hormone.

In pregnancy, the insulin requirements also vary with the phase of the pregnancy. Insulin requirements may increase very early in pregnancy and then decrease in the second half of the first trimester into the early second trimester. Later in the second and then in third trimester, insulin requirement increases steadily, possibly by a factor of 2 or 3 in type 1 diabetes or even more markedly in type 2 diabetes and occasionally in women with gestational diabetes mellitus (GDM) treated with insulin. However, after 32 weeks, insulin requirements may plateau or in fact decline. This late decline may present as hypoglycemia.[8–10] This may be normal, although the mechanisms are not clear. It can signal maternal disease.[11] Previously, decreasing insulin requirements were thought to indicate fetal compromise, but, as outlined previously, this is no longer considered to be correct in most cases. However, it seems prudent to assess fetal well-being with any significant reduction in insulin requirements.

These daily and weekly changes must be considered in managing diabetes in pregnancy, anticipating the trends rather than reacting to the changes, often belatedly.

INSULIN USE IN PREGNANCY: AN INCREASINGLY COMMON REQUIREMENT

Insulin use in pregnancy is increasing rapidly as the nature of diabetes in pregnancy changes. Whereas in the past, insulin use would have been almost exclusively confined to women with type 1 diabetes, the majority of insulin use now is undoubtedly in women with GDM and type 2 diabetes.

The number of women with type 1 diabetes in pregnancy should approximate the background rate of type 1 diabetes in the community.[12] However, in general terms, it is actually less. This is because of a decreased fertility rate associated with diabetes-related ill health[13] as well as a conscious decision of women with type 1 diabetes to restrict family size.

The total number of women with pregestational diabetes is increasing. Whereas about 20 years ago it was around 0.2% to 0.5% of the pregnant population,[14] it has recently at least doubled.[15] Although there has been an absolute increase in the number of women with type 1 diabetes, this increase has been overwhelmed and surpassed by the rapid increase in the number of women with type 2 diabetes. This is related to the increasing rates of obesity, the earlier onset of type 2 diabetes, and the later age of pregnancy in many communities. GDM is increasing for the same reasons as well as because of an increased rate of screening with detection of previously undiagnosed cases.

Into this mixture, it is also necessary to consider the changing nature of GDM. The prevalence has increased over the last 20 years,[16] possibly related to increased rates of testing as well as a genuine increase in prevalence. Although a lack of international consensus about the diagnosis of GDM has bedeviled past attempts to compare prevalence and outcomes, it is possible the new International Association of Diabetes in Pregnancy Study Groups[17] criteria will overcome some of these concerns. A prospective study,[18] a post hoc analysis[19] of the Hyperglycemia Adverse Pregnancy Outcome (HAPO) study data, and a retrospective review of 2 large metropolitan hospitals in Sydney[20] indicate that adoption of the new criteria will increase the prevalence of GDM by 20% to 50%. This increase will likely lead to an increase in insulin use in GDM to meet the glycemic targets.[21]

The types and regimens of insulin used in pregnancy have to take into account the diversity of clinical conditions being managed.

INSULIN USE

As discussed, the introduction of insulin into clinical practice in 1922 resulted in a significant improvement in pregnancy outcomes because of improved glycemic control. At present, soluble human insulin and neutral protamine Hagedorn (NPH) are considered the gold standard for the treatment of diabetes in pregnancy.

RISKS OF INSULIN THERAPY: HYPOGLYCEMIA AND RETINOPATHY

The major limitation to insulin therapy is hypoglycemia, especially in type 1 diabetes. A Danish population survey of pregnancy in women with type 1 diabetes[22] reported a maternal mortality rate of 0.3% caused by hypoglycemia. Balancing tight control to optimize fetal and maternal outcomes with the risk of hypoglycemia is difficult. Hypoglycemia occurs most commonly in the first half of pregnancy when insulin sensitivity increases, and nausea may reduce intake.

Rapid improvement in glycemic control early in pregnancy can exacerbate or precipitate diabetic retinopathy as occurs in the nonpregnant state. The risk during pregnancy may be higher because pregnancy per se may also induce retinopathy.

A current question is if the new insulin analogues are safe for use in pregnancy and if they offer any advantages.

RAPID-ACTING INSULIN ANALOGUES AND PREGNANCY

During pregnancy, control of the postprandial glucose excursions can reduce fetal macrosomia, although overtight control can increase the small-for-gestational-age rate.[23] Insulin analogues, made by modification of human insulin, have a more rapid onset of action than the regular insulin preparations and thus have a potential theoretical advantage in controlling the postprandial glucose excursions. The first available of these was insulin lispro in 1996, followed by insulin aspart and more recently by insulin glulisine.

A relatively early study to assess the safety and efficacy of the insulin analogue lispro was reported by Persson and colleagues.[24] This was a multicenter study conducted in Sweden and included 33 women with type 1 diabetes who were receiving treatment with NPH insulin and a multiple dose regimen with regular insulin. They had to have had type 1 diabetes for a minimum of 2 years and an initial HbA_{1c} level less than 9%. At 15 weeks of gestation, the women were randomized to continue with their regular insulin (Humulin Regular/Actrapid, n = 17) or lispro (Humalog, n = 16) administered before or within 30 minutes of eating. NPH insulin was used at bedtime and in some patients in the morning as well. The dose of regular insulin was adjusted by preprandial glucose values, and the participants were reviewed every 1 to 2 weeks.

The monitored blood glucose level was lower after breakfast in the lispro group, but there were no significant differences with daily glycemic control between the 2 groups for the rest of the day. The HbA1c level was similar in both groups at recruitment and at randomization and did not differ during the course of the study. Two patients in the regular group had 3 episodes of severe hypoglycemia. The pregnancy and perinatal outcomes were similar in both groups. The conclusion from this study was that lispro could be considered an effective alternative to regular insulin.

A retrospective multicenter Italian study[25] (Lapolla, 2008) of insulin lispro at least 3 months before and 3 months after conception in 72 women with type 1 diabetes demonstrated no safety issues during pregnancy compared with women using regular insulin. A trend toward less hypoglycemia was observed in the lispro group.

A multinational retrospective review[26] of more than 500 women who received insulin lispro immediately before conception and in the fist trimester did not show any increased rate of either major or minor congenital malformations.

Two studies have examined the use of lispro in women with GDM. The retrospective cohort study of Bhattacharyya and colleagues[27] reported data on 68 women with GDM compared with 89 treated with regular insulin. The mean daily dose of quick-acting insulin preparations was similar in both groups, but there was a lower HbA1c level in the women treated with lispro. In another study,[28] women with GDM were randomly assigned to treatment with either regular or lispro insulin. The postprandial glucose levels in the lispro group were lower, and there was no significant difference in the pregnancy outcomes.

A recent systematic review and meta-analysis[29] of lispro versus regular insulin identified a higher rate of large-for-gestational-age infants (>90th percentile) despite similar HbA1c levels in the lispro group (relative risk, 1.38; 95% confidence interval, 1.14–1.16) but no differences in the rate of small-for-gestational-age infants. No differences were observed in other fetal or maternal outcomes, although the severe maternal hypoglycemia rate was not specifically identified.

Insulin aspart (NovoRapid) has been examined in a large multicenter multinational clinical trial.[30] This study randomized 412 (for 322 in the final report) women with type 1 diabetes diagnosed for at least 1 year or longer who had an HbA1c level of 8% or less at confirmation of pregnancy. There were 223 women enrolled who were pregnant and 189 women who were planning a pregnancy, of whom 99 became pregnant during the study. Although the study was conducted at 63 centers, the difficulty in conducting studies of this kind can be appreciated because it took 5 years for recruitment and completion. At randomization, women received either mealtime aspart (n = 201) or regular insulin (n = 211), both in combination with NPH insulin. The final report had 157 women in the aspart arm divided between those using the insulin before conception (44) and those commencing the insulin at less than 10 weeks' gestation (113).

The postprandial glucose levels were significantly lower in the aspart group, mainly because of lower levels after breakfast. However, there was no significant difference in the HbA1c level between the 2 groups. There were also no significant differences between either group with respect to maternal or fetal outcomes and the rate of congenital malformations. This study demonstrated that the use of aspart was safe and effective during pregnancy but not superior to regular insulin.

In both the aspart-treated and lispro-treated groups, there was a trend toward less hypoglycemia. In the aspart study, the reduction was more obvious in women who commenced aspart before conception. The aspart data suggest that initiation of insulin analogue treatment before conception rather than during early pregnancy may result in a lower risk of severe hypoglycemia in women with type 1 diabetes.[31] If this positive attribute can be confirmed, it would likely influence insulin selection in planned pregnancies. However, it is possible that in nonblinded studies this may relate to patient education rather than the insulin type.

Both these rapid-acting insulin analogues are accepted for use in pregnancy in Europe and the United States.

LONG-ACTING ANALOGUES

The situation with the long-acting analogues is not as well advanced. Novo Nordisk conducted a randomized, parallel, open-label, controlled, multinational study of a basal/bolus regimen comparing insulin detemir (Levemir) with NPH, both in combination with insulin aspart in pregnant women with type 1 diabetes (http://www.clinicaltrials.gov/ct2). The numbers were not large, 142 women in the detemir arm divided between those using the insulin before conception (73) and those commencing the insulin at less than 12 weeks' gestation (79). There were 130 control women. The results so far have been published in abstract form. No safety issues were raised. The fetal and perinatal outcomes were not significantly different between the 2 treatment regimens.

Insulin detemir seemed to lower the HbA1c level by approximately 0.3% in the preconception "run in" period. This result, although not statistically significant, would be clinically relevant if correct.[32]

Anecdotal reports of the use of both detemir and glargine in pregnancy have raised no safety concerns. They are widely used off-label in pregnancy.[33]

A typical clinical situation is a woman planning a pregnancy or in early pregnancy, on either of these long-acting analogues, who reports better glycemic control and/or less hypoglycemia since commencing the long-acting analogue. Most clinicians consider that this clinical benefit outweighs the risk of any theoretical side effect and would continue the long-acting analogue.

HOW TO ADMINISTER THE INSULIN

Another question often considered by patients is "should I be on a pump for my pregnancy?" We quote from the Cochrane Database of Systematic Reviews, Farrar and colleagues,[34] "there is a dearth of robust evidence to support the use of one particular form of insulin administration over another for pregnant women with diabetes." The investigators conclude that there was no level 1 evidence to answer the patient's question. Pumps (continuous subcutaneous insulin infusion [CSII]) are widely used in pregnancy without obvious problems. Two small studies (61 participants) suggested CSII was associated with increased birth weight but not macrosomia, defined as birth weight less than 4 kg, when compared with multiple daily injections. Once again, this suggests an important outcome difference that would require a large randomized controlled trial (RCT) to confirm or refute.

There is no strong evidence that pump therapy improves glycemic control beyond the increased patient education and/or a change in lifestyle often associated with pump therapy. At present, pump therapy should be viewed as a lifestyle choice.

WHEN TO ADMINISTER: BEFORE OR AFTER MEALS

One small study of women with type 1 diabetes[35] examined the effect of insulin lispro given before or after a meal, and there was no difference in the glycemic excursion. This study suggests that insulin lispro can be taken after meals in pregnancy without altering the glycemic response to the meal. This finding has clinical relevance in early pregnancy when nausea is common and women find it difficult to predict how much they will eat.

HOW OFTEN TO ADMINISTER

Another RCT compared 2 basal/bolus regimens using Actrapid and Insulatard (Novo Nordisk),[36] one with 4 times a day Actrapid and one with twice daily Actrapid. The study was reasonably large, with 274 women with GDM and 118 women with pregestational diabetes. Randomization was based on a computer-generated list of numbers, sealed in numbered opaque envelopes, which were opened sequentially. The 4-times daily regimen resulted in higher daily insulin doses and better glycemic control with lower HbA1c and fructosamine levels. There was no increase in severe maternal hypoglycemia. The significant improvements in pregnancy outcomes were modest and restricted to neonatal hypoglycemia and hyperbilirubinemia in the GDM group, possibly because of power considerations. The open-labeled nature of such studies always leaves open the possibility of bias in the treatment arms.

It seems fair to say that insulin use in pregnancy generally has a very small level 1 evidence base. Insulin analogues can be viewed as a minor advance with no specific problems identified relating to pregnancy based on a relatively small number of studies.

A list of RCTs is shown in **Table 1**.

HOW TO INITIATE INSULIN THERAPY: GDM

Most women with GDM can be well controlled on a diet and exercise regimen suitable for pregnancy. For most women requiring insulin therapy, it will be easy to optimize glycemic control, especially when compared with women with type 1 diabetes. The insulin regimens used in the Australian Carbohydrate Intolerance Study in Pregnant Women[37] and the Maternal-Fetal Medicine Units Network study[38] were left to individual units but consisted of either a short-acting insulin alone or a short-acting insulin and an NPH in a basal/bolus regimen. Some units utilized premixed insulin preparations. Insulin preparations were administered as required to control fasting or postprandial hyperglycemia. For example, a woman with isolated postbreakfast hyperglycemia (a common problem) would require only prebreakfast short-acting insulin. The choice of that insulin is likely to be the short-acting insulin most commonly used by the practitioner involved. Other preprandial doses of short-acting insulin are added as required for postprandial hyperglycemia. The initial dose is chosen arbitrarily depending on the degree of hyperglycemia and then quickly titrated depending on the

Table 1			
RCTs of insulin therapy in diabetes mellitus			
Reference	**Comparison**	**N**	**Diabetes Type**
Nachum et al,[36] 1999	4 vs twice daily Actrapid	392	GDM, 274; type 1 diabetes mellitus, 118
Hod et al,[30] 2008	Aspart vs Actrapid	322	Type 1 diabetes mellitus
Persson et al,[24] 2002	Lispro vs Actrapid/Humulin R	33	Type 1 diabetes mellitus
Jovanovic et al,[57] 1999	Lispro vs Humulin R	42	GDM
Mecacci et al,[28] 2003	Lispro vs regular	49	GDM
Carr et al,[35] 2004	Premeal vs postmeal lispro	9 women, 27 meals	Mainly type 1 diabetes mellitus
Hod et al,[32] 2011	Levemir vs NPH	—	Type 1 diabetes mellitus
Farrar et al,[34] 2007	CSII (pump) vs multiple daily insulin injections	61	Type 1 diabetes mellitus
Rosenberg et al,[56] 2006	Intrapartum fluids vs intravenous insulin	26	Mainly GDM
Ismail et al,[58] 2007	Actrapid vs Insulatard	68	Mainly GDM

initial response. Usually, dose variations are meal specific (ie, more insulin is required for a meal that previously caused more significant hyperglycemia) rather than more complex carbohydrate or portion counting as for preexisting diabetes.

In GDM, the predominant long-acting insulin used is NPH.[39] NPH is usually given at a fixed time before bed and adjusted to normalize the fasting glucose.

Following HAPO[40] and with the increasing knowledge base of the normal range of glycemia in pregnancy,[41] the target for fasting glucose is decreasing. This means that in the future, many more women may require long-acting insulin than is currently the case.

The less common situation of woman diagnosed with GDM with hyperglycemic levels similar to those with preexisting diabetes should be managed as for preexisting diabetes.

WHEN TO INTENSIFY OR INITIATE INSULIN THERAPY

Before discussing glycemic targets, it is worthwhile to remember that good/tight glycemic control is achieved with a complex treatment program involving diet, exercise, and utilization of a difficult-to-acquire knowledge base that is used by the woman to adjust her insulin therapy, taking into account, at least, the distribution and timing of carbohydrate intake, which will be related to food availability and cultural patterns of eating; the varying glycemic index of the carbohydrates; exercise/activity; stressful life, work, or family issues; and the many problems, great and small, which accompany virtually every pregnancy.

The total daily dose needs adjustment on a regular basis as insulin requirements vary at different stages of gestation. The dynamic mixture of basal and prandial insulin preparations depends on the results of home glucose monitoring. The HbA1c level reflects the overall glycemic control.

GLYCEMIC TARGETS

The targets for glycemic control suggested by the American Diabetes Association,[42] the International Diabetes Federation,[43] the UK National Institute for Health and

Clinical Excellence,[44] and the Australasian Diabetes in Pregnancy Society[45] are shown in **Table 2**. These targets are similar but not identical. They are based on expert opinion rather than on RCTs. Recent studies of glycemia in normal and obese pregnancies have led to a push to tighten these targets.[21,46] At some point, RCTs are required to decide how tight the glycemic control should be in pregnancy. Regardless, at present in women already receiving insulin, it seems logical to aim for the middle or lower portion of the target range rather than the upper limit of that range. Thus, tightening the target range will have a lesser effect on treatment approaches in women already receiving insulin. This is particularly true in type 1 diabetes where achieving the current targets is already difficult. The problem area will be in GDM and the initiation of insulin therapy. Lower targets increase the number of women receiving insulin. Careful risk-benefit analysis is required, and this ideally should have an evidence base.

It must be remembered that if subcutaneous insulin therapy is utilized to produce normal circulating glucose levels measured by any technique involving capillary or subcutaneous glucose monitoring, the physiology of the whole body is not the same as normal physiology, whereby insulin secretion is from the pancreas into the portal circulation. Tighter and tighter glycemic control produces decreasing maternal and fetal benefits, particularly in GDM. The currently available RCTs already show very good outcomes with the current albeit arbitrary treatment thresholds.[47] At some point, risk may outweigh benefit. Langer and colleagues[48] and Combs and colleagues[23] have shown that lower circulating glucose levels are associated with an increased frequency of small-for-gestational-age infants.

This issue will remain contentious. We quote from the authors' conclusion from a recent Cochrane analysis of tight versus less tight glycemic control, "In a very limited body of evidence, few differences in outcomes were seen between very tight and tight-moderate glycemic control targets in pregnant women with pre-existing type 1 diabetes, including actual glycemic control achieved. There is evidence of harm (increased pre-eclampsia, caesareans and birth weights greater than 90th centile) for 'loose' control (FBG above 126 mg/dL)."[49]

WHEN TO MONITOR

One randomized study[50] of 66 women with GDM found that better neonatal outcomes were achieved by targeting a 1-hour postprandial glucose level of less than 140 mg/dL rather than a premeal target of 59 to 106 mg/dL. A similar small study[51] (N = 61) on

Table 2
Recommended targets for home-monitored capillary glucose levels during pregnancy

Source	Fasting	1 h	Peak	2 h	Premeal
ADA GDM[42]	5.3	7.8	—	6.7	—
ADA[42] preexisting	3.3–5.5	—	5.5–7.2	—	3.3–5.5[a]
IDF[43]	5.5	—	8.0	—	—
NICE[44]	3.5–5.9	7.8	—	—	—
ADIPS[45]	5.5	8.0	7.0	7.0	—
Mathiesen[46]	4.0–6.0	7.8	4–8 ??	—	4–6

Abbreviations: ADA, American Diabetes Association; ADIPS, Australasian Diabetes in Pregnancy Society; IDF, International Diabetes Federation; NICE, National Institute for Health and Clinical Excellence; ?, or possibly.
[a] Bedtime/overnight.

type 1 diabetes demonstrated a reduction in preeclampsia in women randomly assigned to monitor postprandially. These studies have been criticized for not using comparably tight measures for the pretargets and posttargets.

Regardless, most experts in the area use postprandial testing in part because of the physiologic changes discussed earlier.

INSULIN THERAPY DURING LABOR, DELIVERY, AND THE IMMEDIATE POSTPARTUM PERIOD

The intensity of observation and treatment is related to the type of maternal diabetes and the facilities and staffing available. The spectrum ranges from women with GDM receiving no or very small doses of insulin to women with type 1 diabetes who may be ketosis prone.

For women with type 1 diabetes, the major goals of therapy at the time of delivery are to prevent ketoacidosis in the mother and neonatal acidemia and hypoglycemia. For this purpose, maintaining the maternal glucose level between 70 to 140 mg/dL is generally recommended. Although good glycemic control throughout pregnancy, with less development of fetal beta cells, is likely to reduce the capacity to develop neonatal hypoglycemia, maternal glucose control at the time of delivery is critical.[52–54]

Depending on the facilities available, the standard management during labor and delivery relates to the use of an insulin infusion. The methods used and the protocol followed must be determined for each center and based on the resources and expertise available. Medical and nursing staff must feel comfortable with the protocol. Most protocols are based on consensus and personal experience[55] because it is not an area that lends itself to the conduct of large-scale RCTs.

There are 2 components to the insulin infusion regime. Dextrose should be used to ensure that the maternal glucose level does not decrease less than predetermined levels, and insulin should be used to ensure that the maternal glucose does not exceed predetermined levels. Maternal glucose levels should be monitored with capillary samples every hour.

An intravenous line with a 5% dextrose infusion should be established as soon as practical, and capillary glucose monitoring is initiated on an hourly basis. The initial rate of the dextrose infusion could be 80 mL/h with the intention of keeping the capillary glucose more than 70 mg/dL. The infusion rate can be adjusted, up or down, by 20- to 40-mL/h increments.

Another infusion should be prepared using either a local protocol or normal saline containing 50 U of human soluble insulin (50 U for 500 mL = 1 U for each 10 mL). Depending on the delivery device used, this should be "charged" by running through some of this infusion so that when connected and activated, the patient receives a known concentration of insulin immediately. The starting rate should be 1 to 2 U/h, and the rate should be adjusted upward or downward by 0.5 to 1.0 U/h to keep glucose levels within the target range. A minimum rate of 0.5 U/h should be continued and glucose levels maintained by adjustments of the dextrose infusion.

With spontaneous labor or after induction, the earlier-mentioned infusions should be established and used once oral intake is curtailed. With an elective section, it would be reasonable to administer the usual evening dose of insulin and start the infusions in the morning. For women receiving CSII, this administration can be continued during labor and delivery, with good outcomes, provided a prepregnancy plan is in place and staff, at all hours, are familiar and comfortable with this practice.

Women with known type 2 diabetes who are receiving insulin treatment during the pregnancy should be managed with an insulin infusion.

At the other end of the spectrum are women with GDM receiving only a small dose of insulin. The primary purpose of the insulin treatment for these women is to help control potential abnormal fetal growth and to prevent adverse intrauterine programming. By the time labor is established, the purpose for which insulin has been used would have been achieved. Under these circumstances, no special requirements are necessary during labor and no insulin is required. This suggestion is supported by a recent RCT (N = 16) that suggested a rotating intravenous fluid protocol gave identical results to an insulin infusion in insulin-treated GDM.[56]

Women on a high dose of insulin who may have previously undiagnosed type 1 or type 2 diabetes should, depending on clinical judgment, be managed with an insulin infusion.

After delivery (the decline commences during labor), insulin requirements decrease sharply and a significant reduction in the insulin dose can be expected. These reductions are most marked in the first 24 to 48 hours. For women with type 1 diabetes, returning to the prepregnancy dose as often recommended is usually not appropriate, particularly in women who had tight glycemic control before and in anticipation of pregnancy. It is most important to reduce the risk of hypoglycemia during this period of adjustment. It is vital that the mother feels confident about a low risk of hypoglycemia when nursing. For this purpose, some compromise with diabetic control is required. We suggest, as a guideline, that no more than 75% of the prepregnancy dose should be used. Home glucose monitoring and access to medical advice should be maintained.

For women with type 2 diabetes, who felt comfortable with the use of insulin during pregnancy, this could be continued, at a much lower dose if their control before conception on diet and/or oral agents was less than optimal. For women, who may have had previously undiagnosed diabetes detected during pregnancy, their insulin dose should be significantly reduced and ongoing use based on clinical assessment. This postpregnancy counseling is almost as important as prepregnancy counseling.

WHAT TO DO IN PRACTICE

The proceeding information makes it clear that there is no strong evidence base to recommend one insulin therapeutic strategy over another. It is clear from the literature that units with experience in managing diabetes in pregnancy do better than those without experience. We recommend a basal/bolus approach using the insulin types with which the physician is familiar and which suit the patient. There is no evidence base to recommend the newer analogues over regular soluble human insulin and NPH, although individual patients seem to do better with the analogues, particularly with regard to a reduction in the frequency/severity of hypoglycemia. Home glucose monitoring is required frequently, at least 4 to 5 times daily, targeting both fasting and postprandial results. The recommended targets are shown in **Table 1**. Achieving these targets must be balanced against the risk of hypoglycemia, particularly in women with type 1 diabetes. Addressing patient education and motivation are important determinants of glycemic control. Insulin regimens should be assessed on the basis of glycemic control achieved in each individual patient. No universal regimen exists.

REFERENCES

1. Joslin EP. Treatment of diabetes mellitus. 3rd edition. London: H. Kimpton; 1924.
2. Henley WE. Diabetes and pregnancy. N Z Med J 1947;46:386–97.

3. Hagbard L. Pregnancy and diabetes mellitus; a clinical study. Acta Obstet Gynecol Scand 1956;35(Suppl 1):1–180.
4. Jervell J, Bjerkedal T, Moe N. Outcome of pregnancies in diabetic mothers in Norway 1967-1976. Diabetologia 1980;18:131–4.
5. Shand AW, Bell J, McElduff A, et al. Diabetes mellitus in pregnancy: a population based study of pre-gestational diabetes mellitus and gestational diabetes mellitus in New South Wales, Australia. Diabet Med 2008;25:708–15.
6. Confidential Enquiry into Maternal and Child Health. Pregnancy in women with type 1 and type 2 diabetes in 2002–03, England, Wales and Northern Ireland. London: CEMACH; 2005. 134.
7. Kenshole AB. Diabetes and pregnancy. In: Burrow GN, Duffy TP, Copel JA, editors. Medical complications in pregnancy. 6th edition. Philadelphia: Elsevier Saunders; 2004. p. 16.
8. Pedersen J. Course of diabetes during pregnancy. Acta Endocrinol 1952;9: 342–64.
9. Steel JM, Johnstone FD, Hume R, et al. Insulin requirements during pregnancy in women with type I diabetes. Obstet Gynecol 1994;83:253–8.
10. McManus RM, Ryan EA. Insulin requirements in insulin-dependent and insulin-requiring GDM women during final month of pregnancy. Diabetes Care 1992; 15:1323–7.
11. Flynn MD, Cundy TF, Watkins PJ. Antepartum pituitary necrosis in diabetes mellitus. Diabet Med 1988;5:295–7.
12. IDF diabetes atlas, Brussels. Brussels (Belgium): International Diabetes Federation; 2006. Available at: www.eatlas.idg.org/Prevalence. Accessed December 23, 2011.
13. Jonasson JM, Brismar K, Sparen P, et al. Fertility in women with type 1 diabetes. A population based cohort study in Sweden. Diabetes Care 2007;30:2271–6.
14. Engelgau MM, Herman WH, Smith PJ, et al. The epidemiology of diabetes and pregnancy in the US. Diabetes Care 1995;18:1029–33.
15. Lawrence JM, Contreras R, Chen W, et al. Trends in the prevalence of pre-existing diabetes and gestational diabetes among racially/ethnically diverse population of pregnant women 1999-205. Diabetes Care 2008;31:899–904.
16. Ferrara A. Increased prevalence of gestational diabetes mellitus. Diabetes Care 2007;30(Suppl 2):S141–6.
17. International Association of Diabetes and Pregnancy Study Groups Consensus Panel. International Association of Diabetes and Pregnancy study groups recommendations on the diagnosis and classification of hyperglycemia in pregnancy. Diabetes Care 2010;33:676–82.
18. Moses RG, Morris GJ, Petocz P, et al. The impact of potential new diagnostic criteria on the prevalence of gestational diabetes mellitus in Australia. Med J Aust 2010;194:338–40.
19. Hadden DR, Metzger BE, Lowe LP, et al. The Hyperglycemia and Adverse Pregnancy Outcome Study Cooperative Research Group. Screening and prevention of gestational diabetes. Diabetologia 2010;53(Suppl 1):S9.
20. Flack JR, Ross GP, Ho S, et al. Recommended changes to diagnostic criteria for gestational diabetes: impact on workload. Aust N Z J Obstet Gynaecol 2010;50: 439–43.
21. Combs CA, Moses RG. Aiming at new targets to achieve normoglycemia during pregnancy. Diabetes Care 2011;34:2331–2.
22. Evers IM, de Valk HW, Visser GH. Risk of complications of pregnancy in women with type 1 diabetes: nationwide prospective study in the Netherlands. BMJ 2004; 328:915–21.

23. Combs CA, Gunderson E, Kitzmiller JL, et al. Relationship of fetal macrosomia to maternal postprandial glucose control during pregnancy. Diabetes Care 1992;15: 1251–7.

24. Persson B, Swahn ML, Hjertberg R, et al. Insulin lispro therapy in pregnancies complicated by type 1 diabetes mellitus. Diabetes Res Clin Pract 2002;58: 115–21.

25. Lapolla A, Dalfrà MG, Spezia R, et al. Outcome of pregnancy in type 1 diabetic patients treated with insulin lispro or regular insulin: an Italian experience. Acta Diabetol 2008;45:61–6.

26. Wyatt JW, Frias JL, Hoyme HE, et al. Congenital anomaly rate in offspring of pre-gestational diabetic women treated with insulin lispro during pregnancy. Diabet Med 2004;21:2001–7.

27. Bhattacharyya A, Brown S, Huges S, et al. Insulin lispro and regular insulin in pregnancy. QJM 2001;94:255–60.

28. Mecacci F, Carignani L, Cioni R, et al. Maternal metabolic control and perinatal outcome in women with gestational diabetes treated with regular or lispro insulin: comparison with non-diabetic pregnant women. Eur J Obstet Gynecol Reprod Biol 2003;11:19–24.

29. Blanco CG, Ballesteros AC, Saladich IG, et al. Glycemic control and pregnancy outcomes in women with type 1 diabetes mellitus using lispro versus regular insulin: a systematic review and meta-analysis. Diabetes Technol Ther 2011;13: 907–11.

30. Hod M, Damm P, Kaaja R, et al. Fetal and perinatal outcomes in type 1 diabetes pregnancy: a randomized study comparing insulin aspart with human insulin in 322 subjects. Am J Obstet Gynecol 2008;198:186–93.

31. Heller S, Damm P, Mersebach H, et al. Hypoglycaemia in type 1 diabetes preg-nancy: role of preconception insulin aspart treatment in a randomized study. Diabetes Care 2010;33:473–7.

32. Hod M, McCance DR, Ivanisevic M et-al. Perinatal outcome in a randomized trial comparing insulin detemir with NPH insulin in 310 pregnant women with type 1 diabetes. Diabetes 2011;60(Suppl 1):A62.

33. Mathiesen ER, Damm P, Jovanovic L, et al. Basal insulin analogues in diabetic pregnancy: a literature review and baseline results of a randomised, controlled trial in type 1 diabetes. Diabetes Metab Res Rev 2011;27:543–51.

34. Farrar D, Tuffnell DJ, West J. Continuous subcutaneous insulin infusion versus multiple daily injections of insulin for pregnant women with diabetes. Cochrane Database Syst Rev 2007;3:CD005542.

35. Carr KJ, Idama TO, Masson EA, et al. A randomised controlled trial of insulin lis-pro given before or after meals in pregnant women with type 1 diabetes—the effect on glycemic excursion. J Obstet Gynaecol 2004;24:382–6.

36. Nachum Z, Ben-Shlomo I, Weiner E, et al. Twice daily versus four times daily insulin dose regimens for diabetes in pregnancy: randomised controlled trial. BMJ 1999;319:1223–7.

37. Crowther CA, Hiller JE, Moss JR, et al. Effect of treatment of gestational diabetes mellitus on pregnancy outcomes. N Engl J Med 2005;352:2477–86.

38. Landon MB, Spong CY, Thom E, et al. A multicenter, randomized trial of treatment for mild gestational diabetes. N Engl J Med 2009;361:1339–48.

39. Mathiesen ER, Ringholm L, Damm P. Therapeutic management of type 1 diabetes before and during pregnancy. Expert Opin Pharmacother 2011;12:779–86.

40. HAPO Study Cooperative Research Group. Hyperglycemia and adverse preg-nancy outcomes. N Engl J Med 2008;358:1991–2002.

41. Hernandez TL, Friedman JE, Van Pelt RE, et al. Patterns of glycemia in normal pregnancy: should the current therapeutic targets be challenged? Diabetes Care 2011; 34:1660–8.
42. Available at: http://care.diabetesjournals.org/content/32/Supplement_1/S13.full. pdf+html. Accessed December 23, 2011.
43. Available at: http://www.idf.org/webdata/docs/WDC-PC-IDF%20Guidelines% 20launch_FINAL.pdf. Accessed December 23, 2011.
44. Available at: http://www.nice.org.uk/nicemedia/live/11946/41320/41320.pdf. Accessed December 23, 2011.
45. Available at: http://www.adips.org. Accessed December 23, 2011.
46. Mathiesen ER, Vaz JA. Insulin treatment in diabetic pregnancy. Diabetes Metab Res Rev 2008;24(Suppl 2):S3–20.
47. Horvath K, Koch K, Jeitler K, et al. Effects of treatment in women with gestational diabetes mellitus: systematic review and meta-analysis. BMJ 2010;340:c1395. DOI: 10.1136/bmj.c1395.
48. Langer O, Levy J, Brustman L, et al. Glycemic control in gestational diabetes mellitus—how tight is tight enough: small for gestational age versus large for gestational age? Am J Obstet Gynecol 1989;161:646–53.
49. Middleton P, Crowther CA, Simmonds L, et al. Different intensities of glycemic control for pregnant women with pre-existing diabetes. Cochrane Database Syst Rev 2010;9:CD008540.
50. de Veciana M, Major CA, Morgan MA, et al. Postprandial versus preprandial blood glucose monitoring in women with gestational diabetes mellitus requiring insulin therapy. N Engl J Med 1995;333:1237–41.
51. Manderson JG, Patterson CC, Hadden DR, et al. Preprandial versus postprandial blood glucose monitoring in type 1 diabetic pregnancy: a randomized controlled clinical trial. Am J Obstet Gynecol 2003;189:507–12.
52. Taylor R, Lees C, Kyne-Grzebalski D, et al. Clinical outcomes of pregnancy in women with type 1 diabetes. Obstet Gynecol 2002;99:537–41.
53. Curet LB, Izquierdo LA, Gilson GJ, et al. Relative effects of antepartum and intrapartum maternal blood glucose levels on incidence of neonatal hypoglycaemia. J Perinatol 1997;17:162–4.
54. Lean MF, Pearson DW, Sutherland HW. Insulin management during labour and delivery in mothers with diabetes. Diabet Med 1990;7:162–4.
55. Lepercq J, Abbou H, Agostini C, et al. A standardized protocol to achieve normoglycaemia during labour and delivery in women with type 1 diabetes. Diabetes Metab 2008;34:33–7.
56. Rosenberg VA, Eglinton GS, Rauch ER, et al. Intrapartum maternal glycemic control in women with insulin requiring diabetes: a randomized clinical trial of rotating fluids versus insulin drip. Am J Obstet Gynecol 2006;195:1095–9.
57. Jovanovic L, Ilic S, Pettitt DJ, et al. The metabolic and immunologic effects of insulin lispro in gestational diabetes. Diabetes Care 1999;22:1422–6.
58. Ismail NA, Nor NA, Sufian SS, et al. Comparative study of two insulin regimes in pregnancy complicated by diabetes mellitus. Acta Obstet Gynecol 2007;86: 407–8.

Insulin Therapy for the Management of Hyperglycemia in Hospitalized Patients

Marie E. McDonnell, MD[a], Guillermo E. Umpierrez, MD[b],*

KEYWORDS

- Inpatient diabetes • Hyperglycemia • Hypoglycemia
- Critical illness • Hospital • Nutrition

It has long been established that hyperglycemia with or without a prior diagnosis of diabetes increases both mortality and disease-specific morbidity in hospitalized patients[1–4] and that goal-directed insulin therapy can improve outcomes.[5–9] During the past decade, since the widespread institutional adoption of intensified insulin protocols after the publication of a landmark trial,[5,10] the pendulum in the inpatient diabetes literature has swung away from achieving intensive glucose control and toward more moderate and individualized glycemic targets.[11,12] This change in clinical practice is the result of several factors, including challenges faced by hospitals to coordinate glycemic control across all levels of care,[13,14] publication of negative prospective trials,[15,16] revised recommendations from professional organizations,[17,18] and increasing evidence on the deleterious effect of hypoglycemia.[19–22] This article reviews the pathophysiology of hyperglycemia during illness, the mechanisms for increased complications and mortality due to hyperglycemia and hypoglycemia, beneficial mechanistic effects of insulin therapy and provides updated recommendations for the inpatient management of diabetes in the critical care setting and in the general medicine and surgical settings.[23,24]

PREVALENCE OF HYPERGLYCEMIA AND DIABETES IN HOSPITALIZED PATIENTS

The prevalence of diabetes around the world is alarmingly high and is growing. In 2007, it was estimated that approximately 23.6 million people in the United States

Dr Umpierrez is supported by research grants from the National Institutes of Health (UL1 RR025008) (Atlanta Clinical and Translational Science Institute) and American Diabetes Association (7-03-CR-35).

[a] Department of Medicine, Boston University School of Medicine, 88 East Newton Street, Boston, MA 02118, USA

[b] Department of Medicine, Emory University School of Medicine, 49 Jesse Hill Jr. Drive, Atlanta, GA 30303, USA

* Corresponding author.

E-mail address: geumpie@emory.edu

had diabetes, approximately 7.8% of the population, of whom 90% to 95% of these had type 2 diabetes mellitus.[25] Patients with diabetes have a 3-fold greater chance of hospitalization compared with those without diabetes,[26,27] and it is estimated that more than 20% of all adults discharged have diabetes, with 30% of them requiring 2 or more hospitalizations in any given year.[4,26,27]

The exact prevalence of hospital hyperglycemia is not known but it varies based on study populations and definitions used in previous reports. Observational studies have reported a prevalence of hyperglycemia ranging from 32% to 38% in community hospitals[4,28] to approximately 70% of diabetic patients with acute coronary syndrome[29] and approximately 80% of cardiac surgery patients in the perioperative period.[5,30] Patients with newly identified, or "stress," hyperglycemia may be at the highest risk of hyperglycemia-related morbidity and mortality. The American Diabetes Association (ADA) and American Association of Clinical Endocrinologists (AACE) consensus on inpatient hyperglycemia defined stress hyperglycemia or hospital-related hyperglycemia as any blood glucose (BG) concentration greater than 7.8 mmol/L (140 mg/dL). Although stress hyperglycemia typically resolves as the acute illness or surgical stress abates, it is important to identify and track patients because 60% of patients admitted with new hyperglycemia had confirmed diabetes at 1 year.[13] Cross-sectional studies of patients without a known history of diabetes with hyperglycemia revealed that between 30% and 60% of patients have impaired carbohydrate intolerance or diabetes during follow-up.[13] Until recently, clinical guidelines recommended that all patients with stress hyperglycemia should be tested with an oral glucose tolerance test shortly after discharge to assess carbohydrate tolerance.[10] More recently, the use of the hemoglobin A1c (HbA1c) test has been recommended versus the oral glucose tolerance test as the preferred diagnostic testing in hospitalized patients with hyperglycemia.[31] Measurement of HbA1c levels during periods of hospitalization provides an opportunity to differentiate patients with stress hyperglycemia from those with diabetes who were previously undiagnosed and to identify patients with known diabetes who would benefit from intensification of their glycemic management regimen.[32,33] The ADA recommendations indicate that patients with HbA1c level of 6.5% or higher can be identified as having diabetes.

PATHOPHYSIOLOGY OF HYPERGLYCEMIA DURING ILLNESS

Hyperglycemia is a frequent manifestation of critical and surgical illness, resulting from the acute metabolic and hormonal changes associated with the response to injury and stress.[34,35] Acute illness, surgery, and trauma raise levels of stress mediators, namely stress hormones, cytokines, and central nervous system, that interfere with carbohydrate metabolism, leading to excessive hepatic glucose output and reduced glucose uptake in peripheral tissues. In addition, acute illness increases proinflammatory cytokines, which increase insulin resistance by interfering with insulin signaling.

Regulation of Blood Glucose in Healthy Individuals

Maintenance of a constant BG level is essential for normal physiology in the body, particularly for the central nervous system. The brain can neither synthesize nor store the amount of glucose required for normal cellular function.[36] In the postabsorptive state, systemic glucose balance is maintained, and hypoglycemia and hyperglycemia are prevented, by dynamic, minute-to-minute regulation of endogenous glucose production from the liver and kidneys and of glucose use by peripheral tissues (**Fig. 1**).[37,38] Glucose production is accomplished by gluconeogenesis or glycogenolysis. By way of gluconeogenesis, noncarbohydrate precursors, such as lactate,

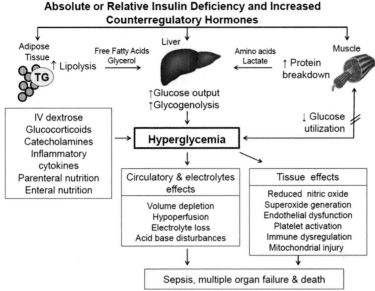

Fig. 1. Pathogenesis of hyperglycemia. Hyperglycemia during acute illness results from increased hepatic glucose production and impaired glucose use in peripheral tissues. Excess counterregulatory hormones (glucagon, cortisol, catecholamines, and growth hormone) increase lipolysis and protein breakdown (proteolysis) and impaired glucose use by peripheral tissues. Hyperglycemia causes osmotic diuresis that leads to hypovolemia decreased glomerular filtration rate and worsening hyperglycemia. At the cellular level, increased BG levels results in mitochondrial injury by generating reaction oxygen species and endothelial dysfunction by inhibiting nitric oxide production. Hyperglycemia increases levels of inflammatory cytokines, such as TNF-α; IL-6, leading to immune system dysfunction; and plasminogen activator inhibitor-1 and fibrinogen, causing platelet aggregation and hypercoagulable state. These changes can eventually lead to increased risk of infection, impaired wound healing, multiple organ failure, prolonged hospital stay, and death.

alanine, and glycerol, are converted to glucose. Excess glucose is polymerized to glycogen, which is mainly stored in the liver and muscle. Glycogenolysis breaks down glycogen to the individual glucose units for mobilization during times of metabolic need. These steps are dependent on the interaction of different mechanisms, including glucoregulatory hormones (insulin and counterregulatory hormones) and gluconeogenic substrate supply (lactate, glycerol, and amino acids). Insulin is the main glucoregulatory hormone and inhibits hepatic glucose production and stimulates peripheral glucose uptake.[36,39] In the liver, insulin directs glucose-6-phosphate to glycogen by increasing the activity of glycogen synthase and decreasing the activity of glycogen phosphorylase, which stimulates the breakdown of glycogen to glucose. In addition, insulin inhibits gluconeogenesis by inhibiting gene transcription and expression of phosphoenolpyruvate carboxykinase, the rate-limiting step in hepatic gluconeogenesis,[40,41] and by increasing the transcription of pyruvate kinase, the main glycolytic enzymes that produces pyruvate molecules, the final product of aerobic glycolysis.[42]

Pathogenesis of Hyperglycemia During Stress and Illness

Given the obligatory role of glucose to maintain normal physical function, it is not surprising that the normal response to stress or illness includes the release of counterregulatory hormones, which counteract insulin to increase the availability of glucose.[43] Counterregulatory hormones leads to several alterations in carbohydrate metabolism, including insulin resistance, increased hepatic glucose production, impaired peripheral glucose use, and relative insulin deficiency. In addition, high epinephrine levels stimulate glucagon secretion and inhibit insulin release by pancreatic β cells (**Table 1**).[44] High cortisol levels increase hepatic glucose production, stimulate protein catabolism, and increase circulating amino acids concentration, providing precursors for gluconeogenesis.[45,46]

Acute stress increases proinflammatory cytokines, such as tumor necrosis factor (TNF)-α, interleukin (IL)-6, and IL-1,[34,47–49] which increase insulin resistance by interfering with insulin signaling. TNF-α activates c-Jun N-terminal kinase, a signaling protein molecule that phosphorylates insulin receptor substrate-1 and prevents insulin-mediated activation of phosphatidylinositol 3-kinase involved in tissue glucose uptake. Downstream effect process decreases insulin stimulation of glucose uptake and causes hyperglycemia.[50,51]

Mechanisms of Detrimental Effects of Hyperglycemia

Although there are still no proved mechanisms to explain the detrimental effects of hyperglycemia in critically ill patients, several mechanisms may explain the higher risk of complications and mortality in hyperglycemic patients in the hospital (see **Fig. 1**). Severe hyperglycemia causes osmotic diuresis that leads to hypovolemia, decreased glomerular filtration rate, and prerenal azotemia. Hyperglycemia has also been shown to increase rate of hospital infections and poor wound healing.[52,53] Hyperglycemia is associated with impaired leukocyte function, including decreased phagocytosis, impaired bacterial killing, and chemotaxis.[54] Hyperglycemia has also been shown to impair collagen synthesis and to impair wound healing among patients with poorly controlled diabetes.[52] In addition, acute hyperglycemia results in nuclear factor κB (NF-κB) activation and production of inflammatory cytokines, such as TNF-α, IL-6, and plasminogen activator inhibitior-1, which cause increased vascular permeability and leukocyte and platelet activation.[55]

Table 1
Important counterregulatory hormones and mediators of inflammation known to be associated with acute hyperglycemia

Glucoregulatory Hormone	Metabolic Effect
Cortisol	↑ Skeletal muscle IR, ↑ lipolysis → ↑ gluconeogenesis
Epinephrine	↑ Skeletal muscle IR, ↑ gluconeogenesis and glycogenolysis, ↑ Lipolysis, ↓ insulin secretion from β cell
Norepinephrine	↑ Gluconeogenesis (at high levels), ↑ lipolysis
Glucagon	↑ Gluconeogenesis and glycogenolysis
Growth hormone	↑ Skeletal muscle IR, ↑ gluconeogenesis, ↑ lipolysis

Inflammation Mediators	Metabolic Effect
TNF-α	↑ Skeletal and hepatic IR
IL-1	↑ Skeletal and hepatic IR
IL-6	↑ Skeletal and hepatic IR
IL-18	↑ Skeletal and hepatic IR
FFAs	↑ Skeletal and hepatic IR, ↑ gluconeogenesis

Abbreviation: IR, insulin resistance.

Acute hyperglycemia activates oxidative pathway through increased generation of reactive oxygen species (ROS). ROS and the cellular redox state are increasingly thought to be responsible for affecting different biologic signaling pathways. ROS are formed from the reduction of molecular oxygen or by oxidation of water to yield products, such as superoxide anion, hydrogen peroxide, and hydroxyl radical; the mitochondria and NADP oxidase are the major sources of ROS production.[56] In moderate amounts, ROS are involved in several physiologic processes that produce desired cellular responses. Large quantities of ROS, however, can lead to cellular damage of lipids, membranes, proteins, and DNA.[57] Oxidative stress activates a series of stress pathways involving a family of serine/threonine kinases, which in turn have a negative effect on insulin signaling. Oxidative stress has also been implicated as a contributor to β-cell and mitochondrial dysfunction, which can lead to the development and worsening of hyperglycemia.[57]

In patients with acute ischemic cardiac events, acute hyperglycemia has been shown to attenuate ischemic preconditioning of the heart, a protective mechanism for ischemic injury, possibly by inhibiting activation of ATP-sensitive potassium channels that activates glycolysis.[58] Increasing evidence indicates that hyperglycemia may induce cardiac myocyte death through apoptosis or by exaggerating ischemia-reperfusion cellular injury.[53,59] High glucose concentrations also have deleterious effect on endothelial function by suppressing formation of nitric oxide and impairing endothelium-dependent flow-mediated dilation.[60] In addition, hyperglycemia induces abnormalities in hemostasis, including increased platelet activation, adhesion, and aggregation[61]; reduced plasma fibrinolytic activity; and increased plasminogen activator inhibitor-1 activity.[62] Adding to the effects of hyperglycemia in acute coronary syndrome, high free fatty acid (FFA) levels seen in diabetes and stress can also aggravate ischemia/reperfusion damage by limiting the ability of cardiac muscle to uptake glucose for anaerobic metabolism.[63,64] Although FFAs are the normal substrate of choice for healthy myocardium, high FFA levels are toxic to an ischemic myocardium,[63,64] leading to cardiac arrhythmias, sympathetic overactivity, increased blood pressure, oxidative stress, and endothelial dysfunction.[65–67] Increased FFAs also produce dose-dependent insulin resistance in peripheral tissues and increase hepatic glucose output in both diabetic and nondiabetic individuals.[35,68]

In patients with ischemic stroke, hyperglycemia has been shown to aggravate neuronal damage after brain ischemia.[53,69–71] During the progression of stroke, the area of ischemic penumbra (the region of the brain tissue surrounding the core of infarcted tissue where neurons still viable) is more sensitive to ischemic injury.[70,72] Studies using animal models of stroke have shown that hyperglycemia decreases reperfusion to the ischemic tissue and increases infarct volumes compared with normoglycemia.[73] Hemispheric cerebral blood flow has been shown reduced by as much as 37% in hyperglycemia compared with normoglycemia.[74] Increased tissue acidosis due to accumulation of lactate in the ischemic brain mediates ischemic injury by enhancing lipid peroxidation and free radical formation, accumulation of intracellular calcium, and impairing mitochondrial function.[70]

HYPERGLYCEMIA IN ACUTE ILLNESS: RATIONALE FOR PROACTIVE TREATMENT

Extensive observational and prospective randomized trials in patients with critical illness indicate a strong association between hyperglycemia and poor clinical outcome, such as mortality, morbidity, length of stay, infections, and overall complications.[4,75] This association is well documented on admission and also for the mean glucose level during the hospital stay.[2,3,76] Cross-sectional studies have shown that the risk of complications and mortality relates to the severity of hyperglycemia, with a higher risk observed in patients without a history of diabetes (new-onset and stress-induced hyperglycemia) compared with those with a known diagnosis of diabetes.

Glycemic Control Trials in Critical Care Setting

A large retrospective cohort study of more than 250,000 veterans admitted to various ICUs in the United States found that the development of hyperglycemia is an independent risk for mortality in individuals with cardiac diagnoses, sepsis, and respiratory failure.[76] In cardiac surgery patients, perioperative hyperglycemia has been associated with increased length of stay, delayed extubation, increased risk of perioperative complications, and mortality.[77] Similarly, several observational studies and meta-analyses in patients with myocardial infarction[29,78] and with stroke and subarachnoid hemorrhage[70,73,79] have consistently reported that hyperglycemia on admission or during the hospital stay is associated with poor clinical outcome and a higher risk of mortality, independently from other predictors of a poor prognosis, such as age and diabetic status. In a nonrandomized, prospective study, Furnary and colleagues[2] followed 3554 patients with diabetes who underwent coronary artery bypass graft and were treated with either subcutaneous insulin or continuous insulin infusion (CII) for hyperglycemia. Compared with patients treated with subcutaneous insulin who had average BG level of 11.9 mmol/L (214 mg/dL), patients treated with CII with average BG level of 9.8 mmol/L (177 mg/dL) had significantly less deep sternal wound infections and a reduction in risk-adjusted mortality by 50%.[7] A follow-up analysis in a subset of this study population revealed that patients with BG levels greater than 11.1 mmol/L (>200 mg/dL) had higher mortality (5.0% vs 1.8%, $P<.001$) than those with BG levels less than 11.1 mmol/L.[2] Similarly, the Leuven surgical ICU study reported that intensive therapy to maintain target glucose levels 4.4 mmol/L to 6.1 mmol/L (80–110 mg/dL) compared with conventional therapy to maintain target levels between 10 mmol/L and 11.1 mmol/L (180–200 mg/dL) significantly reduced the frequency of bacteremia, antibiotic requirements, length of ventilator dependency, number of ICU days, and an an overall mortality (34% reduction).[5] In a different study, these investigators following the same protocol in medical ICU patients also reported less ICU and hospital mortality after 3 days of treatment with CII.[15]

Recent randomized controlled trials, however, have shown that intensive glycemic control (target glucose <110 mg/dL) has been difficult to achieve without increasing the risk for severe hypoglycemia,[16,80–82] causing some to be discontinued early (**Table 2**). In addition, several multicenter trials have failed to show significant improvement in clinical outcome or have resulted in increased mortality risk.[16,80–83] The largest and recent Normoglycemia in Intensive Care Evaluation Survival Using Glucose Algorithm Regulation (NICE-SUGAR) trial, with more than 6000 subjects from different ICUs,[16] randomized patients to receive either conventional glycemic control (<10 mmol/L [<180 mg/dL]) or intensive glycemic control (4.5–6 mmol/L [81–108 mg/dL]) and reported that intensive glycemic control was associated with increased mortality at 90 days (24.9% vs 27.5%, $P = .02$) and higher incidence of hypoglycemia (6.8% vs 0.5%, $P<.001$).[16]

Hyperglycemia and Noncritical Illness

The importance of hyperglycemia also applies to non–critically ill patients admitted to general medicine and surgery services. In such patients, hyperglycemia is associated with poor hospital outcomes, including prolonged hospital stay, infections, disability after hospital discharge, and death.[4,84] In a retrospective study of 1886 patients admitted to a community hospital, mortality was significantly higher in patients with newly diagnosed hyperglycemia and those with known diabetes compared with those with normoglycemia (10% vs 1.7% vs 0.8%, respectively; P<.01).[4] Admission hyperglycemia has also been linked to worse outcomes in patients with community-acquired pneumonia.[85] In a prospective cohort multicenter study of 2471 patients, those with admission glucose levels greater 11 mmol/L (198 mg/dL) had a greater risk of mortality and complications than those with glucose less than 11 mmol/L. The risk of in-hospital complications increased 3% for each 1 mmol/L increase in admission glucose. In a retrospective study of 348 patients with chronic obstructive pulmonary disease and respiratory tract infection, the relative risk of death was 2.10 in those with a BG levels of 7 mmol/L to 8.9 mmol/L (126–160 mg/dL) and 3.42 for those with BG levels greater than 9.0 mmol/L (162 mg/dL) compared with patients with BG levels 6.0 mmol/L (110 mg/dL).[86] Furthermore, each 1 mmol/L increase in BG level was associated with a 15% increase in the risk of an adverse clinical outcome, which was defined as death or length of stay of greater than 9 days.

Several observational studies in general surgery patients admitted to noncritical care areas have also shown that hyperglycemia is associated with increased risks of perioperative complications, length of stay, and mortality.[87–90] Patients with glucose levels of 5.6 mmol/L to 11.1 mmol/L (110–200 mg/dL) and those with glucose levels greater than 11.1 mmol/L (>200 mg/dL) had, respectively, a 1.7-fold and 2.1-fold increased mortality compared with those with glucose levels less than 5.6 mmol/L (<110 mg/dL). General surgery patients with glucose levels greater than 12.2 mmol/L (>220 mg/dL) on the first postoperative day had a 2.7-times increased rate of infection.[89] The risk of postoperative infection rate in patients undergoing noncardiac general surgery was estimated to increase by 30% for every 2.2 mmol/L (40 mg/dL) rise in the presence of hyperglycemia.[91] A recent study in 3184 general surgery patients in non-ICU setting reported a strong association between presurgery and postsurgery hyperglycemia and postoperative cases of pneumonia, systemic blood infection, urinary tract infection, acute renal failure, and acute myocardial infarction.[87] In that study, multivariate analysis adjusted for age, gender, race, and surgery severity found that the risk of death increased in proportion to perioperative glucose levels; however, this association was significant only for patients without a history of diabetes compared with patients with a known history of diabetes.[87] Patients without a history of diabetes (stress hyperglycemia) experiencing worse outcome and higher mortality at a same glucose level than those with known history of diabetes suggests a lack of adaptation to acute hyperglycemia and its associated inflammatory and oxidative state.

Beneficial Mechanistic Effects of Insulin Therapy

The adverse outcomes associated with hyperglycemia may be attributed to the inflammatory and pro-oxidant effects observed with increased glucose levels. Many of the adverse outcomes can be prevented by administration of insulin. The positive effects of insulin administration are attributed to its anti-inflammatory, vasodilatory, and antioxidant effects as well as its ability to inhibit lipolysis and platelet aggregation. Several studies have reported that elevated levels of cytokines and inflammatory markers associated with severe hyperglycemia return to normal shortly after the treatment with insulin and resolution of hyperglycemia.[48] Insulin acts to suppress counterregulatory hormones and proinflammatory transcription factors and may even suppress the formation of ROS.[34,92] Insulin suppresses the proinflammatory transcription factors, NF-κB and early growth response-1.[93–95] Recent

Table 2
Summary of key randomized clinical trials designed to test effect of glycemic control in critical illness

Author	Population	Design/Endpoint	No. of Patients	Achieved Glycemic Endpoints (Mean ± SD [mg/dL])		Hospital Mortality OR (95% CI)[a]	Comments
				Control	Glycemic Control		
Van den Berghe et al[5,15]	Surgical, mechanical ventilation	Randomized 80–110 vs 180–200 mg/dL Research RN-titrated insulin per protocol	1548	Daily 153 ± 33	Daily 103 ± 19 (P<.001)	0.64 (0.45–0.91)	High use of parenteral dextrose (in TPN); stopped early for benefit
Van den Berghe et al[5,15]	Medical, expected ICU stay >72 h	Randomized Bedside RN-titrated per paper protocol	1200	Daily 153 ± 31	Daily 111 ± 29 (P<.001)	0.89 (0.71–1.13)	High use of parenteral dextrose (in TPN)
Presier GLUCONTROL[163]	Medical, surgical	Randomized 80–110 vs 140–180 mg/dL Bedside RN-titrated per protocol	1078	144 (IQR 128–162) median—all values	117 (IQR 108–130) median—all values	1.27 (0.94–1.7)	Stopped early for hypoglycemia; many protocol violations
NICE-SUGAR[16]	Medical, surgical	Randomized 80–110 vs 140–180 mg/dL Adjusted via computerized algorithm	6104	144 ± 23	115 ± 18 (P<.001)	28-Day mortality: 1.09 (0.96–1.23) 90-Day mortality: 1.14 (1.02–1.28)	GC group did not achieve target

Study	Population	Intervention	N	Control glucose	GC glucose	Outcome (OR or rate)	Comments
Brunkhorst et al[80] (VISEP)	Sepsis	Randomized 80–110 vs 180–200 mg/dL Bedside RN-titrated per Van den Berghe protocol	537	Median—daily 138 (IQR 111–184)	Median—daily 130 (IQR 108–167) (P = .05)	28-Day mortality: 0.94 (0.63–1.38)	GC group did not achieve target; study stopped early for hypoglycemia risk; underpowered
De La Rosa et al[81]	Medical, surgical	Randomized 80–110 vs 180–200 mg/dL Bedside RN-titrated per protocol	504	Median— all values 149 (IQR 124–180)	Median— all values 120 (IQR 110–134) (P<.001)	28-Day mortality: 1.09 (0.75–1.54)	GC group did not achieve target; underpowered
Arabi et al[165]	Medical, surgical	Randomized 80–110 vs 180–200 mg/dL Bedside RN-titrated per paper protocol	523	171 ± 34	115 ± 18 (P<.0001)	0.78 (0.53–1.13)	Underpowered
Farah et al[168]	Medical with >3-day LOS	Randomized 110–140 vs 140–200 mg/dL	89	174 ± 20	142 ± 14	28-Day mortality: 54% vs 46% (P>.05)	Underpowered; vascular morbidity lower with GC
Gray and Perdrizet[169]	Surgical, excluded patients with diabetes	Randomized 80–120 mg/dL vs 180–220 mg/dL	61	179 ± 61	125 ± 36 mg/dL; daily mean value lower on each day	21% vs 11% (P = .5)	Underpowered; lower nosocomial infection incidence with GC
Mackenzie et al[170]	Medical, surgical, trauma	Randomized 72–108 vs 180–198 mg/dL	240	144 ± 40 Time-weighted mean	113 ± 22 Time-weighted mean	40% vs 32% (P = .28)	Stopped early due to financial limits

Abbreviations: GC, glycemic control; IQR, interquartile; IV, intravenous; LOS, length of stay; OR, odds ratio; RN, registered nurse; SQ, subcutaneous; TPN, total parenteral nutrition.

[a] Hospital mortality unless otherwise specified. OR <1 indicates benefit due to glycemic control. Outcome prevalence written as control group vs glycemic control.

studies have also shown that insulin administration is associated with a decrease in the concentration of compounds whose gene transcription is modulated by these factors, including plasminogen activator inhibitor-1, intercellular adhesion molecule-1, monocyte chemotactic protein-1, and monocyte chemotactic protein-9.[93,95] Additionally, insulin induces vasodilation and inhibits lipolysis and platelet aggregation. The vasodilation that accompanies insulin administration may be attributed to its ability to stimulate nitric oxide release and induce the expression of endothelial nitric oxide synthase.

GLYCEMIC TARGETS IN ICU AND NON-ICU SETTINGS

The AACE/ADA Task Force on Inpatient Glycemic Control recommended targeting a BG level between 7.8 mmol/L and 10.0 mmol/L (140 and 180 mg/dL) for the majority of ICU patients and lower glucose targets between 6.1 mmol/L and 7.8 mmol/L (110 and 140 mg/dL) in selected ICU patients (ie, centers with extensive experience and appropriate nursing support, cardiac surgical patients, and patients with stable glycemic control without hypoglycemia). Glucose targets greater than 10 mmol/L (>180 mg/dL) or less than 6.1 mmol/L (<110 mg/dL) are not recommended in ICU patients due to lack of proved benefit and potential risk in both large and small prospective randomized trials (see **Table 2**).

In non-ICU settings, the AACE/ADA Practice Guideline[18,96] recommends a premeal glucose level less than 140 mg/dL (7.8 mmol/L) and a random BG level less than 10.0 mmol/L (180 mg/dL) for the majority of non–critically ill patients treated with insulin.[96] To avoid hypoglycemia (<3.9 mmol/L), the total basal and prandial insulin dose should be reduced if glucose levels fall between less than 3.9 mmol/L and 5.6 mmol/L (70–100 mg/dL). In contrast, higher glucose ranges may be acceptable in terminally ill patients or in patients with severe comorbidities as well as in those in patient-care settings where frequent glucose monitoring or close nursing supervision is not feasible.[18,96,97] In such patients, however, it is prudent to maintain a reasonable degree of glycemic control (BG <11.1 mmol/L [200 mg/dL]) as a way of avoiding symptomatic hyperglycemia.

MANAGING HYPERGLYCEMIA IN THE HOSPITAL ENVIRONMENT

Despite solid evidence in support of glycemic control in hospitalized patients, BG control continues to be deficient and is frequently overlooked in critically ill patients and in general medicine and surgery services.[4,98] Many factors could explain the physician's inactivity in addressing in-hospital hyperglycemia. First, hyperglycemia is rarely the focus of care during the hospital stay, because the overwhelming majority of hospitalizations in patients with hyperglycemia occur for comorbid conditions.[4,99] Second, fear of hypoglycemia constitutes a major barrier to efforts to improve glycemic control in hospitalized subjects, especially in patients with poor caloric intake.[100] Third, in the presence of altered nutrition and associated medical illness, physicians frequently hold a patient's previous outpatient diabetes regimen and initiate sliding scale coverage with regular insulin. Finally, the specific morbidities due to secondary causes of hyperglycemia, such as steroid-exacerbated hyperglycemia, remain largely unknown.[101] Hospital care of patients with diabetes and hyperglycemia is complex, involving multiple providers with varying degrees of expertise who are dispersed across many different areas of the hospital. A multidisciplinary systems approach with identifiable hospital champions can help guide meaningful progress away from clinical inertia and toward safe glycemic control, insulin management, and hypoglycemia prevention.[18,102]

Glucose Monitoring in Hospital

Bedside capillary point of care (POC) testing is the preferred method for guiding ongoing glycemic management of individual patients.[18] POC testing is usually performed 4 times a day: before meals and at bedtime for patients who are eating.[53,96] For patients who are restricted to nothing by mouth or are receiving continuous enteral nutrition, POC testing is recommended every 4 to 6 hours. More frequent glucose monitoring is indicated in patients treated with continuous intravenous insulin infusion[103,104] or after a medication change that could alter glycemic control (eg, corticosteroid use or abrupt discontinuation of enteral or parenteral nutrition)[101,105,106] or in patients with frequent episodes of hypoglycemia.[11,53]

Health care workers should keep in mind that the accuracy of most hand-held glucose meters is far from optimal.[107] There is an accepted variance between meter readings and central laboratory results (up to 20% allowed by Food and Drug Administration regulations),[96,108] which can potentially lead to inappropriate therapy. Many patient factors are known to affect the accuracy of the POC testing including pH changes, oxygenation status, and low hematocrit, among others.[107,109]

Medical Nutrition Therapy in Hospitalized Patients with Diabetes

Medical nutrition therapy (MNT) plays an important role in management of hyperglycemia in hospitalized patients with diabetes mellitus and often requires specifically designed insulin programs. The goals of inpatient MNT for patients with diabetes are to help optimize glycemic control, provide adequate calories to meet metabolic demands, address individuals needs based on personal food preferences, and provide a discharge plan for follow-up care.[53,97,110] MNT in the hospital can be challenging in the presence of acute medical illness, poor appetite, inability to eat, increased nutrient and calorie needs due to catabolic stress, and variation in diabetes medications.

The metabolic needs of most hospitalized subjects can be supported by providing 25 to 35 cal/kg/d[111,112] whereas critically ill patients require less caloric intake at 15 to 25 cal/kg/d.[113] This translates into a diet on average containing 1800 to 2000 cal/d[53] or a diet containing approximately 200 g/d of carbohydrates divided between meals.[112] Care must be taken not to overfeed patients because this can exacerbate hyperglycemia. There is no single meal planning system that is ideal for hospitalized patients. It is suggested, however, that hospitals consider implementing a consistent carbohydrate diabetes meal-planning system.[112] This systems uses meal plans without a specific calorie level but with consistency in the carbohydrate content of meals. The carbohydrate components of breakfast, lunch, dinner, and snacks may vary, but the day-to-day carbohydrate content of specific meals and snacks is kept constant.[53,112] It is recommended that the term, *ADA diet*, no longer be used, because the ADA no longer endorses a single nutrition prescription or percentages of macronutrients.[112]

Patients requiring clear or full liquid diets should receive approximately 200 g/day of carbohydrates in equally divided amounts at meal and snack times. Liquids should not all be sugar-free because patients require sufficient carbohydrate and calories, and sugar-free liquids do not meet these nutritional needs. After surgery, food intake should be initiated as quickly as possible with progression from clear liquids to full liquids to solid foods as rapidly as tolerated.[112,114] Increasing evidence, however, indicates that early enteral feeding in the perioperative period is safe and well tolerated and results in reduction of wound morbidity and healing, fewer septic complications, diminished weight loss, and improved protein kinetics.[114]

Enteral Nutrition

Although the majority of non–critically ill hospitalized patients receive nutrition support as 3 discrete meals with or without scheduled snacks each day, some patients may require enteral nutrition support. Standard enteral formulas reflect the reference values for macronutrients and micronutrients for a healthy population and contain 1 to 2 calories per milliliter. Standard diabetes-specific formulas provide low amounts of lipids (30% of total calories) combined with a high carbohydrate content (55%–60% of total calories); however, newer diabetic formulas have replaced part of carbohydrates with monounsaturated fatty acids (up to 35% of total calories), 10 g/L to 15 g/L dietary fiber, and up to 30% fructose.[115,116] Several outpatient and inpatient studies in subjects with type 2 diabetes mellitus have reported better glycemic control (lower mean, fasting, and/or postprandial glucose levels), a trend toward decreased HbA1c levels, and lower insulin requirements with a low-carbohydrate, high–monounsaturated fatty acids (LCHM) formulas compared with a standard high-carbohydrate formulas.[117,118] In a meta-analysis of studies comparing enteral LCHM formulas with standard formulations, the postprandial glucose rise was reduced by 18 mg/dL to 29 mg/dL with the newer formulations.[119]

Parenteral Nutrition

The beneficial effect of parenteral nutrition in improving the nutritional status of critically ill patients is well established.[120] Recent randomized trials and meta-analyses, however, have suggested that parenteral nutrition may be associated with increased risk of infectious complications and mortality in critically ill patients.[120,121] In addition, its use has been linked to aggravation of hyperglycemia independent of a prior history of diabetes.[121,122] BG level measures above 150 mg/dL before and within 24 hours of initiation of parenteral nutrition are predictors of both increased inpatient complications and hospital mortality. Although randomized controlled studies to guide effective and safe administration of insulin during parenteral nutrition are lacking, patients with or without history of diabetes with persistent hyperglycemia (>140 mg/dL) should be treated with insulin therapy. To correct hyperglycemia, regular insulin can be added to parenteral nutrition solutions or can be given as continuous insulin infusion.

PHARMACOLOGIC TREATMENT OF INPATIENT HYPERGLYCEMIA

Insulin, given either intravenously or subcutaneously, is the preferred regimen for effectively treating hyperglycemia in the hospital. The use of oral antidiabetic agents should be avoided in the hospital setting because no data are available on their safety and efficacy in the inpatient setting.[53,98] Major limitations to the use of oral agents for hospital use are their slow onset of action that does not allow rapid glycemic control and dose adjustments to meet the changing needs of acutely ill patients and risk of hypoglycemia with insulin secretagogues. Sulfonylureas may increase the risk of hypoglycemia in hospitalized patients with poor appetite or ordered dietary restrictions. In addition, they may worsen cardiac and cerebral ischemia[123–126] by inhibiting ATP-sensitive potassium channels, resulting in cell membrane depolarization and increased intracellular calcium concentration.[127] Many patients have one or more contraindications to the use of metformin on admission,[128] including acute congestive heart failure, renal or liver dysfunction, and chronic pulmonary disease. The use of thiazolidinediones is limited because they can increase intravascular volume and may precipitate or worsen congestive heart failure and peripheral edema.[129,130] Despite their benign side-effect profile and single oral daily dose of dipeptidyl peptidase-IV inhibitors,[131] these agents have a minor reduction in glucose concentration, and no previous studies have assessed their efficacy and safety in hospitalized patients.

Insulin Therapy in Critical Care

In the critical care setting, a variety of CII protocols have been shown effective in achieving glycemic control and in improving hospital outcome with a low-rate of hypoglycemic events.[2,132] In most patients, CII lowers BG levels to target range in approximately 4 to 8 hours and allows for rapid titration of dose for both anticipated (eg, initiation or discontinuation of vasopressors) or unanticipated (eg, acute deteriorations in clinical status) changes in clinical status. Essential elements that increase protocol success of CII are (1) rate adjustment considers the current and previous glucose value and the current rate of insulin infusion, (2) rate adjustment considers the rate of change (or lack of change) from the previous reading, and (3) frequent glucose monitoring (hourly until stable glycemia is established, and then every 2–3 h) **(Fig. 2)**.[132–134] BG level greater than140 mg/dL should trigger initiation of insulin therapy, titrated to maintain glucose values absolutely between 140 mg/dL and 180 mg/dL while avoiding hypoglycemia. Using a higher trigger value to start insulin treatment could allow excursion to glucose values above 180 mg/dL, which is undesirable with respect to the immunosuppressive effects.

Recently, computer-based algorithms aiming to direct the nursing staff in adjusting insulin infusion rates have become commercially available.[135,136] Controlled trials have reported more rapid and tighter glycemic control with computer-guided algorithms than with standard paper form protocols in ICU patients.[137] Uuse of computer-based algorithms has been associated with lower glycemic variability and a higher percentage of BG level readings within target range than treating patients with the standard regimen. The clinical importance of the degree of variability and rapidity of fluctuations in glucose levels in critically ill patients is a topic of recent interest because it has been identified as an independent contributor to the risk of mortality in critically ill patients.[138] Despite differences in glycemic control between insulin algorithms, no clinical outcome differences have been reported in the frequency of severe hypoglycemic events, length of ICU and hospital stay, or mortality. Thus, most insulin algorithms seem appropriate alternatives for the management of hyperglycemia in critically ill patients, and the choice depends on physician preferences and cost considerations.[132,139,140]

The use of subcutaneous insulin has not been formally studied in ICU patients and should be avoided in critical ill patients, in particular during hypotension or shock. Many factors can affect insulin absorption during critical illness and in the perioperative period.[141] The net of these factors is increased potential for overlapping dose effects, administration timing errors, and unexpected hypoglycemia.

Transition from Intravenous Insulin Infusion to Subcutaneous Insulin

All patients with type 1 diabetes mellitus and most patients with type 2 diabetes mellitus receiving CII in critical care setting require transitioning to a subcutaneous insulin regimen.[9,18,142,143] Several models have been proposed for transition from insulin infusion to subcutaneous insulin therapy.[144–147] In general, the initial dose and distribution of subcutaneous insulin at the time of transition can be determined by extrapolating the intravenous insulin requirement over the preceding 6 to 8 hours to a 24-hour period.[53,146] The total daily dose of insulin can also be calculated based on body weight, which could emulate general subcutaneous weight-based insulin guidelines. It is important that consideration be given to a patient's nutritional status and

Continuous Insulin Infusion Protocol
Target BG =110 – 180 mg/dL

If bolus is ordered by MD, give 0.1 unit/Kg (IV push). Calculate initial IV Insulin infusion rate as follows

BG/ 100 = units/hour = mL/hour (round to nearest 0.1 Unit)
Check BG in 1 hour, titrate per protocol below. (Insulin drip= 1 unit/mL)

Did the BG increase or change by 30 mg/dL from the prior BG?			
BG (mg/dL)	**WITH ANY INCREASE** in BG from prior BG	**BG DECREASE** LESS than 30 mg/dL from prior BG	**BG DECREASE** GREATER than or EQUAL to 30 mg/dL from prior BG
241 or greater	Increase rate by 3 units/hr	Increase rate by 3 units/hr	NO CHANGE
211 – 240	Increase rate by 2 units/hr	Increase rate by 2 units/hr	NO CHANGE
181 – 210	Increase rate by 1 unit/hr	Increase rate by 1 unit/hr	NO CHANGE
141 – 180	NO CHANGE	NO CHANGE	NO CHANGE
110 – 140	NO CHANGE	NO CHANGE	Decrease rate by 1/2
91 – 109	Decrease rate by 1/2	Decrease rate by 1/2	1.HOLD insulin drip. 2.Check BG q 1 hour: Restart infusion rate at 1/2 prior infusion rate when BG greater than 180 mg/dL

71 – 90	1. HOLD insulin drip. 2. Check BG q 30 minutes until BG is greater than 90mg/dL then check BG q 1 hour. 3. Restart prior infusion rate at 1/2 rate when BG greater than180 mg/dL
70 or Less	1. HOLD insulin drip 2. Give IV D50 • BG 41 – 70 mg/dL: give 1/2 amp D50 IV or 8 ounce juice PO • BG 40 mg/dL or less: give 1 amp D50 IV 3. Repeat BG q 15 minutes until BG greater than 70 mg/dL, then check BG q 30 minutes until BG greater than 90 mg/dL 4. BG greater than 90 mg/dL,, Check BG q 1 hour; Restart infusion at 1/2 prior infusion rate when BG greater than 180 mg/dL

When BG reaches target (BG=110-180 mg/dL) for 2 consecutive readings, check BG q 2 hours

Critical Values: Treat for BG less than 45 mg/dL or greater than 450 mg/dL per protocol then Notify MD.

If patient's BG levels continue to increase after 2 interventions, notify MD.

Fig. 2. Example of insulin infusion protocol. Essential elements that increase protocol success of CII are (1) rate adjustment considers the current and previous glucose value and the current rate of insulin infusion, (2) rate adjustment considers the rate of change (or lack of change) from the previous reading, and (3) frequent glucose monitoring.

medications, with continuation of glucose monitoring to guide ongoing adjustments in the insulin dose, because changes in insulin sensitivity can occur during acute illness.

Recent literature on transition methodology discusses 2 general principles behind safe and effective transition from intravenous to subcutaneous insulin: (1) the 24-hour insulin requirement is extrapolated from an appropriately selected hourly insulin rate and (2) the subcutaneous insulin program is designed to fit a patient's nutrition program.[146,148] Strategies to find the basal dose include taking 80% of the total amount of insulin used in the preceding 24 hours and splitting it into basal and prandial insulin to maintain glucose in the optimal range.[146] To prevent recurrence of hyperglycemia during the transition to subcutaneous insulin, it is important to allow an overlap of 1 to 2 hours between discontinuation of intravenous insulin and the administration of subcutaneous insulin. For patients who are not receiving significant amount of calories, the basal dose can be given in 1 single, long-acting, daily insulin (eg, glargine or detemir) dose or 2 intermediate-acting insulin (neutral protamine Hagedorn [NPH]) doses every 12 hours. Short-acting insulins (regular) or rapid-acting insulins (aspart, glulisine, and lispro) can be added as needed depending on nutritional intake and glucose levels.

Most patients with stress hyperglycemia and with normal HbA1c levels who have been on CII in the ICU at rates less than or equal to 1 to 2 U/h at the time of transition do not require a scheduled subcutaneous insulin regimen. Many of these patients can be treated with correction insulin to determine if they require scheduled subcutaneous insulin.

Insulin Therapy in the Non–Critical Care Setting

Subcutaneous insulin is the preferred therapeutic agent for BG control in the non-ICU setting. No single insulin regimen meets the needs for all subjects with hyperglycemia. Scheduled subcutaneous insulin therapy with basal or intermediate acting insulin given once or twice a day in combination with short-acting or rapid-acting insulin administered before meals is preferred as an effective and safe strategy for glycemic management in non–critically ill patients.[18,149] Subcutaneous insulin programs should address the 3 components of insulin requirement: basal (what is required in the fasting state), nutritional (what is required for glucose elevations or to dispose of glucose in hyperglycemia) **(Fig. 3)**.[149]

The practice of discontinuing oral diabetes medications and/or insulin therapy and starting sliding scale insulin (SSI) results in undesirable levels of hypoglycemia and hyperglycemia.[150,151] The SSI regimen, although straightforward and easy to use, is faced with several challenges that include inadequate coverage of glycemic excursions and insulin stacking.[152] The authors recently reported the results of a prospective, randomized multicenter trial comparing the efficacy and safety of a basal/bolus insulin regimen with basal bolus regimen and SSI in patients with type 2 diabetes mellitus admitted to general medicine wards.[153] The authors found that among 130 insulin-naïve patients with an admission BG level between 140 mg/dL and 400 mg/dL, the use of basal-bolus insulin had greater improvement in BG control than sliding scale alone. A BG target of less than 140 mg/dL was achieved in 66% of patients in the glargine plus glulisine group and 38% in the sliding scale group. One-fifth of patients treated with an SSI without a basal component had persistently elevated BG level greater than 240 mg/dL during the hospital stay. The incidence of hypoglycemia, defined as a BG level less than 3.3 mmol/L (<60 mg/dL), was low in this study. In general surgery patients, the recent RAndomized Study of Basal Bolus Insulin Therapy in the Inpatient Management of Patients with Type 2 Diabetes Undergoing General Surgery (RABBIT 2 Surgery) trial[154] compared the efficacy and safety of basal bolus regimen to SSI in 211 patients with type 2 diabetes mellitus. Study outcomes included differences in daily glucose levels and a composite of postoperative complications, including wound infection, pneumonia, respiratory failure, acute renal failure, and bacteremia. Patients were randomized to receive basal bolus regimen with glargine and glulisine (starting dose of 0.5 U/kg/d) or SSI (4 times/d). The basal bolus regimen resulted in significant improvement in glucose control and a reduction in the frequency of the composite complications. The results of these trials indicate that basal bolus regimen is preferred to SSI and results in improved glycemic control and lower rate of hospital complications in general medical and surgical patients with type 2 diabetes mellitus.

An open-label, controlled, multicenter trial randomly assigned 130 medical patients with type 2 diabetes mellitus to receive detemir once daily and aspart before meals with NPH and regular insulin twice daily.[155] Both treatment regimens resulted in

Subcutaneous Insulin orders

1. **Check capillary blood glucose (BG)**
   - ☐ Before meals and at bedtime   ☐ Before meals, bedtime, and 03:00
   - ☐ Every 6 hours (patients on continuous tube feeds or NPO)

2. **Scheduled Subcutaneous Insulin** *(Recommend use ½ daily dose as basal and other ½ as prandial)*

Basal Insulin*	BREAKFAST	LUNCH	DINNER	BEDTIME
	Give ____ units ☐ NPH ☐ Glargine ☐ Determir		Give ____ units ☐ NPH ☐ Glargine ☐ Determir	Give ____ units ☐ NPH ☐ Glargine ☐ Determir
Prandial Insulin**†	BREAKFAST Give ____ units ☐ Lispro ☐ Aspart ☐ Glulisine ☐ Regular	LUNCH Give ____ units ☐ Lispro ☐ Aspart ☐ Glulisine ☐ Regular	DINNER Give ____ units ☐ Lispro ☐ Aspart ☐ Glulisine ☐ Regular	BEDTIME
Continuous feeds or NPO (q6h)	0600 Give ____ units Regular insulin	1200 Give ____ units Regular insulin	1800 Give ____ units Regular insulin	2400 Give ____ units Regular insulin

*Give NPH insulin: twice daily, Glargine: once daily, and Detemir: Once or twice daily
** Give lispro/Aspart immediately before or after meals. Give regular insulin 30 minutes prior to meals
† Patients with inconsistent oral intake: RN may reduce prandial dose of aspart based on the percent of meal ingested (e.g. if 50% of calories are ingested, give 50% of the dose)

3. **Supplemental/Correction Insulin (regular, lispro, aspart, glulisine) ADD to dose of scheduled insulin.**
   *** Check appropriate column below and cross out other columns

<u>BEFORE MEALS</u> add supplemental insulin dose (# of units) from table below to the scheduled insulin dose.

<u>BEDTIME</u>. Give ½ of supplemental sliding scale Insulin dose at bedtime

Blood Glucose (mg/dL)	☐ Insulin Sensitive	☐ Usual	☐ Insulin Resistant
<141	0	0	0
>141-180	1	2	4
181-220	2	4	6
221-260	4	6	8
261-300	6	8	10
301-350	8	10	12
351-400	10	12	14
> 400	12	14	16

Physician: _____   ID#: _____   Pager#: _____
Nurse Signature: _____   Title: _____   Time: _____

Fig. 3. Use of insulin ordering forms to prescribe basal/bolus insulin programs. Insulin order forms are useful to illustrate and encourage the use of the 3 components of a patient-tailored insulin program (eg, basal, nutritional, and supplemental/correction).

significant improvements in inpatient glycemic control with a glucose target of less than 140 mg/dL before meals achieved in 45% in the detemir/aspart group and in 48% of NPH/regular insulin group. Hypoglycemia (<60 mg/dL) was observed in approximately one-fourth of patients treated with detemir/aspart and NPH/regular insulin during the hospital stay. There were no differences in length of hospital stay or mortality between groups. Thus, it seems that similar improvement in glycemic control can be achieved with either basal bolus therapy with detemir/aspart or with NPH/regular insulin in general medical patients with type 2 diabetes mellitus.

Initial insulin doses of basal bolus protocols vary widely from 0.3 U/kg/d to 1.5 U/kg/d,[53,153,156,157] although only the initial starting dose range between 0.4 U/kg/d and 0.5 U/kg/d, divided into a balanced basal bolus regimen, has been studied prospectively.[153,154] A case-control analysis of 1990 patients with diabetes using hypoglycemia as a tool to identify insulin dose ranges based on risk reported that a total daily dose of 0.6 U/kg seems to be the threshold below which the odds of hypogly-cemia are low and that doses more than 0.79 U/kg/d are associated with a 3-fold higher odds of hypoglycemia than doses lower than 0.2 U/kg/d. Thus, it may be reasonable to consider lower initial daily doses ($\leq$0.3 U/kg) in patients with hypogly-cemia risk factors (eg, elderly patients and those with renal insufficiency). Approxi-mately 50% of the calculated dose can be administered as basal insulin and 50% as prandial or nutritional insulin in divided doses administered with meals. Daily or twice-daily adjustment of the initial insulin doses is required to achieve and maintain glucose targets and to avoid hypoglycemia in nearly all cases of hyperglycemia during hospitalization.

RECOGNITION AND MANAGEMENT OF HYPOGLYCEMIA IN THE HOSPITAL SETTING

Hypoglycemia is defined as any glucose level less than 3.9 mmol/L (70 mg/dL).[106,158] Severe hypoglycemia has been defined by many investigators as less than 2.2 mmol/L (40 mg/dL).[158] The incidence of severe hypoglycemia among the different trials ranged between 5% and 28%, depending on the intensity of glycemic control in the ICU,[133] whereas rates from trials using subcutaneous insulin in non–critically ill patients range from less than 1% to 33%.[153,154] The key predictors of hypoglycemic events in hospitalized patients include older age, greater illness severity, diabetes, and the use of oral glucose-lowering medications and insulin.[159,160] In-hospital processes of care that contribute to risk for hypoglycemia include unexpected changes in nutritional intake that are not accompanied by associated changes in the glycemic management regimen (eg, cessation of nutrition for procedures and adjustment in the amount of nutritional support), interruption of the established routine for glucose monitoring, deviations from the established glucose control protocols, and failure to adjust therapy when glucose is trending down or steroid therapy is tapered.[156,161]

Increasing evidence from observational studies and clinical trials indicates that the development of severe hypoglycemia is independently associated with increased risk of mortality.[15,20,22,83,162–166] The odds ratio (95% CI) for mortality associated with 1 or more episodes was 2.28 (1.41–3.70, $P = .0008$) among a cohort of 5365 patients admitted to a mixed medical-surgical ICU.[159] In a larger cohort of more than 60,000 patients, hypoglycemia was associated with longer ICU stay and greater hospital mortality, especially for patients with more than 1 episode of hypoglycemia. In patients with acute myocardial infarction, those with hypoglycemia had higher mortality compared with patients without hypoglycemic event (12.7% vs 9.6%, $P = .03$), and the relationship between hypoglycemia and mortality was similar in patients with and without known history of diabetes.[22] Despite these observations, the direct causal effect of iatrogenic hypoglycemia on adverse outcome is still debatable. In a recent study assessing the impact of iatrogenic versus spontaneous hypoglycemia in critical illness, Kosiborod and colleagues[22] reported that spontaneous hypoglycemia is asso-ciated with higher in-hospital mortality and that insulin-induced hypoglycemia was not associated with increased risk of death compared with subjects without hypogly-cemia. Similarly, a recent study of 31,970 patients also reported that hypoglycemia is associated with increased in-hospital mortality (hazard ratio 1.67; 95% CI, 1.33–2.09); however, the greater risk was limited to patients with spontaneous hypogly-cemia and not to patients with drug-associated hypoglycemia.[167] After adjustment for patient comorbidities, the association between spontaneous hypoglycemia and mortality was eliminated. These studies raised the possibility that hypoglycemia is a marker of disease burden rather than a direct cause of death.[22,162,167]

SUMMARY

Based on currently available literature, insulin should not be viewed passively as an optional therapy in the hospital. Current evidence supports proactive, scheduled insulin regimens for any patient with consistent hyperglycemia, not only patients with known diabetes and/or who were taking insulin before hospitalization. The proactive approach considers that hyperglycemia is at once both deleterious and related to the endocrinology of the stressed state and requires patient-tailored and situation-tailored insulin therapy. Exposed patients with newly identified hyperglycemia may be at the highest risk of hyperglycemia-related morbidity and mortality. In consideration of the hospital environment, namely unpredictable changes in care and patient condition, imprecision of glucose monitoring, and the variable effects of interventions and nutrition therapy on glycemia, moderate glycemic goals that seek to control glucose while avoiding hypoglycemia are prudent for the majority of hospitalized patients.

REFERENCES

1. Capes SE, Hunt D, Malmberg K, et al. Stress hyperglycaemia and increased risk of death after myocardial infarction in patients with and without diabetes: a systematic overview. Lancet 2000;355(9206):773–8.
2. Furnary AP, Zerr KJ, Grunkemeier GL, et al. Continuous intravenous insulin infusion reduces the incidence of deep sternal wound infection in diabetic patients after cardiac surgical procedures. Ann Thorac Surg 1999;67(2):352–60 [discussion: 360–2].
3. Krinsley JS. Association between hyperglycemia and increased hospital mortality in a heterogeneous population of critically ill patients. Mayo Clin Proc 2003; 78(12):1471–8.
4. Umpierrez GE, Isaacs SD, Bazargan N, et al. Hyperglycemia: an independent marker of in-hospital mortality in patients with undiagnosed diabetes. J Clin Endocrinol Metab 2002;87(3):978–82.
5. van den Berghe G, Wouters P, Weekers F, et al. Intensive insulin therapy in critically ill patients. N Engl J Med 2001;345(19):1359–67.
6. Weekers F, Giulietti AP, Michalaki M, et al. Metabolic, endocrine, and immune effects of stress hyperglycemia in a rabbit model of prolonged critical illness. Endocrinology 2003;144(12):5329–38.
7. Furnary AP, Gao G, Grunkemeier GL, et al. Continuous insulin infusion reduces mortality in patients with diabetes undergoing coronary artery bypass grafting. J Thorac Cardiovasc Surg 2003;125(5):1007–21.
8. Jovanovic L, Peterson CM. Insulin and glucose requirements during the first stage of labor in insulin-dependent diabetic women. Am J Med 1983;75(4): 607–12.
9. Malmberg K, Ryden L, Efendic S, et al. Randomized trial of insulin-glucose infusion followed by subcutaneous insulin treatment in diabetic patients with acute myocardial infarction (DIGAMI study): effects on mortality at 1 year. J Am Coll Cardiol 1995;26(1):57–65.
10. Garber AJ, Moghissi ES, Bransome ED Jr, et al. American College of Endocrinology position statement on inpatient diabetes and metabolic control. Endocr Pract 2004;10(Suppl 2):4–9.
11. Inzucchi SE. Clinical practice. Management of hyperglycemia in the hospital setting. N Engl J Med 2006;355(18):1903–11.

12. Kavanagh BP, McCowen KC. Clinical practice. Glycemic control in the ICU. N Engl J Med 2010;363(26):2540–6.
13. Greci LS, Kailasam M, Malkani S, et al. Utility of HbA(1c) levels for diabetes case finding in hospitalized patients with hyperglycemia. Diabetes Care 2003;26(4): 1064–8.
14. Moghissi ES, Hirsch IB. Hospital management of diabetes. Endocrinol Metab Clin North Am 2005;34(1):99–116.
15. Van den Berghe G, Wilmer A, Hermans G, et al. Intensive insulin therapy in the medical ICU. N Engl J Med 2006;354(5):449–61.
16. Finfer S, Chittock DR, Su SY, et al. Intensive versus conventional glucose control in critically ill patients. N Engl J Med 2009;360(13):1283–97.
17. Qaseem A, Humphrey LL, Chou R, et al. Use of intensive insulin therapy for the management of glycemic control in hospitalized patients: a clinical practice guideline from the American College of Physicians. Ann Intern Med 2011;154(4):260–7.
18. Moghissi ES, Korytkowski MT, DiNardo M, et al. American Association of Clinical Endocrinologists and American Diabetes Association consensus statement on inpatient glycemic control. Diabetes Care 2009;32(6):1119–31.
19. Turchin A, Matheny ME, Shubina M, et al. Hypoglycemia and clinical outcomes in patients with diabetes hospitalized in the general ward. Diabetes Care 2009; 32(7):1153–7.
20. Vriesendorp TM, DeVries JH, van Santen S, et al. Evaluation of short-term consequences of hypoglycemia in an intensive care unit. Crit Care Med 2006; 34(11):2714–8.
21. Egi M, Bellomo R, Stachowski E, et al. Hypoglycemia and outcome in critically ill patients. Mayo Clin Proc 2010;85(3):217–24.
22. Kosiborod M, Inzucchi SE, Goyal A, et al. Relationship between spontaneous and iatrogenic hypoglycemia and mortality in patients hospitalized with acute myocardial infarction. JAMA 2009;301(15):1556–64.
23. Braithwaite SS, Magee M, Sharretts JM, et al. The case for supporting inpatient glycemic control programs now: the evidence and beyond. J Hosp Med 2008; 3(Suppl 5):6–16.
24. Magee MF, Clement S. Subcutaneous insulin therapy in the hospital setting: issues, concerns, and implementation. Endocr Pract 2004;10(Suppl 2):81–8.
25. Association AD. Diabetes Statistics. Diabetes Basics. Available at: http://www. diabetes.org/diabetes-basics/diabetes-statistics/. Accessed June 11, 2010.
26. Jiang HJ, Stryer D, Friedman B, et al. Multiple hospitalizations for patients with diabetes. Diabetes Care 2003;26(5):1421–6.
27. Donnan PT, Leese GP, Morris AD. Hospitalizations for people with type 1 and type 2 diabetes compared with the nondiabetic population of Tayside, Scotland: a retrospective cohort study of resource use. Diabetes Care 2000;23(12):1774–9.
28. Cook CB, Kongable GL, Potter DJ, et al. Inpatient glucose control: a glycemic survey of 126 U.S. hospitals. J Hosp Med 2009;4(9):E7–14.
29. Kosiborod M, Inzucchi SE, Spertus JA, et al. Elevated admission glucose and mortality in elderly patients hospitalized with heart failure. Circulation 2009; 119(14):1899–907.
30. Schmeltz LR, DeSantis AJ, Thiyagarajan V, et al. Reduction of surgical mortality and morbidity in diabetic patients undergoing cardiac surgery with a combined intravenous and subcutaneous insulin glucose management strategy. Diabetes Care 2007;30(4):823–8.
31. Sonksen PH. Home monitoring of blood glucose by diabetic patients. Acta Endocrinol Suppl (Copenh) 1980;238:145–55.

32. Mazurek JA, Hailpern SM, Goring T, et al. Prevalence of hemoglobin A1c greater than 6.5% and 7.0% among hospitalized patients without known diagnosis of diabetes at an urban inner city hospital. J Clin Endocrinol Metab 2010;95(3):1344–8.

33. Baldwin D, Villanueva G, McNutt R, et al. Eliminating inpatient sliding-scale insulin: a reeducation project with medical house staff. Diabetes Care 2005; 28(5):1008–11.

34. Umpierrez GE, Kitabchi AE. ICU care for patients with diabetes. Curr Opin Endocrinol 2004;11:75–81.

35. McCowen KC, Malhotra A, Bistrian BR. Stress-induced hyperglycemia. Crit Care Clin 2001;17(1):107–24.

36. Corssmit EP, Romijn JA, Sauerwein HP. Review article: regulation of glucose production with special attention to nonclassical regulatory mechanisms: a review. Metabolism 2001;50(7):742–55.

37. Cryer PE. Hypoglycemia, functional brain failure, and brain death. J Clin Invest 2007;117(4):868–70.

38. Boden G. Gluconeogenesis and glycogenolysis in health and diabetes. J Investig Med 2004;52(6):375–8.

39. Rizza RA, Mandarino LJ, Gerich JE. Dose-response characteristics for effects of insulin on production and utilization of glucose in man. Am J Physiol 1981; 240(6):E630–9.

40. Edgerton DS, Ramnanan CJ, Grueter CA, et al. Effects of insulin on the metabolic control of hepatic gluconeogenesis in vivo. Diabetes 2009;58(12): 2766–75.

41. Gabbay RA, Sutherland C, Gnudi L, et al. Insulin regulation of phosphoenolpyruvate carboxykinase gene expression does not require activation of the Ras/ mitogen-activated protein kinase signaling pathway. J Biol Chem 1996;271(4): 1890–7.

42. Parks WC, Drake RL. Insulin mediates the stimulation of pyruvate kinase by a dual mechanism. Biochem J 1982;208(2):333–7.

43. Losser MR, Damoisel C, Payen D. Bench-to-bedside review: glucose and stress conditions in the intensive care unit. Crit Care 2010;14(4):231.

44. Scherpereel PA, Tavernier B. Perioperative care of diabetic patients. Eur J Anaesthesiol 2001;18(5):277–94.

45. Chan TM. The permissive effects of glucocorticoid on hepatic gluconeogenesis. Glucagon stimulation of glucose-suppressed gluconeogenesis and inhibition of 6-phosphofructo-1-kinase in hepatocytes from fasted rats. J Biol Chem 1984; 259(12):7426–32.

46. McMahon M, Gerich J, Rizza R. Effects of glucocorticoids on carbohydrate metabolism. Diabetes Metab Rev 1988;4(1):17–30.

47. Esposito K, Nappo F, Marfella R, et al. Inflammatory cytokine concentrations are acutely increased by hyperglycemia in humans: role of oxidative stress. Circulation 2002;106(16):2067–72.

48. Stentz FB, Umpierrez GE, Cuervo R, et al. Proinflammatory cytokines, markers of cardiovascular risks, oxidative stress, and lipid peroxidation in patients with hyperglycemic crises. Diabetes 2004;53(8):2079–86.

49. Lang CH, Dobrescu C, Bagby GJ. Tumor necrosis factor impairs insulin action on peripheral glucose disposal and hepatic glucose output. Endocrinology 1992;130(1):43–52.

50. Fan J, Li YH, Wojnar MM, et al. Endotoxin-induced alterations in insulin-stimulated phosphorylation of insulin receptor, IRS-1, and MAP kinase in skeletal muscle. Shock 1996;6(3):164–70.

51. del Aguila LF, Claffey KP, Kirwan JP. TNF-alpha impairs insulin signaling and insulin stimulation of glucose uptake in C2C12 muscle cells. Am J Physiol 1999;276(5 Pt 1):E849–55.

52. Edwards FH, Grover FL, Shroyer AL, et al. The Society of Thoracic Surgeons National Cardiac Surgery Database: current risk assessment. Ann Thorac Surg 1997;63(3):903–8.

53. Clement S, Braithwaite SS, Magee MF, et al. Management of diabetes and hyperglycemia in hospitals. Diabetes Care 2004;27(2):553–97.

54. Bagdade JD, Root RK, Bulger RJ. Impaired leukocyte function in patients with poorly controlled diabetes. Diabetes 1974;23(1):9–15.

55. Garg R, Chaudhuri A, Munschauer F, et al. Hyperglycemia, insulin, and acute ischemic stroke: a mechanistic justification for a trial of insulin infusion therapy. Stroke 2006;37(1):267–73.

56. Valko M, Leibfritz D, Moncol J, et al. Free radicals and antioxidants in normal physiological functions and human disease. Int J Biochem Cell Biol 2007; 39(1):44–84.

57. Rains JL, Jain SK. Oxidative stress, insulin signaling, and diabetes. Free Radic Biol Med 2011;50(5):567–75.

58. Kersten JR, Montgomery MW, Ghassemi T, et al. Diabetes and hyperglycemia impair activation of mitochondrial K(ATP) channels. Am J Physiol Heart Circ Physiol 2001;280(4):H1744–50.

59. Ceriello A, Quagliaro L, D'Amico M, et al. Acute hyperglycemia induces nitrotyrosine formation and apoptosis in perfused heart from rat. Diabetes 2002;51(4): 1076–82.

60. Title LM, Cummings PM, Giddens K, et al. Oral glucose loading acutely attenuates endothelium-dependent vasodilation in healthy adults without diabetes: an effect prevented by vitamins C and E. J Am Coll Cardiol 2000; 36(7):2185–91.

61. Gresele P, Guglielmini G, De Angelis M, et al. Acute, short-term hyperglycemia enhances shear stress-induced platelet activation in patients with type II diabetes mellitus. J Am Coll Cardiol 2003;41(6):1013–20.

62. Pandolfi A, Giaccari A, Cilli C, et al. Acute hyperglycemia and acute hyperinsulinemia decrease plasma fibrinolytic activity and increase plasminogen activator inhibitor type 1 in the rat. Acta Diabetol 2001;38(2):71–6.

63. Oswald GA, Smith CC, Betteridge DJ, et al. Determinants and importance of stress hyperglycaemia in non-diabetic patients with myocardial infarction. Br Med J (Clin Res Ed) 1986;293(6552):917–22.

64. Norhammar AM, Ryden L, Malmberg K. Admission plasma glucose. Independent risk factor for long-term prognosis after myocardial infarction even in nondiabetic patients. Diabetes Care 1999;22(11):1827–31.

65. Trence DL, Kelly JL, Hirsch IB. The rationale and management of hyperglycemia for in-patients with cardiovascular disease: time for change. J Clin Endocrinol Metab 2003;88(6):2430–7.

66. Steinberg HO, Tarshoby M, Monestel R, et al. Elevated circulating free fatty acid levels impair endothelium-dependent vasodilation. J Clin Invest 1997;100(5): 1230–9.

67. Oliver MF, Opie LH. Effects of glucose and fatty acids on myocardial ischaemia and arrhythmias. Lancet 1994;343(8890):155–8.

68. Robinson LE, van Soeren MH. Insulin resistance and hyperglycemia in critical illness: role of insulin in glycemic control. AACN Clin Issues 2004;15(1): 45–62.

69. Pulsinelli WA, Levy DE, Sigsbee B, et al. Increased damage after ischemic stroke in patients with hyperglycemia with or without established diabetes mellitus. Am J Med 1983;74(4):540–4.

70. Capes SE, Hunt D, Malmberg K, et al. Stress hyperglycemia and prognosis of stroke in nondiabetic and diabetic patients: a systematic overview. Stroke 2001;32(10):2426–32.

71. Kawai N, Keep RF, Betz AL. Hyperglycemia and the vascular effects of cerebral ischemia. Stroke 1997;28(1):149–54.

72. Prado R, Ginsberg MD, Dietrich WD, et al. Hyperglycemia increases infarct size in collaterally perfused but not end-arterial vascular territories. J Cereb Blood Flow Metab 1988;8(2):186–92.

73. Kruyt ND, Biessels GJ, Devries JH, et al. Hyperglycemia in acute ischemic stroke: pathophysiology and clinical management. Nat Rev Neurol 2010;6(3): 145–55.

74. Quast MJ, Wei J, Huang NC, et al. Perfusion deficit parallels exacerbation of cerebral ischemia/reperfusion injury in hyperglycemic rats. J Cereb Blood Flow Metab 1997;17(5):553–9.

75. Furnary AP, Wu Y, Bookin SO. Effect of hyperglycemia and continuous intravenous insulin infusions on outcomes of cardiac surgical procedures: the Portland Diabetic Project. Endocr Pract 2004;10(Suppl 2):21–33.

76. Falciglia M, Freyberg RW, Almenoff PL, et al. Hyperglycemia-related mortality in critically ill patients varies with admission diagnosis. Crit Care Med 2009;37(12): 3001–9.

77. Lazar HL, Chipkin SR, Fitzgerald CA, et al. Tight glycemic control in diabetic coronary artery bypass graft patients improves perioperative outcomes and decreases recurrent ischemic events. Circulation 2004;109(12): 1497–502.

78. Goyal A, Mahaffey KW, Garg J, et al. Prognostic significance of the change in glucose level in the first 24 h after acute myocardial infarction: results from the CARDINAL study. Eur Heart J 2006;27(11):1289–97.

79. Mazighi M, Labreuche J, Amarenco P. Glucose level and brain infarction: a prospective case-control study and prospective study. Int J Stroke 2009; 4(5):346–51.

80. Brunkhorst FM, Engel C, Bloos F, et al. Intensive insulin therapy and pentastarch resuscitation in severe sepsis. N Engl J Med 2008;358(2):125–39.

81. De La Rosa Gdel C, Donado JH, Restrepo AH, et al. Strict glycaemic control in patients hospitalised in a mixed medical and surgical intensive care unit: a randomised clinical trial. Crit Care 2008;12(5):R120.

82. Preiser JC, Brunkhorst F. Tight glucose control and hypoglycemia. Crit Care Med 2008;36(4):1391 [author reply: 1391–2].

83. Griesdale DE, de Souza RJ, van Dam RM, et al. Intensive insulin therapy and mortality among critically ill patients: a meta-analysis including NICE-SUGAR study data. CMAJ 2009;180(8):821–7.

84. Montori VM, Bistrian BR, McMahon MM. Hyperglycemia in acutely ill patients. JAMA 2002;288(17):2167–9.

85. McAlister FA, Majumdar SR, Blitz S, et al. The relation between hyperglycemia and outcomes in 2,471 patients admitted to the hospital with community-acquired pneumonia. Diabetes Care 2005;28(4):810–5.

86. Baker EH, Janaway CH, Philips BJ, et al. Hyperglycaemia is associated with poor outcomes in patients admitted to hospital with acute exacerbations of chronic obstructive pulmonary disease. Thorax 2006;61(4):284–9.

87. Frisch A, Chandra P, Smiley D, et al. Prevalence and clinical outcome of hyperglycemia in the perioperative period in noncardiac surgery. Diabetes Care 2010; 33(8):1783–8.
88. Turnbull PJ, Sinclair AJ. Evaluation of nutritional status and its relationship with functional status in older citizens with diabetes mellitus using the mini nutritional assessment (MNA) tool—a preliminary investigation. J Nutr Health Aging 2002; 6(3):185–9.
89. Pomposelli JJ, Baxter JK 3rd, Babineau TJ, et al. Early postoperative glucose control predicts nosocomial infection rate in diabetic patients. JPEN J Parenter Enteral Nutr 1998;22(2):77–81.
90. Noordzij PG, Boersma E, Schreiner F, et al. Increased preoperative glucose levels are associated with perioperative mortality in patients undergoing noncardiac, nonvascular surgery. Eur J Endocrinol 2007;156(1):137–42.
91. Ramos M, Khalpey Z, Lipsitz S, et al. Relationship of perioperative hyperglycemia and postoperative infections in patients who undergo general and vascular surgery. Ann Surg 2008;248(4):585–91.
92. Hirsch IB, McGill JB. Role of insulin in management of surgical patients with diabetes mellitus. Diabetes Care 1990;13(9):980–91.
93. Dandona P, Aljada A, Mohanty P, et al. Insulin inhibits intranuclear nuclear factor kappaB and stimulates IkappaB in mononuclear cells in obese subjects: evidence for an anti-inflammatory effect? J Clin Endocrinol Metab 2001;86(7): 3257–65.
94. Aljada A, Ghanim H, Mohanty P, et al. Insulin inhibits the pro-inflammatory transcription factor early growth response gene-1 (Egr)-1 expression in mononuclear cells (MNC) and reduces plasma tissue factor (TF) and plasminogen activator inhibitor-1 (PAI-1) concentrations. J Clin Endocrinol Metab 2002; 87(3):1419–22.
95. Dandona P, Aljada A, Bandyopadhyay A. The potential therapeutic role of insulin in acute myocardial infarction in patients admitted to intensive care and in those with unspecified hyperglycemia. Diabetes Care 2003;26(2):516–9.
96. Moghissi ES, Korytkowski MT, DiNardo M, et al. American Association of Clinical Endocrinologists and American Diabetes Association consensus statement on inpatient glycemic control. Endocr Pract 2009;15(4):353–69.
97. American Diabetes Association. Standards of medical care in diabetes—2011. Diabetes Care 2011;34(Suppl 1):S11–61.
98. Levetan CS, Magee MF. Hospital management of diabetes. Endocrinol Metab Clin North Am 2000;29(4):745–70.
99. Levetan CS, Passaro M, Jablonski K, et al. Unrecognized diabetes among hospitalized patients. Diabetes Care 1998;21(2):246–9.
100. Ben-Ami H, Nagachandran P, Mendelson A, et al. Drug-induced hypoglycemic coma in 102 diabetic patients. Arch Intern Med 1999;159(3):281–4.
101. Donihi AC, Raval D, Saul M, et al. Prevalence and predictors of corticosteroid-related hyperglycemia in hospitalized patients. Endocr Pract 2006;12(4): 358–62.
102. Korytkowski M, Dinardo M, Donihi AC, et al. Evolution of a diabetes inpatient safety committee. Endocr Pract 2006;12(Suppl 3):91–9.
103. Juneja R, Foster SA, Whiteman D, et al. The nuts and bolts of subcutaneous insulin therapy in non-critical care hospital settings. Postgrad Med 2010; 122(1):153–62.
104. Smiley D, Rhee M, Peng L, et al. Safety and efficacy of continuous insulin infusion in noncritical care settings. J Hosp Med 2010;5(4):212–7.

105. Seley JJ, D'Hondt N, Longo R, et al. Position statement: inpatient glycemic control. Diabetes Educ 2009;35(Suppl 3):65–9.
106. American Diabetes Association. Standards of medical care in diabetes–2010. Diabetes Care 2010;33(Suppl 1):S11–61.
107. Dungan K, Chapman J, Braithwaite SS, et al. Glucose measurement: confounding issues in setting targets for inpatient management. Diabetes Care 2007; 30(2):403–9.
108. Scott MG, Bruns DE, Boyd JC, et al. Tight glucose control in the intensive care unit: are glucose meters up to the task? Clin Chem 2009;55(1):18–20.
109. Kanji S, Buffie J, Hutton B, et al. Reliability of point-of-care testing for glucose measurement in critically ill adults. Crit Care Med 2005;33(12):2778–85.
110. Schafer RG, Bohannon B, Franz MJ, et al. Diabetes nutrition recommendations for health care institutions. Diabetes Care 2004;27(Suppl 1):S55–7.
111. McMahon MM, Rizza RA. Nutrition support in hospitalized patients with diabetes mellitus. Mayo Clin Proc 1996;71(6):587–94.
112. Bantle JP, Wylie-Rosett J, Albright AL, et al. Nutrition recommendations and interventions for diabetes: a position statement of the American Diabetes Association. Diabetes Care 2008;31(Suppl 1):S61–78.
113. McClave SA, Martindale RG, Vanek VW, et al. Guidelines for the Provision and Assessment of Nutrition Support Therapy in the Adult Critically Ill Patient: Society of Critical Care Medicine (SCCM) and American Society for Parenteral and Enteral Nutrition (A.S.P.E.N.). JPEN J Parenter Enteral Nutr 2009;33(3): 277–316.
114. Warren J, Bhalla V, Cresci G. Postoperative diet advancement: surgical dogma vs evidence-based medicine. Nutr Clin Pract 2011;26(2):115–25.
115. Kreymann KG, Berger MM, Deutz NE, et al. ESPEN guidelines on enteral nutrition: intensive care. Clin Nutr 2006;25(2):210–23.
116. Via MA, Mechanick JI. Inpatient enteral and parental nutrition for patients with diabetes. Curr Diab Rep 2010;11(2):99–105.
117. Craig LD, Nicholson S, SilVerstone FA, et al. Use of a reduced-carbohydrate, modified-fat enteral formula for improving metabolic control and clinical outcomes in long-term care residents with type 2 diabetes: results of a pilot trial. Nutrition 1998;14(6):529–34.
118. Leon-Sanz M, Garcia-Luna PP, Sanz-Paris A, et al. Glycemic and lipid control in hospitalized type 2 diabetic patients: evaluation of 2 enteral nutrition formulas (low carbohydrate-high monounsaturated fat vs high carbohydrate). JPEN J Parenter Enteral Nutr 2005;29(1):21–9.
119. Elia M, Ceriello A, Laube H, et al. Enteral nutritional support and use of diabetes-specific formulas for patients with diabetes: a systematic review and meta-analysis. Diabetes Care 2005;28(9):2267–79.
120. Heyland DK, Montalvo M, MacDonald S, et al. Total parenteral nutrition in the surgical patient: a meta-analysis. Can J Surg 2001;44(2):102–11.
121. Ziegler TR. Parenteral nutrition in the critically ill patient. N Engl J Med 2009; 361(11):1088–97.
122. Muller JM, Brenner U, Dienst C, et al. Preoperative parenteral feeding in patients with gastrointestinal carcinoma. Lancet 1982;1(8263):68–71.
123. Brady PA, Terzic A. The sulfonylurea controversy: more questions from the heart. J Am Coll Cardiol 1998;31(5):950–6.
124. Meinert CL, Knatterud GL, Prout TE, et al. A study of the effects of hypoglycemic agents on vascular complications in patients with adult-onset diabetes. II. Mortality results. Diabetes 1970;19(Suppl):789–830.

125. Murry CE, Jennings RB, Reimer KA. Preconditioning with ischemia: a delay of lethal cell injury in ischemic myocardium. Circulation 1986;74(5):1124–36.

126. Deutsch E, Berger M, Kussmaul WG, et al. Adaptation to ischemia during percutaneous transluminal coronary angioplasty. Clinical, hemodynamic, and metabolic features. Circulation 1990;82(6):2044–51.

127. Terzic A, Jahangir A, Kurachi Y. Cardiac ATP-sensitive K+ channels: regulation by intracellular nucleotides and K+ channel-opening drugs. Am J Physiol 1995; 269(3 Pt 1):C525–45.

128. Horlen C, Malone R, Bryant B, et al. Frequency of inappropriate metformin prescriptions. JAMA 2002;287(19):2504–5.

129. Delea TE, Edelsberg JS, Hagiwara M, et al. Use of thiazolidinediones and risk of heart failure in people with type 2 diabetes: a retrospective cohort study. Diabetes Care 2003;26(11):2983–9.

130. Nesto RW, Bell D, Bonow RO, et al. Thiazolidinedione use, fluid retention, and congestive heart failure: a consensus statement from the American Heart Association and American Diabetes Association. Diabetes Care 2004;27(1): 256–63.

131. Drucker DJ, Nauck MA. The incretin system: glucagon-like peptide-1 receptor agonists and dipeptidyl peptidase-4 inhibitors in type 2 diabetes. Lancet 2006;368(9548):1696–705.

132. Goldberg PA, Siegel MD, Sherwin RS, et al. Implementation of a safe and effective insulin infusion protocol in a medical intensive care unit. Diabetes Care 2004;27(2):461–7.

133. Krikorian A, Ismail-Beigi F, Moghissi ES. Comparisons of different insulin infusion protocols: a review of recent literature. Curr Opin Clin Nutr Metab Care 2010; 13(2):198–204.

134. Donihi A, Rea R, Haas L, et al. Safety and effectiveness of a standardized 80-150mg/dl iv insulin infusion protocol in the Medical Intensive care unit: >11,000 hours of experience. Diabetes 2006;55(Suppl 1):459-P.

135. Davidson PC, Steed RD, Bode BW. Glucommander: a computer-directed intravenous insulin system shown to be safe, simple, and effective in 120,618 h of operation. Diabetes Care 2005;28(10):2418–23.

136. Juneja R, Roudebush C, Kumar N, et al. Utilization of a computerized intravenous insulin infusion program to control blood glucose in the intensive care unit. Diabetes Technol Ther 2007;9(3):232–40.

137. Newton CA, Smiley D, Bode BW, et al. A comparison study of continuous insulin infusion protocols in the medical intensive care unit: computer-guided vs. standard column-based algorithms. J Hosp Med 2010;5(8):432–7.

138. Dossett LA, Cao H, Mowery NT, et al. Blood glucose variability is associated with mortality in the surgical intensive care unit. Am Surg 2008;74(8):679–85 [discussion: 685].

139. DeSantis AJ, Schmeltz LR, Schmidt K, et al. Inpatient management of hyperglycemia: the Northwestern experience. Endocr Pract 2006;12(5):491–505.

140. Rea RS, Donihi AC, Bobeck M, et al. Implementing an intravenous insulin infusion protocol in the intensive care unit. Am J Health Syst Pharm 2007;64(4): 385–95.

141. Akhtar S, Barash PG, Inzucchi SE. Scientific principles and clinical implications of perioperative glucose regulation and control. Anesth Analg 2010;110(2): 478–97.

142. Kitabchi AE, Umpierrez GE, Miles JM, et al. Hyperglycemic crises in adult patients with diabetes. Diabetes Care 2009;32(7):1335–43.

143. Mao CS, Riegelhuth ME, Van Gundy D, et al. An overnight insulin infusion algorithm provides morning normoglycemia and can be used to predict insulin requirements in noninsulin-dependent diabetes mellitus. J Clin Endocrinol Metab 1997;82(8):2466–70.

144. O'Malley CW, Emanuele M, Halasyamani L, et al. Bridge over troubled waters: safe and effective transitions of the inpatient with hyperglycemia. J Hosp Med 2008;3(Suppl 5):55–65.

145. Donaldson S, Villanuueva G, Rondinelli L, et al. Rush University guidelines and protocols for the management of hyperglycemia in hospitalized patients: elimination of the sliding scale and improvement of glycemic control throughout the hospital. Diabetes Educ 2006;32(6):954–62.

146. Schmeltz LR, DeSantis AJ, Schmidt K, et al. Conversion of intravenous insulin infusions to subcutaneously administered insulin glargine in patients with hyperglycemia. Endocr Pract 2006;12(6):641–50.

147. Grainger A, Eiden K, Kemper J, et al. A pilot study to evaluate the effectiveness of glargine and multiple injections of lispro in patients with type 2 diabetes receiving tube feedings in a cardiovascular intensive care unit. Nutr Clin Pract 2007;22(5):545–52.

148. Avanzini F, Marelli G, Donzelli W, et al. Transition from intravenous to subcutaneous insulin: effectiveness and safety of a standardized protocol and predictors of outcome in patients with acute coronary syndrome. Diabetes Care 2011;34(7):1445–50.

149. King AB, Armstrong DU. Basal bolus dosing: a clinical experience. Curr Diabetes Rev 2005;1(2):215–20.

150. Umpierrez G, Maynard G. Glycemic chaos (not glycemic control) still the rule for inpatient care: how do we stop the insanity? J Hosp Med 2006;1(3):141–4.

151. Hirsch IB. Sliding scale insulin–time to stop sliding. JAMA 2009;301(2):213–4.

152. Umpierrez GE, Palacio A, Smiley D. Sliding scale insulin use: myth or insanity? Am J Med 2007;120(7):563–7.

153. Umpierrez GE, Smiley D, Zisman A, et al. Randomized study of basal-bolus insulin therapy in the inpatient management of patients with type 2 diabetes (RABBIT 2 trial). Diabetes Care 2007;30(9):2181–6.

154. Umpierrez E, Smiley D, Jacobs S, et al. Randomized study of basal bolus insulin therapy in the inpatient management of patients with type 2 diabetes undergoing general surgery (RABBIT 2 surgery). Diabetes Care 2011;34(2):256–61.

155. Hor T, Smiley D, Munoz C, et al. Comparison of inpatient insulin regimens: DEtemir plus Aspart vs. NPH plus regular in Medical Patients with Type 2 Diabetes (DEAN Trial). Diabetes 2008;57(Suppl 1):458A.

156. Maynard G, Lee J, Phillips G, et al. Improved inpatient use of basal insulin, reduced hypoglycemia, and improved glycemic control: effect of structured subcutaneous insulin orders and an insulin management algorithm. J Hosp Med 2009;4(1):3–15.

157. Pietras SM, Hanrahan P, Arnold LM, et al. State-of-the-art inpatient diabetes care: the evolution of an academic hospital. Endocr Pract 2010;16(3):512–21.

158. Cryer PE, Axelrod L, Grossman AB, et al. Evaluation and management of adult hypoglycemic disorders: an Endocrine Society Clinical Practice Guideline. J Clin Endocrinol Metab 2009;94(3):709–28.

159. Krinsley JS, Grover A. Severe hypoglycemia in critically ill patients: risk factors and outcomes. Crit Care Med 2007;35(10):2262–7.

160. Kagansky N, Levy S, Rimon E, et al. Hypoglycemia as a predictor of mortality in hospitalized elderly patients. Arch Intern Med 2003;163(15):1825–9.

161. Smith WD, Winterstein AG, Johns T, et al. Causes of hyperglycemia and hypo-glycemia in adult inpatients. Am J Health Syst Pharm 2005;62(7):714–9.
162. Zoungas S, Patel A, Chalmers J, et al. Severe hypoglycemia and risks of vascular events and death. N Engl J Med 2010;363(15):1410–8.
163. Preiser JC, Devos P, Ruiz-Santana S, et al. A prospective randomised multi-centre controlled trial on tight glucose control by intensive insulin therapy in adult intensive care units: the Glucontrol study. Intensive Care Med 2009; 35(10):1738–48.
164. Wiener RS, Wiener DC, Larson RJ. Benefits and risks of tight glucose control in critically ill adults: a meta-analysis. JAMA 2008;300(8):933–44.
165. Arabi YM, Tamim HM, Rishu AH. Hypoglycemia with intensive insulin therapy in critically ill patients: predisposing factors and association with mortality. Crit Care Med 2009;37(9):2536–44.
166. Krinsley JS, Schultz MJ, Spronk PE, et al. Mild hypoglycemia is independently associated with increased mortality in the critically ill. Crit Care 2011;15(4):R173.
167. Boucai L, Southern WN, Zonszein J. Hypoglycemia-associated mortality is not drug-associated but linked to comorbidities. Am J Med 2011;124(11):1028–35.
168. Farah R, Samokhvalov A, Zviebel F, et al. Insulin therapy of hyperglycemia in intensive care. Isr Med Assoc J 2007;9(3):140–2.
169. Grey NJ, Perdrizet GA. Reduction of nosocomial infections in the surgical inten-sive-care unit by strict glycemic control. Endocr Pract 2004;10(Suppl 2):46–52.
170. Mackenzie IM, Ercole A, Blunt M, et al. Glycaemic control and outcome in general intensive care: the East Anglian GLYCOGENIC study. Br J Intensive Care 2008;18:121–6.

Index

Note: Page numbers of article titles are in **boldface** type.

A

A$_{1c}$. See *Hemoglobin A$_{1c}$ (HgbA$_{1c}$).*
ACCORD (Action to Control Cardiovascular Risk) trial, insulin therapy and hypoglycemia
    in, 57, 62–63
    insulin therapy goal reevaluation from, 44–45, 47, 49
Activation times of insulin action, endogenous glucose output and, 31–32
Acute illness, hyperglycemia related to. See *Hospitalized patients.*
Adolescents, insulin therapy in, **145–160**. See also *Pediatric insulin therapy.*
    pregnant, insulin therapy for, 151. See also *Pregnancy.*
ADVANCE (Action in Diabetes and Vascular Disease: Preterax and Diamacron
    MR Controlled Evaluation) trial, insulin therapy and hypoglycemia in, 57, 62–63
    insulin therapy goal reevaluation from, 44–45, 47
Age/aging, hypoglycemia and, 64–65, 71
α cells. See *Pancreatic α cells.*
American Association of Clinical Endocrinologists (AACE), on inpatient hyperglycemia,
    176, 184
American Diabetes Association (ADA), epidemiologic examination of hyperglycemia
    association with diabetic complications, 41–43
    glycemic goal recommendations of, 57–58
        for pediatric patients, 145
        for pregnant patients, 167–168
    on inpatient hyperglycemia, 176, 184
Amylin receptor agonists, 50
Antecedent hypoglycemia, 64–65
Anti-GAD antibodies, in type 1 diabetes, 90
        late-onset, 50
Anti-islet antibodies, in late-onset type 1 diabetes, 50
Artificial pancreas prototypes, in closed-loop insulin delivery, for pediatric insulin
    therapy, 158
        for type 1 diabetes, 105–106, 108–109
Aspart insulin, amino acid structure of, 95
    description of, 8, 10
    for type 1 diabetes, 95
    for type 2 diabetes, 123, 126–127
        in hospitalized patients, 189–190
        with incretin-based therapy, 128
    in pediatric insulin therapy, 146, 148
    pharmacokinetic parameters of, 6
    use during pregnancy, 164–165
Australasian Diabetes in Pregnancy Society, 168
Australian Carbohydrate Intolerance Study in Pregnant Women, 166

Endocrinol Metab Clin N Am 41 (2012) 203–230
doi:10.1016/S0889-8529(12)00020-5
0889-8529/12/$ – see front matter © 2012 Elsevier Inc. All rights reserved.

endo.theclinics.com

Moving?

Make sure your subscription moves with you!

To notify us of your new address, find your **Clinics Account Number** (located on your mailing label above your name), and contact customer service at:

Email: journalscustomerservice-usa@elsevier.com

800-654-2452 (subscribers in the U.S. & Canada)
314-447-8871 (subscribers outside of the U.S. & Canada)

Fax number: 314-447-8029

Elsevier Health Sciences Division
Subscription Customer Service
3251 Riverport Lane
Maryland Heights, MO 63043

*To ensure uninterrupted delivery of your subscription, please notify us at least 4 weeks in advance of move.

ELSEVIER

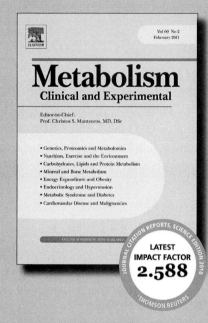
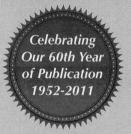

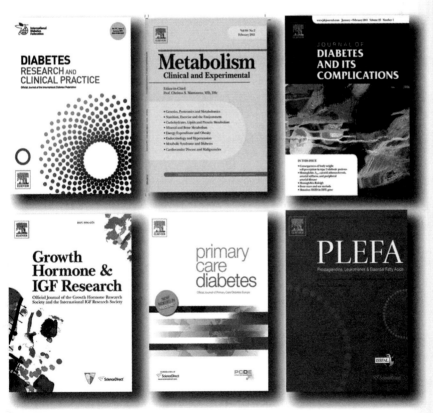